Cases in Bioethics

SELECTIONS FROM THE HASTINGS CENTER REPORT

Cases in Bioethics

SELECTIONS FROM THE HASTINGS CENTER REPORT

Edited by

Carol Levine

Formerly, Editor,
The Hastings Center Report
Currently, Executive Director,
Citizens Commission on AIDS

St. Martin's Press, Inc.
New York

Editor: Don Reisman
Project Management: Publication Services, Inc.
Cover Design: Ben Santora

Library of Congress Catalog Card Number: 88-60530

Manufactured in the United States of America.

3 2 1 0 9

f e d c b a

For information, write:
St. Martin's Press, Inc.
175 Fifth Avenue
New York, NY 10010

ISBN: 0-312-01278-0

Note to the Reader

The purpose of this book is not to report actual incidents, but to pose ethical dilemmas. A few of the cases are nevertheless drawn from the public record. These are "The Unwanted Child: Caring for the Fetus Born Alive After an Abortion"; "A Demand to Die"; "Parental Consent and a Teenage Sex Survey"; "Mrs. X and the Bone Marrow Transplant"; "The Woman Who Died in a Box"; "Sterilizing the Retarded Child"; "Refusing an Amputation: Who Should Pay for the Extra Care?"; "In Organ Transplants, Americans First?"; "A Prisoner in Need of a Bone Marrow Transplant"; and "Mentally Retarded Hepatitis B Carriers in Public Schools." Even in some of these cases, the names are omitted or altered. The remaining cases are not intended to be and should not be read as reports of actual incidents. Some of these cases were inspired by actual incidents, but the names and many of the facts have been changed to provide both anonymity and greater clarity in presenting the ethical issues. The others were designed as paradigmatic examples of common ethical dilemmas or composites of a number of cases posing similar problems, and thus were not derived from any particular incidents. None of these cases should be read as reports of actual events.

Acknowledgments

Acknowledgments and copyrights are continued at the back of the book on page 291, which constitutes an extension of the copyright page. All citations refer to the *Hastings Center Report.*

1. Vol. 13, No. 6, December 1983, pp. 21–22
2. Vol. 16, No. 3, June 1986, pp. 28–29
3. Vol. 14, No. 6, December 1984, pp. 30–31
4. Vol. 17, No. 2, April 1987, pp. 25–26
5. Vol. 17, No. 3, June 1987, pp. 11–12
6. Vol. 12, No. 1, February 1982, pp. 27–28
7. Vol. 10, No. 3, June 1980, pp. 22–24
8. Vol. 11, No. 1, February 1981, pp. 10–11
9. Vol. 15, No. 6, December 1985, pp. 13–15
10. Vol. 17, No. 1, February 1987, pp. 22–23

Contributors

VIRGINIA ABERNETHY is Professor of Psychiatry (Anthropology), Vanderbilt University Medical School

LORI B. ANDREWS is a Research Fellow at the American Bar Foundation.

B. JAYE ANNO is Vice President, National Commission on Correctional Health Care, Chicago.

PAUL S. APPELBAUM is A.F. Zeleznik Professor of Psychiatry and Director of the Law and Psychiatry Program, University of Massachusetts Medical School.

HENRY ARANOW, Jr. (deceased) was Lambert Professor Emeritus of Medicine, College of Physicians and Surgeons, Columbia University.

MILA ANN AROSKAR is Associate Professor, School of Public Health, University of Minnesota.

MARC D. BASSON is Postdoctoral Research Fellow, Department of Surgery, Yale University.

MARGARET BATTIN is Professor of Philosophy, University of Utah.

ROBERT C. BENFARI is a lecturer in Psychology in the Department of Behavioral Sciences, Harvard School of Public Health.

JOYCE BERMEL is Director of Media Relations, State University of New York at Purchase.

ELLEN W. BERNAL is Assistant Professor of Nursing and the Humanities, School of Nursing, Medical College of Ohio.

J. DAVID BLEICH is Talmud Professor of Jewish Law and Ethics, Cordoza School of Law, Yeshiva University.

SISSELA BOK is Associate Professor of Philosophy, Brandeis University.

RICHARD B. BRANDT is Professor Emeritus of Philosophy, University of Michigan.

ANTHONY BREUER is a contributor to this volume.

DAN W. BROCK is Professor of Philosophy and Professor of Human Values in Medicine, Brown University.

BARUCH BRODY is Leon Jaworski Professor of Biomedical Ethics, Baylor College of Medicine.

SIDNEY CALLAHAN is Professor of Psychology, Mercy College, Dobbs Ferry, N.Y.

MICHAEL L. CALLEN is a founding member of People with AIDS Coalition and Community Research Initiative.

ARTHUR L. CAPLAN is Director of the Center for Biomedical Ethics, University of Minnesota.

HOWARD CAPLAN is a physician (geriatrics) in private practice in Los Angeles.

RONALD A. CARSON is Kempner Professor and Director, Institute for the Medical Humanities, University of Texas Medical Branch at Galveston.

ERIC J. CASSELL is Clinical Professor of Public Health, Cornell University Medical College.

JAMES F. CHILDRESS is Kyle Professor of Religious Studies and Professor of Medical Education, University of Virginia.

ALAN W. CHILDS is Associate Professor of Psychology and Dean of Academic Services, Lafayette College.

LUTHER A. CLOUD is former Director, Alcholism Rehabilitation Center, St. Mary's General Hospital, Lewiston, Maine.

ROBERT L. COHEN is former Vice President for Medical Operations, New York Health and Hospital Corporation.

MORRIS F. COLLEN is a consultant in the Division of Research, Kaiser Permanente, Oakland.

CHARLES M. CULVER is Professor of Psychiatry, Dartmouth Medical School, and Adjunct Professor of Philosophy, Dartmouth College.

NANCY DICKEY is Associate Professor, University of Texas Medical School at Houston.

STRACHAN DONNELLEY is Director of Education, The Hastings Center.

NANCY NEVELOFF DUBLER is Director, Division of Legal and Ethical Issues in the Health Care Department of Epidemiology and Social Medicine, Montefiore Medical Center/The Albert Einstein College of Medicine.

GERALD DWORKIN is Professor of Philosophy, University of Illinois at Chicago.

HAROLD EDGAR is Julius Silver Professor of Law, Science, and Technology, Columbia University School of Law.

EBUN O. EKUNWE is Senior Research Fellow, Institute of Child Health and Primary Care, College of Medicine of the University of Lagos, Nigeria.

H. TRISTRAM ENGELHARDT, Jr. is Professor of Medicine and Community Medicine and Member, Center for Ethics & Public Issues, Baylor College of Medicine.

CHERYL ETH is Assistant to the Director, Emanuel Streisand School, Venice, California.

SPENCER ETH is Associate Chief of Psychiatry, VA Medical Center, West Los Angeles, California.

DAVID FASSLER is Clinical Director, Otter Creek Associates, Burlington, Vermont, and Instructor in Psychiatry, Cambridge Hospital, Harvard Medical School.

HERBERT FINGARETTE is Professor of Philosophy, University of California, Santa Barbara.

PHILIPPA FOOT is Griffin Professor of Philosophy, University of California at Los Angeles, and Seminar Research Fellow, Somerville College, Oxford.

CORY FRANKLIN is Director of Medical Intensive Care, Cook County Hospital, and Assistant Professor of Medicine and Medical Ethics, University of Health Sciences, Chicago Medical School.

BENJAMIN FREEDMAN is Associate Professor, McGill Centre for Medicine, Ethics and Law, and Clinical Ethicist, Jewish General Hospital, Montreal.

CHARLES FRIED is Professor of Law, Harvard University, and former Solicitor General, Department of Justice, Washington D.C.

WILLARD GAYLIN is President of The Hastings Center.

JAMES M. GUSTAFSON is Henry R. Luce Professor of Humanities and Comparative Studies, Emory University.

SALLY GUTTMACHER is Assistant Professor of Urban Studies, Rutgers University.

MICHAEL R. HARRISON is Director, Fetal Treatment Program, Department of Surgery, University of California at San Francisco.

MARY SUE HENIFIN is a lawyer with the firm Debevoise & Plimpton, New York City, Editor of *Women & Health*, and a member of the Reproductive Rights Law and Policy Project, Rutgers University.

STANLEY S. HERR is Associate Professor of Law, University of Maryland Law School.

LAWRENCE HESSMAN is Clinical Instructor in Medicine and Community Medicine, Tufts University School of Medicine.

ANGELA R. HOLDER is Clinical Professor of Pediatrics (Law), Yale University School of Medicine, and Counsel for Medicolegal Affairs, Yale-New Haven Hospital and Yale University School of Medicine.

PATRICIA S. HOOVER is Assistant Professor of Nursing, Medical College of Ohio, School of Nursing.

KIM HOPPER is Assistant Professor, City University of New York Medical School.

KENNETH V. ISERSON is Associate Professor of Surgery and Residency Director of Emergency Medicine, Section of Emergency Medicine, University of Arizona College of Medicine.

DAVID L. JACKSON is Clinical Professor of Preventive Medicine, Ohio State University.

MICHAEL JELLINEK is Chief of Child Psychiatry Service and Director of Outpatient Psychiatry, Massachusetts General Hospital.

DEBORAH G. JOHNSON is Associate Professor of Philosophy, Department of Science and Technology Studies, Rensselaer Polytechnic Institute.

OLGA JONASSON is Professor and Chair, Department of Surgery, Ohio State University Hospital.

GEORGE A. KANOTI is Director of the Office of Bioethics, Cleveland Clinic Foundation.

M. MARGARET KEMENY is Chief of Surgical Oncology, St. Vincent's Hospital and Medical Center, and Associate Professor of Surgery, New York Medical College.

ROSS KESSEL is former Acting Dean of Graduate and Interprofessional Studies and Research, University of Maryland at Baltimore.

NICHOLAS N. KITTRIE is Edwin A. Moders Scholar and Professor of Law, The American University.

HOWARD KLAR is former Director of Inpatient Psychiatrics, VA Medical Center, Bronx, NY.

JOHN I. KLEINIG is Professor of Philosophy, Department of Law and Police Science, John Jay College of Criminal Justice, City University of New York.

HANS-GEORG KOCH is Research Associate and Director of the Department of Law and Medicine, Max Planck Institute for Foreign and International Criminal Law in Freiburg, West Germany.

DOUGLAS P. LACKEY is Professor of Philosophy, Baruch College and the Graduate Center, City University of New York.

STEPHEN E. LAMMERS is Professor of Religion, Lafayette College.

SHELDON H. LANDESMAN is Associate Professor of Medicine and Director of AIDS Study Group, State University of New York—Health Science Center at Brooklyn.

HUNTER C. LEAKE III is a pediatrician formerly with the Franklin Foundation, Franklin, Louisiana.

DANIEL H. LEDERER is Clinical Assistant Professor of Medicine, Brown University.

CAROL LEVINE is Executive Director of the Citizens Commission on AIDS.

ROBERT J. LEVINE is Professor of Medicine and Lecturer in Pharmacology, Yale University School of Medicine.

A-J ROCK LEVINSON is former Executive Director, Concern for Dying, New York.

CHARLES W. LIDZ is Professor of Psychiatry and Sociology, Western Psychiatric Institute and Clinic, Department of Psychiatry, University of Pittsburgh.

E. JAMES LIEBERMAN is Adjunct Professor, Family and Community Development, University of Maryland.

ROBERT E. LITMAN is Co-Director of the Suicide Prevention Center in Los Angeles.

JOANNE LYNN is Associate Professor of Geriatric Medicine and Director of the Center for Aging Studies and Services, George Washington University, and Medical Director, The Washington Home and Hospice of Washington.

THOMAS B. MACKENZIE is Associate Professor of Psychiatry and Medicine, Department of Psychiatry, University of Minnesota.

RUTH MACKLIN is Professor of Bioethics, Albert Einstein College of Medicine.

DANIEL C. MAGUIRE is Professor of Moral Theology, Marquette University.

MARY MAHOWALD is Associate Professor, Case Western Reserve University.

DON MARQUIS is Associate Professor of Philosophy, The University of Kansas.

J. JOEL MAY is Senior Consultant, The Pennington Group, Titusville, New Jersey.

MICHAEL McDONALD is Associate Professor of Philosophy, University of Waterloo, Ontario.

KEVIN M. McINTYRE is Associate Clinical Professor of Medicine, Harvard Medical School.

GILBERT MEILAENDER is Professor of Religion, Oberlin College.

ALAN MEISEL is Professor of Law and Psychiatry and Co-Director of the Center for Medical Ethics, University of Pittsburgh.

MITCHEL H. MERNICK is Clinical Instructor, Mount Sinai School of Medicine, and Assistant, Department of Medicine, Hematology-Oncology, Beth Israel Medical Center.

ROBERT MICHELS is Professor and Chairman, Department of Psychiatry, Cornell University Medical College, and Psychiatrist-in-Chief, The New York Hospital.

CAROL KLAPERMAN MORROW is Director of Administrative Policy Studies and Funded Research, Faculty of Arts and Science, New York University.

THEODORE C. NAGEL is Associate Professor of Obstetrics and Gynecology, University of Minnesota.

DAVID C. NATHAN is Physician-in-Chief, Children's Hospital, and Ronald A. Strandhan Professor of Pediatrics, Harvard Medical School.

BERNARD N. NATHANSON is Clinical Assistant Professor of Obstetrics and Gynecology, Cornell University Medical College.

RICHARD H. NICHOLSON is Deputy Director, Institute of Medical Ethics in London, and Editor of *IME Bulletin*.

DONALD RICHARD NILSON is Director, The Sun School, and Co-Director, Peace and Conflict Resolution Program, Hiroshima International School, Japan.

THEODORA OOMS is Director, Family Impact Seminar, American Association for Marriage and Family Therapy, Research and Education Foundation.

JEFFREY PAUL is Associate Director and Professor of Philosophy, Social Philosophy and Policy Center, Bowling Green State University.

RICHARD M. PAULI is Associate Professor of Pediatrics and Medical Genetics, University of Wisconsin at Madison.

JOY HINSON PENTICUFF is Associate Professor and Coordinator, High-Risk Perinatal Clinical Specialist Program, The University of Texas at Austin School of Nursing.

FRANCIS C. PIZZULLI is an attorney in Santa Monica, California.

ROBERT PLOTKIN is a partner with the law firm Laxalt, Washington, Perito, & Dubuc.

JEFFREY M. PROTTAS is Deputy Director, Bigel Institute for Health Policy, Heller Graduate School, Brandeis University.

REN-ZONG QIU is Associate Professor, Department of Philosophy of Science and Director of the Program in Bioethics, Institute of Philosophy of the Chinese Academy of Social Sciences in Beijing.

JAMES RACHELS is Professor of Philosophy, University of Alabama at Birmingham.

FREDERIC G. REAMER is Professor, School of Social Work, Rhode Island College.

ROBERT REDMON is Associate Professor of Philosophy, Virginia Commonwealth University.

NANCY K. RHODEN is Professor of Law, University of North Carolina School of Law.

LINDA M. RHODES is Secretary of Aging, Commonwealth of Pennsylvania.

KNUT RINGEN is Technical Advisor Coordinator, Labor's Health and Safety Fund, Washington, D.C.

LOREN H. ROTH is Professor of Psychiatry, University of Pittsburgh, Western Psychiatric Institute and Clinic.

BARBARA KATZ ROTHMAN is Professor of Sociology, Baruch College, and the Graduate Center, City University of New York.

WILLIAM RUDDICK is Professor of Philosophy, New York University.

DENNIS F. SAVER is a physician in private practice in Newburg, West Virginia.

SYLVAN J. SCHAFFER is Assistant Professor of Psychiatry, Albert Einstein Medical School, and Coordinator of Law and Psychiatry Services, Long Island Jewish Medical Center.

KENNETH F. SCHAFFNER is Co-Director, Center for Medical Ethics, University of Pittsburgh.

R. B. SCHIFFER is Associate Professor of Psychiatry and Neurology, University of Rochester.

LAWRENCE J. SCHNEIDERMAN is Professor in the Department of Community & Family Medicine, University of California at San Diego, School of Medicine.

DANIEL H. SCHWARTZ is Associate Vice President and Director, Office of Risk Management, Montefiore Medical Center.

EDITH T. SHAPIRO is a physician in private practice, and Clinical Associate Professor of Psychiatry, New Jersey Medical School of the University of Medicine and Dentistry of New Jersey.

MARK SHELDON is Associate Professor of Philosophy, Indiana University, and Adjunct Associate Professor of Medicine, Indiana University School of Medicine.

MARK SIEGLER is Professor of Medicine and Director, Center for Clinical Medical Ethics, The University of Chicago.

STEVEN SIEVERTS is former Vice President of Blue Cross and Blue Shield of Greater New York.

ETHEL S. SIRIS is Associate Professor of Clinical Medicine, Department of Medicine, Columbia University College of Physicians and Surgeons.

PETER P. SORDILLO is Associate Professor of Medicine, Mount Sinai School of Medicine.

GRANT E. STEFFEN is a member of the Ethics Committee, Swedish Medical Center, Englewood, Colorado.

MARGARET O'BRIEN STEINFELS is Editor of *Commonweal*.

RON STEPHENS is Professor of Medicine, Division Director, University of Kansas Medical Center.

ROBERT E. STEVENSON is Director, American Type Culture Collection, Rockville, Maryland.

CAROL A. TAUER is Professor of Philosophy, The College of St. Catherine, St. Paul, Minnesota.

KIM MARIE THORBURN is Health Care Director, Hawaii Department of Corrections, and Associate Professor of Medicine, University of Hawaii, John A. Burns School of Medicine.

JOE E. THORNTON is former Professor of Psychiatry, Stanford University Medical Center.

HANS O. TIEFEL is Professor of Religion, The College of William and Mary.

TATJANA ULSHOEFER is Scientific Collaborator, Department of Law and Medicine, Max Planck Institute for Foreign and International Criminal Law, Freiburg, West Germany.

JAN VAN EYS is Mosbacher Chair in Pediatrics and Head, Division of Pediatrics, University of Texas, M.D. Anderson Cancer Center, and Interim Chairman, Department of Pediatrics, University of Texas Medical School at Houston.

ROBERT M. VEATCH is Professor of Medical Ethics, Kennedy Institute of Ethics, Georgetown University.

SOPHIA VINOGRADOV is Research Fellow, Biological Psychiatry, Department of Psychiatry, Stanford University Medical Center.

LEROY WALTERS is Director, Center for Bioethics at the Kennedy Institute of Ethics, Georgetown University.

MARY ANNE WARREN is a Lecturer in Philosophy, San Francisco State University.

JEFFREY WASSERMAN is Pew Health Policy Fellow, The RAND Graduate School.

ROBERT WEIKART is Substance Abuse Therapist, Chelsea Hospital, Chelsea, Michigan.

ROBERT B. WHITE is Marie B. Gale Professor of Psychiatry, Department of Psychiatry and Behavioral Sciences, The University of Texas Medical Branch at Galveston.

MORTON E. WINSTON is Associate Professor of Philosophy, Trenton State College and Adjunct Professor of Ethics, Johns Hopkins University School of Continuing Studies.

SALLY M. WINSTON is Director, Anxiety Disorders Program, Sheppard and Enoch Pratt Hospital, Towson, Maryland.

STUART J. YOUNGNER is Associate Professor of Psychiatry and Medicine, Case Western Reserve University School of Medicine.

DAVID ZIMMERMAN is Associate Professor of Philsophy, Simon Fraser University, Burnaby, British Columbia.

Preface

Since its founding in 1969, The Hastings Center has been committed to the idea that good work in applied ethics requires serious attention to both basic questions of ethical theory and real-life, day-to-day problems of ethical decision making. Beginning with the first issue of the *Hastings Center Report* in 1971, case studies in bioethics and related fields of applied ethics have been a regular feature of the publication. Teachers, students, clinicians, workshop leaders, and many others have used these cases; many more have used the first two editions of *Cases in Bioethics from the Hastings Center Report,* the collected case studies originally published by The Hastings Center. This volume is a completely revised and updated edition; it includes a selection of cases published from 1975 through 1988, as well as several new features.

All the cases were inspired by the experiences of people who have to make critical decisions. Sometimes health care professionals—physicians, nurses, administrators, and others—make these decisions; but often the ethical dilemmas are posed for laypersons—patients, their families, judges, public officials, and others. A few of the cases, listed in the "Note to the Reader" on the copyright page, are drawn from material in the public record. The names and details in the other cases are fictional. The purpose of the book is to pose the kinds of ethical dilemmas that arise in real life, and not to report actual incidents.

The objective of presenting the cases has never been to expose ethical outrages or to point to a clear ethical solution to a problem. Both categories exist. However, in selecting material for case studies, the editorial staff of the *Hastings Center Report* has been drawn to more difficult cases, where there appears to be room for reasonable people to disagree.

The commentators on the cases were selected to illustrate how thoughtful people from various ethical traditions and frameworks and from different academic and professional disciplines analyze the issues. Many times commentators, on first reading the cases presented to them, have pleaded that they seem irresolvable. When pressed to probe more deeply, they have gone on to work toward a resolution and give the reasons that led them to their conclusions. The goal of these case studies is to illustrate that pursuit of reflective, well-thought-out solutions to real human dilemmas.

For this volume the case studies are organized into categories chosen to provide some continuity for the reader, and to emphasize the primary focus of the case. Still, as in any case collection, the groupings are somewhat arbitrary. Many cases have more than one ethical dimension and are included under the thematic headings that seem most appropriate.

For some cases the authors are identified with bylines. Cases not otherwise identified were written by the editorial staff, or by individuals who have chosen to remain anonymous.

The cases and commentaries in this volume are reprinted as they appeared in the *Hastings Center Report,* with a few minor changes. All supplementary material that appeared on the *Report* pages has been deleted. The identifications of contributors have been updated and combined in a single list on pp. v-xi. A *Selected Bibliography* follows each Part, and a *Glossary* (pp. 287-90) defines basic terms in bioethics. Though not intended to be definitive, the glossary covers the important terms that appear regularly in the cases.

Over the years many people at The Hastings Center have contributed to the development of the case studies: chief among them are Daniel Callahan, Director of the Center; Robert M. Veatch, who originated the case study format when he was a staff member of the Center; Peter Steinfels and Margaret O'Brien Steinfels, former editors of the *Hastings Center Report*; and Arthur Caplan, former Assoicate for the Humanities. I was managing editor of the *Report* from 1976–1980, and editor from 1980–87. Margaret Fletcher Stack and Courtney Campbell prepared the case studies published after I left the Center.

Many others have contributed editorial, research, and administrative skills to the case studies; listing only a few—Nancy deKoven and Joyce Bermel, the current and former managing editors; Bette-Jane Crigger, associate editor—is not meant to minimize the debt owed to all the others. Special thanks are due to Marna Howarth, the Center's librarian, who has provided indispensable assistance at many points. Paul Homer, Courtney Campbell, and Lauri Posner skillfully assisted in the preparation of this volume. I also want to thank the individuals who offered valuable suggestions to St. Martin's Press for the final selection and organization of the case studies: Marilyn Bennett, University of Minnesota; Dan W. Brock, Brown University; Baruch Brody, Baylor College of Medicine; Marjorie Clay, Bloomsburg University; and James Rachels, University of Alabama at Birmingham.

My greatest debt, as editor of this volume, is to all the contributors—those authors and commentators who have reflected on the hard cases and have shared their deliberations with the readers of the *Hastings Center Report* and now with the readers of this collection.

C.L.

Topical Contents in Brief

Contents

Part One: Health Care Professionals' Responsibilities and Patients' Rights

Part Three: Death and Dying

Part Four: Research with Living Subjects

Part Five: Mental Incompetence

Part Six: Allocation and Health Care Policy

Cases in Bioethics

SELECTIONS FROM THE HASTINGS CENTER REPORT

PART ONE

Health Care Professionals' Responsibilities and Patients' Rights

INTRODUCTION

In their most classic forms, medicine and biomedical ethics begin with one doctor, one patient. Since ancient times physicians have had a unique and privileged relationship with their patients, one in which physicians' powers derive not only from technical expertise in treatment but also from the special moral authority of their role. Beginning with the ancient Greeks, and the Hippocratic Oath, professional codes of ethics have defined the terms of the relationship. Ethical questions concerned largely what the physician should or should not do in the service of what he (only rarely she) considered to be in the patient's best interests.

In the modern era patients have begun to assert a stronger claim to a more balanced relationship. In addition, health care workers other than physicians have taken a more active role in defining their own professional rights and responsibilities. Moreover, changes in the health care system have radically restructured the physician-patient relationship. These changes have created a peculiarly modern set of ethical dilemmas. The case studies in Part One illustrate those quandaries.

Cases in the first section—"Professional Conduct"—derive from the historical concern with the special roles of professionals. They discuss questions such as the physician's right to withhold information that he or she considers unsuitable for a patient, the use of cadavers for practice and teaching, and the touchy subject of a professional relationship that includes sex. The section also examines concerns of other professionals, such as nurses and ministers.

The second section—"Informed Consent"—reveals the complexities of the seemingly straightforward idea that physicians should not treat patients without their consent. Questions in this area include how much information patients should have about a physician's experience and how decisions are made for persons who are not competent to decide for themselves, such as children and persons with severe neurological impairments.

The final section—"Privacy and Confidentiality"—reflects one of the basic proscriptions of the Hippocratic Oath: not to divulge the patient's secrets. How do professionals balance their primary responsibilities to their patients with the interests of others who may be threatened or otherwise affected?

All these cases reveal the interplay between patients' rights and professionals' responsibilities, carried out in a modern, highly technological health care setting.

PROFESSIONAL CONDUCT

1

"I Want to See My Mother's Picture!"

Barbara Bello, seventeen years old, has lived in foster care since infancy following her mother's death from systemic lupus erythematosis. Her mother was unmarried, and Barbara does not know the whereabouts of her natural father. She somehow learned that her mother had been a patient at the local city hospital during her terminal illness.

Coincidentally, Barbara herself frequently receives treatment at the same hospital for severe asthma. In fact, although lupus and asthma are quite different, Barbara takes the same steroid drug—prednisone—that her mother had received. As a result of her illness and the medication Barbara's growth has been significantly stunted. She also has a history of psychiatric treatment.

After investigating, Barbara discovered that her mother's physician, Dr. Phyllis Stein, is still in practice at the hospital. Barbara requested a meeting to discuss whatever information Dr. Stein might have about Barbara's late mother. Dr. Stein agreed, and in preparation for that discussion she recovered Barbara's mother's hospital record. There she found a color photograph of Barbara's mother taken shortly before her death, dramatically illustrating the ravages of her disease.

During their meeting Barbara told Dr. Stein that she wanted to learn as much about her mother as she could. In addition to her recollections, Dr. Stein mentioned that a picture of Barbara's mother existed, warning Barbara that the picture was quite unflattering. Barbara declared that she wished to have the picture anyway, since she had no other likeness of her mother. Dr. Stein gave the photograph to Barbara and shortly afterwards the meeting ended.

All that evening Barbara stared at her mother's picture, becoming increasingly depressed. Convinced that she would share her mother's fate of an early and painful death, Barbara made her first serious but nonlethal suicide attempt.

Was Dr. Stein correct in releasing the photo to Barbara? What is the nature of her relationship to Barbara, and what obligation does she owe to her?

COMMENTARY

Spencer Eth

Here we face a series of moral decisions concerning disclosure of information to Barbara Bello, an emotionally unstable young woman. Dr. Stein, who treated Barbara's mother during her terminal illness many years earlier, is confronted by an insistent daughter demanding to learn everything possible about her mother.

I maintain that Dr. Stein should keep secret the existence of the morbid picture of Barbara's mother. Barbara insists on learning everything possible about her deceased mother, and her request seems legitimate. We sympathize with her deprivation and, although we cannot restore her mother, we would like to provide some additional information so that Barbara can flesh out a memory of her.

But Dr. Stein has no specific duty to disclose to Barbara all clinical data, as she might be obliged to do on request from her own patient. She must decide whether the photo of Barbara's mother is a memento or a medical document. Clearly Dr. Stein would not consider providing Barbara with X rays, slides, or other comparable material. These are not appropriate, relevant, or informative for nonmedical personnel. Since the photo in question was evidently taken to illustrate the ravages of the disease, it is in essence a medical document.

The unspoken understanding between the two parties is that Dr. Stein will act honestly in helping Barbara to restore an image of her mother as a person. There can be no expectation of total openness, especially with regard to recreating Barbara's mother as an organism riddled with pathology. Keeping the photo secret is not intended to deceive. It is a professional judgment that certain material is provocative medical information whose value is exclusively clinical.

Suppose, however, that somehow Barbara learns that Dr. Stein possesses a picture of her mother. Then Barbara would approach Dr. Stein not with a general request for information, but with a specific demand to view the photo. Under these circumstances I would suggest that Dr. Stein release the picture to Barbara, after following certain prudential precautions.

Dr. Stein cannot deny the existence of the photo (an outright lie), nor should she withhold the photo despite Barbara's pleas. To do so would unleash Barbara's morbid fantasies. The implicit message would be that no matter how awful she could imagine her mother looking, the photo was in reality worse and must remain hidden. Thus, withholding the photo would be intrinsically countertherapeutic, validating unseen dangers and promoting fearful helplessness.

The preferred alternative in this situation is to release the photo. But first Dr. Stein must assess whether Barbara can tolerate viewing the picture. Barbara's behavior seems to indicate mental illness, but that suspicion is relevant only insofar as showing her the photo could be harmful. The mere presence or absence of a psychiatric disorder does not concern us; rather, we need to decide whether the disclosure will lead to severe distress or self-destructive activity. Given Barbara's mental state, it would seem necessary that Dr. Stein defer releasing the photo until a subsequent meeting. Meanwhile, Dr. Stein should refer Barbara for psychiatric care, thereby facilitating the release of the photo at a later date.

By performing an informal clinical evaluation of Barbara prior to releasing the photo, Dr. Stein has not established a true doctor-patient relationship. Interactions with family members constitute the ill-defined, though closely related category of the doctor-collateral relationship. In this professional role, the physician is not contracting for diagnostic and treatment services. However, as in traditional doctor-patient interactions, there is a fiduciary relationship governed by the same ethical norms of respect for autonomy and beneficence, with one crucial difference: the interests of the identified patient supersede those of the family member. For example, if Barbara's mother had instructed that the photo never be shown to her daughter, the doctor must honor that wish.

COMMENTARY

Mark Sheldon

Any suicide attempt is depressing, and to encounter a suicide attempt by a seventeen-year-old, orphaned when very young and suffering from illness, is even more depressing. The picture is complex: on the one hand, an isolated young woman, frightened of her condition and of what she may learn about her mother; on the other, a person courageous enough to attempt to confront a reality about her life.

The suicide attempt appears to be the result of Dr. Stein's having given the photograph to Barbara, though this is not certain. Dr. Stein knew nothing of Barbara's prior psychiatric history, and there seems to be no reason why she should have suspected such a history. Barbara contacted Dr. Stein for information about her mother, who was Dr. Stein's patient. Did Dr. Stein act correctly in showing the photograph to Barbara?

Barbara is not Dr. Stein's patient. Thus we cannot discuss the obligation to disclose information to Barbara within the context of the physician/patient relationship. The two central questions seem to be whether Dr. Stein, having access to particular information because of her professional position, acted in an acceptable and appropriate manner when she released the information; and whether she was, in particular, correct to release it to Barbara.

On the first count, it is clear that physicians in their professional capacity have access to different sorts of information about patients. It seems fair to say that perhaps some information should never be released. For instance, various sorts of psychiatric information about particular patients that do not put at risk any other individual or society ought to be kept confidential, even if the patient in question is dead.

This practice protects the trust that the public has invested in the profession and allows the profession to operate with maximum efficiency. But it does seem reasonable, in certain situations, for physicians to release information about their patients to others. I am not here concerned only with cases where harm might come to individuals or society. Rather, I am concerned with cases like Barbara's, where the individual requesting information appears to have a reasonable right to expect to be taken seriously.

On the second question, Barbara is seventeen years old and has come to Dr. Stein seeking information about her mother. Clearly the photograph is information. Seventeen is not very old, but Barbara appears emancipated enough to have a right to negotiate for information that pertains to her. From Dr. Stein's perspective, nothing would indicate that a suicide attempt might be likely, or that such a notion even exists in the young woman's mind.

To withhold from Barbara what appears to be the only existing photograph of her mother seems to be not only paternalistic, but unfeeling as well. It would also be very difficult to argue that it was Dr. Stein's responsibility to investigate Barbara's background before the meeting. This would have involved her in matters not hers professionally or personally. To investigate records of a person who is not one's own patient is a violation of privacy. It is also, in most places, illegal.

Did Dr. Stein act with any impropriety in disclosing these records and passing on the photograph to Barbara? I do not think that she did. Barbara's mother is dead, and apparently no living person is subject to possible harm or violation of privacy. Dr. Stein met privately with Barbara, answered her questions, and thoughtfully warned Barbara of her mother's appearance. What additional precautionary actions were necessary is not clear.

Barbara's suicide attempt is very unfortunate, but there is no sense in which it is due to any negligence on the part of Dr. Stein.

2

Using a Cadaver to Practice and Teach

A paramedic unit brings a man in cardiac arrest who appears to be in his mid-fifties into the Emergency Room (ER). The paramedics have already intubated the patient (passed a breathing tube into his trachea) and begun an intravenous line to administer drugs. Since both appear to be working well at the time the patient arrives, the emergency room physician and a resident continue to use them during the resuscitation. Ninety minutes later, the patient still cannot be converted from asystolic (flat line) cardiac rhythm and is declared dead.

The patient's family, contacted earlier by the police, have just arrived. They have told the nurse that the patient had a longstanding history of heart disease. However, since the cardiac arrest was an unanticipated event that occurred in a public place, the medical examiner's office has been notified.

Before the body is removed, the ER physician would like to instruct the resident and practice two procedures: intubation and starting a central venous line. Must he notify the family and obtain consent?

COMMENTARY

Kenneth V. Iserson

Establishing a definitive airway and obtaining access to the vascular system are the keys to resuscitating all critically ill patients. The safest and easiest method is to pass an endotracheal tube through the patient's mouth while manipulating the tongue and laryngeal structures with an illuminating blade. Once the tube is in place, ventilation and suctioning can be accomplished. While this is not a difficult procedure in most cases, frequent practice eliminates the tendency to hesitate and increases the chance for success.

Obtaining access to the venous circulation (via an intravenous line) becomes a difficult task in the critically ill patient. Access must be gained via the large veins in the neck, shoulders, or groin area. These central veins are also utilized to insert both catheters that monitor the internal pressures of the heart and temporary cardiac pacemakers. Technically, these are more complicated procedures. Again, frequent practice is essential to master the skill. Access must be gained and with little trauma to the patient.

In the past, physicians working in emergency care areas had little need to be concerned about getting practice in performing endotracheal intubation or beginning central line IVs. Because patients arrived frequently in critical condition, these procedures were performed daily. Nowadays highly trained personnel often begin intubation and peripheral IV lines prior to arrival at the hospital. Despite recent advances in prehospital and hospital care of the critical patient, skill in certain life-supporting procedures must be maintained. And the only patients to reach hospitals without successful prehospital intervention are the most critically ill. These patients are also the most difficult ones on whom to perform life-supporting measures.

The physician-patient relationship that exists during resuscitation of the critical patient mandates that the most complicated procedures should be performed by the most experienced person present. These complicated procedures include intubation and central venous line placement. Since both time and safety are critical factors in the unstable patient, this is not the proper setting to teach these exacting procedures. However, once the patient has been pronounced dead the physician-patient relationship is over. A responsibility now exists to prepare the clinician and future clinicians to care for the next critically ill patient, with whom a prospective physician-patient relationship exists.

A patient who is pronounced dead is a duplicate of the next potential patient. Unlike the plastic models or stiff or embalmed cadavers available in pathology, this cadaver has anatomic flexibility. In many minds, practicing procedures on cadavers connotes horrible mutilation of the body. But neither intubation nor percutaneous central line placement significantly disfigures the deceased patient. Endotracheal intubation, even if done repeatedly, leaves no visible marks on the body. Placement of a central IV line leaves a barely discernible needle puncture mark at the practice site.

The question now becomes: Should permission be obtained first from the next of kin who now owns the body? During the resuscitation a relationship develops between family and staff. Because of this relationship and the unexpected nature of the death, requesting this type of permission becomes difficult. Unlike autopsy, corneal transplantation, or some other cadaver organ transplants, these invasive procedures need to be performed immediately after the pronouncement of death. Permission must be obtained immediately to avoid changes that take place with *rigor mortis*, and before the patient is removed (usually quickly) to the morgue.

Medical examiner laws are the most significant deterrence to postmortem practice. These laws, prevalent in the United States, generally prevent physicians from performing procedures or removing resuscitation equipment in cases of sudden, unexplained, or violent death. Since virtually every patient who dies in the emergency department meets these criteria, postmortem practice becomes impossible. Such laws specifically prohibit removal and reintroduction of the endotracheal tube and introduction of any needles into the cadaver. The rationale for this is sound: to insure optimal medical and legal postmortem evaluation of the body. However, more than anything else, this has prevented adequate training and continued practice in vital procedures.

Religious attitudes and medical examiner laws are having a negative impact on our ability to save lives. All attempts should be made, in every case, to train and keep medical personnel up-to-date in life-saving procedures. To this end, staff physicians and trainees participating in resuscitations should be allowed, and encouraged, to practice these procedures in the brief period immediately following death.

COMMENTARY

Charles M. Culver

It would be seriously immoral for the physician to proceed. To practice these procedures might cause great psychological pain to the family, were they aware of the situation. To do the procedures without telling the family would be deceptive, and the deception cannot be morally justified.

Families almost always have a strong emotional interest in the respectful care and handling of their loved one's newly dead body. In many cases they would strongly object to the body's being used as an object on which students might practice. For some families, objections would be based on important religious beliefs. Orthodox Jews, for example, have explicit beliefs forbidding any kind of action that derives benefit from the dead body. Mutilation of the corpse is considered a serious desecration, and is permissible only in the extremely rare case where such mutilation (for example, an autopsy) will probably save the life of another seriously ill patient immediately at hand. Intubation, even if the resident's practice goes well, could slightly mutilate the body; installing a central venous line would always be mutilating. Have these physicians inquired about the family's religious or other beliefs covering the treatment of the newly dead?

To practice procedures on a newly dead body without telling the family would clearly be deceptive. Suppose the family discovered later, perhaps from an Emergency Room nurse, that the body had been used for practice. The family would certainly be justified in feeling that something significant had happened, about which they had a right to know but had not been told.

Would the deception be morally justified? Truthtelling is not an absolute duty: there are rare occasions when health care workers are not acting immorally if they withhold information from patients or survivors. For deception to be justified, however, fairly stringent criteria must be met: Rational persons must agree that everyone should be allowed to deceive in all cases with morally similar circumstances. If there are circumstances in which one would advocate deception for some but not others, one is not acting impartially, and it is universally agreed that morality requires impartiality.

In what kinds of cases would rational persons agree that deception could be universally allowed? Only when deception would certainly or very probably prevent much greater harm than it would cause. In the case at hand, deception prevents no harm at all: If the resident cannot practice, he has not been deprived of anything that is his due. No one has any duty to give over his or her body, dead or alive, for the practice of students or residents. Doing so might be virtuous or meritorious, but declining does not harm anyone and thus is not immoral.

By contrast, what harm might the deception cause? Here we must weigh not only the harm caused by this particular act of deception, but also the harm that would ensue if deception were universally allowed under these circumstances. Secrets in a hospital have a way of becoming known, and practicing on dead bodies without survivors' knowledge or consent is news that would and should spread. Suppose community members came to know, or suspect on good grounds, that a hospital's doctors engaged in such activities. That could easily lead to great anxiety for many people, and a justified decrease in the trust that patients have for their doctors. Thus great harm could follow from these practices, affecting many more persons than the family in question.

Residents do need to obtain supervised practice for the benefit of their own future patients. But that practice, whether on live bodies or dead, should never be carried out without the consent of the parties concerned.

3

When the Doctor and the Minister Disagree

Mary Clarkson is fifty-five years old; for the past eight months her husband, Bill, has been in California settling the estate of a relative. He comes home once every two months for a weekend visit and then returns to California. Mrs. Clarkson has been feeling depressed and lethargic; she voluntarily admits herself to the psychiatric unit of a community hospital seventy-five miles from home.

Mrs. Clarkson is very religious and has been attending church with her sister and brother-in-law. Upon admission to the hospital Mrs. Clarkson calls her minister, Rev. Tark, and asks him to visit her.

During the visit Mrs. Clarkson tells him about her marital problems: she and her husband constantly argue about his absences and how to deal with their thirty-year-old son who has had recurrent emotional and financial problems. Mrs. Clarkson feels guilty about not having given her son more money and support, and she wants to help him solve his problems. Her husband, however, wants nothing more to do with him. Rev. Tark offers her absolution after her "confession," and prays with her for strength to get well and to return home.

The next day Rev. Tark receives a call from Mrs. Clarkson's psychiatrist, Dr. Vern. Dr. Vern wants to know if Rev. Tark has visited Mrs. Clarkson and what was said. Rev. Tark explains that he saw Mrs. Clarkson at her request and that he heard her confession and offered her absolution.

Dr. Vern states that Mrs. Clarkson would be better off if she saw only him for counseling during her three-week stay as an inpatient. He feels that her depession is the result of a failed marriage and that she can only recover when she acknowledges that fact and begins proceedings for separation. Rev. Tark disagrees that the marriage should be ended. His goal is to help resolve the difficulties, which he thinks began when Mr. Clarkson retired from his factory job, at the age of fifty-five, about a year and a half earlier.

A few days later Rev. Tark's superior receives a letter from Dr. Vern, in which he states that Rev. Tark "must get clearance from the attending psychiatrist for any contact he is to have with the patient during hospitalization." After Mrs. Clarkson is sent home she will be free to choose whom she wants to see for counseling, the letter continues, but in the hospital the presence of her minister will only undermine her medical treatment.

Should Rev. Tark return to see Mrs. Clarkson in spite of Dr. Vern's ban? Does Mrs. Clarkson have the right to choose her counselor? Do patients "belong" to any professionals?

COMMENTARY

Robert Weikart

The case suggests several ethical issues: informed consent, autonomy vs. paternalism, beneficence, and respect for differing belief systems. The patient is directly involved in the first and last issues, while the psychiatrist and clergyman are involved in the middle two.

In considering informed consent, it would be helpful to know what Mrs. Clarkson was told upon admission to the hospital. Was she told that her visitors would be limited? Was she told that the psychiatrist would determine whom she could see? The case does state that Mrs. Clarkson called Rev. Tark "upon admission to the hospital" and requested a visit. Either she was informed of a visitor rule and had disregarded it or was not informed and subsequently invited specific people to visit her. Since she was depressed and lethargic upon admission, it could be a positive sign if she has called upon those who can offer her support with or without the approval of her psychiatrist.

Assuming that Mrs. Clarkson is competent and was not told that her visitors would be restricted, she was treated paternalistically. Paternalism usually protects someone from hurting himself or herself or others or protects the individual who is incompetent to make decisions. Paternalism presupposes that the physician will act only in the patient's best interests. It also gives the patient the right to negotiate the bounds of such paternalism. But in this case the patient's best interests were not served when her minister was asked not to return, with no negotiation about the extent of paternalism.

Those who would favor paternalism in this case might argue that Mrs. Clarkson does not know what is good for her and needs the guidance of a professional. However, if we accept this argument, was she competent to admit herself initially to the hospital and to ask her minister to visit? If she is conditionally or intermittently competent, who makes that diagnosis?

The psychiatrist also faced a conflict of interest. Can a psychiatrist who works for a hospital psychiatric unit be beneficent toward patients while also being an agent of the institution? If the institution prohibits visitors for new patients but the psychiatrist deems visitors helpful for patients, which side will he uphold?

At the crux of this discussion are Mrs. Clarkson's religious beliefs. Since she has been attending church with her relatives, it appears that religion is important to her. She also seems to believe in the sacrament since she participated in confession and absolution with Rev. Tark.

Her faith raises several questions. How does Mrs. Clarkson view divorce? If she views it as a sin, and is encouraged by Dr. Vern to leave her husband, she may have feelings of guilt and a sense that she has lost grace with God.

There is some overlap between what clergy and psychiatrists do, and this seems to be part of the problem. In this instance, the minister is dealing with the sacramental aspect of her life, which affects how she lives her life. The psychiatrist is concerned with her marital situation, but needs to consider her religious values as well.

After the inpatient treatment is finished Mrs. Clarkson will need ongoing support. She will probably see Rev. Tark as she did before. There is some question, however, about whether she will continue to see Dr. Vern since he is affiliated with a hospital far from her home. Rev. Tark can provide continuity of care as well as support for her religious beliefs.

If Dr. Vern thinks it unwise for Mrs. Clarkson to see Rev. Tark, he should meet with Rev. Tark and explain his reasons. Dr. Vern also should enlist Rev. Tark's help in resolving any guilt generated by Mrs. Clarkson's decision, if she makes it, to divorce her husband.

I believe that Mrs. Clarkson has the right, especially if she was not previously informed otherwise, to see the professionals she chooses. Her beliefs are important to her and need to be sustained as a resource both for the present and the future.

COMMENTARY

Howard Klar

Psychiatric disorders, more than any other group of medical problems, are shaped and influenced by the social and cultural milieu in which they occur. When changes in a person's emotional life lead that person to seek treatment, the psychiatrist's obligation is to consider sociocultural factors, as well as many others that may be contributing to the patient's problem. After carefully assessing the problem from these different frames of reference, the physician can integrate biological, social, and psychodynamic factors in order to arrive at a plausible explanation. Then, with the patient's consent, effective treatment can begin.

Dr. Vern did not fulfill this responsibility to his patient and Rev. Tark could not, due to a different orientation, fulfill this responsibility either. As a result, a travesty of clinical care occurred.

Mrs. Clarkson is a woman with a shaky marriage, a troubled son, a guilt-ridden conscience, and perhaps, a biologic propensity toward depression. Given the turmoil in her personal life, it would not be surprising if Mrs. Clarkson were also troubled by thoughts and feelings that are at odds with her strong religious beliefs. Despite her regular attendance at church services, she is unable to find solace from her depression solely through religion. She then voluntarily seeks medical care in a hospital. Implicit in this decision is Mrs. Clarkson's belief that Rev. Tark's counseling alone could not help her overcome her depression.

When patients enter the hospital they have the right to expect that the medicine practiced there will be grounded in science and that the practitioners in the hospital will be credentialed professionals. They further have the right to assume, in most cases, that they will participate in all decisions regarding their care, including decisions about who can and cannot provide care in the hospital. Patients do not retain the right to choose anyone to treat them in a hospital, particularly if they seek a treatment not acceptable by the hospital's standards.

We never know if Rev. Tark views himself as a practitioner, only that Dr. Vern finds him intrusive. Interestingly, both men seem to have a point of view regarding Mrs. Clarkson's marriage. One wants to save the marriage, the other seeks to end it. What does the patient want? Neither Rev. Tark nor Dr. Vern seems to care. Mrs. Clarkson is not mentally incompetent, therefore she does not need to be told what to do. She may require time to struggle toward a decision about her marriage, but it is *her* decision to make. The two men are engaged in a struggle to impose their points of view on Mrs. Clarkson, not in a discussion of how to help the patient.

Banning the minister from seeing Mrs. Clarkson is Dr. Vern's trump card in this test of wills. There is no question regarding a hospital's right to restrict visitors if the visit is harmful to the patient's condition. Whether Dr. Vern was correct in interpreting Rev. Tark's visit as harmful is another matter. Certainly, "confession and absolution" are not medical treatments for depression. However, religious beliefs obviously play an important role in understanding Mrs. Clarkson's problems, and the potentially positive role Rev. Tark could play in her treatment should not be underestimated.

Rev. Tark was fulfilling his professional role and attempting to help his congregant. We should not expect him to be aware of the complex issues involved in the treatment of depression, that is, to behave like a physician.

We may even be inclined toward a more forgiving stance toward his trying to "save the marriage," without placing Mrs. Clarkson's wishes first.

Dr. Vern was wrong to deny the minister his right to visit Mrs. Clarkson. While the minister may have been misguided, he was clearly not dangerous or harmful to the patient. As a psychiatrist, Dr. Vern's professional obligation to his patient is to be aware of the multiple factors impinging on her clinical condition. To suddenly deny her access to her minister, without even consulting her, is clearly an abridgment of her rights.

Physicians in the hospital setting are granted enormous authority over the care and management of their patients. It is reasonable to expect that this authority will be used fairly and in the interests of the patient, not to prevent the patient from hearing points of view that differ from the physician's.

Hospitals rightly impose limitations on the freedom of patients to choose both treatments and "treaters." While this restriction protects patients from snake-oils and charlatans, it also requires that the physician in charge exercise judgment regarding the role of "nonscientific" factors, like religion, in a patient's treatment. If Rev. Tark and Dr. Vern cannot work out their differences, then Rev. Tark should call Mrs. Clarkson and explain the dilemma. Mrs. Clarkson would then be free to discuss it with Dr. Vern and seek another medical opinion, or even to leave the hospital.

Every profession carries with it a set of values and obligations. The conflict in this case occurred when the professional values of Rev. Tark collided with those of Dr. Vern. While both men lost sight of the patient's right to find her own way, even within the constraints of being in a hospital, Dr. Vern lost sight of the values of his profession—namely, to make use of the patient's values and psychosocial supports in her care, rather than to further alienate her from them.

4

The Nurse's Appeal to Conscience

Alice Howard is a registered nurse at Hillside Nursing Home where she cares for Jane Barnes, a sixty-three-year-old woman who has terminal colon cancer. Mrs. Barnes is in considerable pain, which has been increasingly difficult to control. The attending physician, Dr. Jones, has ordered moderate doses of morphine. The family understands that at these doses morphine may depress respiratory effort, thus hastening death.

In the past months Mrs. Barnes and her family have moved toward acceptance of death. Some member of her family is with her constantly to comfort her. She is receiving morphine as often as every three hours and her sleeping respiratory rate is now very slow.

Most of the nurses see no problem with giving morphine to Mrs. Barnes. However, Nurse Howard disagrees. She believes that the morphine will cause

Mrs. Barnes to die earlier than she would have otherwise; thus she cannot, in good conscience, give the injection. The other nurses resent interrrupting their busy schedules to "cover" for Nurse Howard. Dr. Jones regards her refusal as a potentially serious form of disobedience.

One night, Nurse Howard is the only R.N. on duty. Mrs. Barnes has been very restless, and unable to sleep, even though she received her medication. In obvious discomfort, Mrs. Barnes presses the call button and asks for more medication. Her daughter pleads with Nurse Howard to help her mother. Nurse Howard hesitates. She is the only person on the night shift who is legally qualified to give this injection; if she refuses, she will have to bother Dr. Jones with a late-night call and suffer the consequences.

Do nurses have the right to refuse medical orders or to ignore the wishes of the patient and family on grounds of conscience?

COMMENTARY

Ellen W. Bernal and Patricia S. Hoover

Alice Howard has made an appeal to conscience the basis for her ongoing refusal to administer the morphine. Such an appeal should be founded on a prior judgment of the rightness or wrongness of an action. The action, if taken, will violate one's integrity; thus the deciding factor is personal rather than external sanction. For the nurse, an appeal to conscience also requires consideration of professional obligations. Nurse Howard believes that giving morphine injections is wrong because it may hasten Mrs. Barnes's death.

Nurse Howard should examine the factual basis for this belief and current nursing practice recommendations with respect to pain control. In order to give competent care, the nurse must understand the pharmacology of the medications she administers. Respiratory distress is an important potential side effect to consider when administering morphine. It is difficult to say with absolute certainty how much morphine might lead to severe respiratory distress or the death of a patient.

Nurse Howard can decrease this risk by carefully assessing Mrs. Barnes's condition *each time* the analgesic is to be given. She needs to consider the following: When did Mrs. Barnes get the last dose of morphine? How has she responded to previous doses? What is her mental status? What are her vital signs, especially respiratory rate and depth? What subjective and objective symptoms of pain does she exhibit? The answers will guide Nurse Howard in deciding whether giving the morphine is safe. However, no blanket assurance can be given that the morphine she administers will not hasten Mrs. Barnes's death.

Nurse Howard should also consider the American Nurses' Association Code for Nurses (1985). The Code states that nurses have a moral obligation to "take all reasonable means to protect and preserve human life when there is a hope of recovery or reasonable hope of benefit from life-prolonging treatment." But nurses also "may provide interventions to relieve symptoms in the dying client even when the interventions entail substantial risks of hastening death." When analgesics such as morphine are administered for alleviating pain, this should be done on a regularly scheduled basis and before the pain occurs or increases significantly. We see no indication that Nurse Howard attempted to assess or anticipate her patient's need for morphine or to explore other means of pain relief such as positioning, relaxation exercises, or imagery.

It is the nurse's duty to remain faithful to the implicit promises she has made to her patient. One implicit promise is Nurse Howard's obligation to respect Mrs. Barnes's autonomy. At the beginning of this illness and at her admission to the nursing home, Mrs. Barnes could have expressed her values and plans. Nurse Howard should have based nursing treatment on the informed decisions of her patient. Allowing Mrs. Barnes to be as fully involved as possible in planning for pain relief can have an added benefit; increasing Mrs. Barnes's control over the situation may reduce her perceived pain.

If after such discussions Nurse Howard finds that she cannot give the morphine, she should explain, nonjudgmentally, her own moral position regarding the use of morphine. She should then assure Mrs. Barnes that another nurse will give the medication. Nurse Howard is also obligated to make her refusal known to the nursing home, "in advance and in time for other appropriate arrangements to be made for the client's nursing care" (ANA Code, 1985).

A second implicit promise is the obligation to "be with" the patient both physically and psychologially. But Nurse Howard's conscientious objection to administering morphine seems to stand in the way of a trusting, healing relationship; perhaps she should remove herself from Mrs. Barnes's care. She should also persist in her attempt to resolve the situation with Dr. Jones and the nursing home administration. If she is unable to reach an understanding, then she may have to consider employment elsewhere.

While Nurse Howard hesitates, Mrs. Barnes suffers. We believe her basic nursing duty should override her appeal to conscience in the immediate situation. It is inexcusable that she has allowed herself to be placed in this avoidable position. She should formulate a plan of action before other such emergencies occur.

COMMENTARY

Mila Ann Aroskar

Nurses (and the public) agree that nurses have a primary obligation to relieve the pain and suffering of dying patients. Such a position is supported by the American Nurses' Association Code for Nurses (1985). Meeting this obligation is one way of demonstrating respect for persons and advocacy in support of a dying patient's comfort and best interests.

Alice Howard cannot appeal to external authority such as the nursing code to support her position and she has not done so. Her appeal is to her own conscience and her concepts of right and wrong. This also assumes that she is basing her refusal on accurate and complete information about Mrs. Barnes's clincial situation, knowledge about drugs such as morphine, and so forth.

Nurses who refuse to participate in certain patient care procedures or treatments and who base their refusals on an appeal to conscience are still responsible for the consequences to patients of their decisions. They are responsible for assuring that patients' lives and safety are not jeopardized by such decisions. Simply abandoning indentified patients is never morally justifiable.

At the same time, patient advocacy has some limits. Nurses do not have an absolute moral obligation to do unquestioningly whatever is requested by patients, families, or other health professionals or to take actions that violate deeply held moral beliefs. (Legally, nurses and other health professionals cannot be required to participate in abortions or sterilizations.) If such an absolute obligation existed, it would negate the idea of nurses as moral agents who are responsible for making decisions and taking into account the possible consequences of those decisions.

Nurses, like patients, are persons worthy of respect. As such, they should never be treated solely as means to the ends of others even if the "others" are patients or clients to whom nurses are primarily accountable. Nurses may be subjected to various forms of coercion ranging from threats to peer pressure if they refuse to carry out the physician's "orders," particularly when other nurses do not question them. Such actions or an environment that condones such actions may jeopardize an individual nurse's personal and professional integrity in any practice setting and require change.

Alice Howard has several obligations as a moral agent, including explicit consideration of both positive and negative consequences of her decision. No one can guarantee that there will be no negative consequences for refusing to carry out patient care that other nurses in a similar situation do perform. She must also be aware that nurses have moral obligations for advance planning to assure that Mrs. Barnes's welfare is not jeopardized by her refusal to give the morphine as ordered.

Mrs. Barnes's situation clearly requires effective pain relief. If Alice Howard has used every available nursing means to reduce Mrs. Barnes's pain and suffering without effect, then the injection of morphine is a last resort, which has been ordered by Mrs. Barnes's physician with the support of her family. We do not know if the patient has made any specific choices about pain control or if she is able to participate in such planning. Since Alice Howard is the only one who can legally give the morphine, she must either give it herself, find someone else who can give it legally (unlikely at 2:00 A.M.), or notify Dr. Jones and accept the consequences of doing so—possibly at serious risk of losing her job.

While patient care institutions would be unable to continue providing services if everyone refused to carry out standard interventions designed to reduce pain and suffering of dying patients, there should be mechanisms by which staff can be heard if they disagree with patient care decisions based on an appeal to conscience. Institutions should develop an explicit policy for managing such situations. Nurses do not have an obligation to carry out "orders" that jeopardize patients' safety and welfare. In fact, they clearly have a professional and moral obligation to question such written or verbal orders to stop such actions.

Nursing practice or ethics committees can discuss this and similar issues before they end up in the courts. Nurses should be allowed to refuse to carry out particular procedures or treatments based on an appeal to personal conscience and ideas of right and wrong if the decision is founded on accurate and complete information, acceptance of consequences, and advance planning. The patient's safety and welfare remain the primary consideration.

5

Sex in the MD's Office

Over several days, Dr. Jones, a psychiatrist, receives several anonymous phone calls from a woman who sounds confused, frightened, and threatens to kill herself. Finally, he persuades her to make an appointment as Miss X.

During her visit, Miss X. paces up and down, and mumbles. When she reaches into her pocketbook and pulls out a gun, Dr. Jones gives his secretary a prearranged signal for help. Minutes later the police arrive. Miss X. begs Dr. Jones to let her stay. It was not him she meant to kill, she says, but herself.

She tells Dr. Jones that an internist in the same small town—whose name she refuses to reveal—has had sexual relations with her in his office many times. In addition, he has beaten her and she believes him capable of killing her, as he has threatened to do, if she lodges a complaint. She feels vengeful. Nevertheless, she admires him as a doctor, continues to have sex with him, and wants to protect him.

Dr. Jones feels she is telling the truth. What is more, he thinks he knows who the colleague is. Over the years, a few patients have confided to him that they had voluntarily had sex in the office of a physician—Dr. Smith. Dr. Jones has no reason to question Dr. Smith's standard of care in other regards. What steps, if any, should Dr. Jones take?

COMMENTARY

Edith T. Shapiro

Dr. Jones has an array of treatment and other interventions from which to choose. Some of these are mandated by the physician-patient relationship, by a general right to privacy implicit in the Fourth Amendment, by the rules of confidentiality, and by state laws.

To begin with, once Dr. Jones has decided that Miss X. is credible, he needs to determine her psychological state and the extent of the abuse. If, after consulting with Dr. Jones, Miss X. decides to terminate her relationship with Dr. Smith or to file civil or criminal charges, her interests are protected. Unless Dr. Jones believes that Dr. Smith is dangerous to others, he has no further obligation.

However, if Miss X. persists in continuing her relationship with Dr. Smith, and if Dr. Jones decides that her life is in imminent danger but that she lacks the judgment to understand this, he may feel morally compelled to report his suspicions to the ethics committee of the state medical society, and probably to the police. Since this may jeopardize the therapeutic relationship, Dr. Jones will have to weigh the dangers Dr. Smith poses to Miss X. against the consequences of her dropping out of treatment. In a suicidal patient, the latter course could have serious consequences and even could lead to the patient's death.

If Dr. Jones believes there is no threat to life, he should provide the appropriate psychiatric treatment to Miss X., which may include exploring her relationship with Dr. Smith. However, he should not take any action against Dr. Smith since his patient is a competent adult who does not wish to waive confidentiality.

It is far less clear whether and how Dr. Jones should have reacted to earlier information from patients that Dr. Smith used his office for sexual liasions. Did Dr. Smith behave illegally, unprofessionally, immorally, or unethically in this regard? Which of these charges calls for intervention?

According to the reports Dr. Jones received, Dr. Smith did not misrepresent his sexual activities as medical treatment, and did not intimidate his patients. Both civil and criminal penalties have been applied against physicians who exploit patients sexually under the pretext of treatment.

In 1987 we do not peek in other peoples' beds. But where the beds are situated is the issue. In England adultery or an improper association with patients is expressly prohibited by the General Medical Council (1977). In the United States no such ban exists. Dr. Smith has also not breached any tenet of the AMA Principles of Medical Ethics; only psychiatrists are specifically prohibited from engaging in sexual relationships with patients through the APA code of ethics. However, the absence of a prohibition does not mean approval of consensual sexual relations in a physician's office.

In the Hippocratic Oath the prohibition against consensual sex is stated explicitly: "I . . . will abstain . . . from the seduction of females or males." Although not all physicians swear to the Oath, for most physicians the precepts of the Oath define medical ethics. At the very least consensual sex between physician and patient gives the appearance of wrongdoing.

Galen said of Hippocrates: "With purity and holiness he lived his life and practiced his art." It would be difficult today to make such demands of a physician in private life. However, in professional life it is appropriate to hold a physician to a higher standard of morality than is prevalent in the community. A major prerogative of a profession is its freedom from scrutiny by outsiders, but to maintain this freedom it must police itself effectively. Internal review bodies have disciplinary powers, which have been repeatedly upheld by courts. And physicians have a fraternal obligation to take responsibility for each other's behavior.

Dr. Jones had a powerful moral and fraternal obligation to inform Dr. Smith that his sexual practices, even if consensual, violated the spirit of medical practice. If he decided that Dr. Smith's behavior is the result of physical or psychological impairment, he should have also contacted an Impaired Physicians Committee.

In a recent study of sexual misconduct among psychiatrists, the researchers suggest that physicians need to be educated about sexual ethics (N. Gartrell, et al., "Psychiatrist-Patient Sexual Contact: Results of a National Survey," *American Journal of Psychiatry,* Sept. 1986). I believe that the problem is not lack of knowledge about right or wrong, but a lack of consensus about which interventions or sanctions to choose. Uncertainty about the activities of professional disciplinary bodies and their scope of powers further restrains physicians from reporting delinquent colleagues. Given the unique and complex nature of the physician-patient relationship, consensual sex in the context of a professional relationship needs to be unambiguously prohibited. At the same time procedures need to be developed that assure a just review of facts and safeguard the physician's civil rights.

COMMENTARY

Carol Klaperman Morrow

Like most professionals, Dr. Jones is reluctant to judge a colleague's conduct and take measures that could embarrass him, undermine his reputation, and even curtail his practice. Miss X.'s dramatic plea for help should persuade him of his responsibility to prevent further encounters and effectively discipline or rehabilitate Dr. Smith.

Because Miss X. is a new patient, Dr. Jones probably has a blurred impression of a distraught woman who threatens suicide, threatens others as well, and shows strong ambivalence about her relationship with Dr. Smith. Her confusion and reluctance to identify herself greatly undermine her credibility. However, given similar reports from other patients, Dr. Jones has good reason to suspect unprofessional conduct and to be concerned about Miss X.'s well-being, and the welfare of others. It is difficult to argue that a pattern of sexual encounters within the context of the doctor-patient relationship will not affect Dr. Smith's ability to function dependably and to exercise good judgment.

Given a reasonable possibility that professional performance is compromised and patients are being endangered, Dr. Jones is morally obligated to intervene. Quite aside from harm to patients, Dr. Jones's responsibilities to his colleagues obligate him to intervene where problem doctors threaten to undermine public trust and cast doubt on the integrity and competence of the profession.

Dr. Jones might confront Dr. Smith, giving a straightforward account of the problem as he believes it to exist, and urging Dr. Smith to desist from further sexual encounters with patients in his office. While well intended, interpersonal efforts of this kind are often ineffective. Dr. Jones may not be sufficiently knowledgeable about the full extent of Dr. Smith's misconduct. He may not be sufficiently firm, resourceful, or tactful to influence Dr. Smith.

Apart from listening for reports from patients they both treat, how will Dr. Jones monitor Dr. Smith's conduct? And how will Dr. Jones learn anything of Dr. Smith's overall pattern of care with other patients?

What of Dr. Jones's legal obligation to report problem doctors to state disciplinary authorities? Under his state's mandatory reporting law, Dr. Jones must report any case in which there is reason to believe a physician is either incompetent or impaired. Physicians may be incriminated for failing to report and are offered immunity when reports are made in good faith and without malice.

For all these reasons, Dr. Jones would do better to report what he knows to a special agency (within or outside the profession) that has been organized and charged with controlling problem doctors.

In reporting what he knows, Dr. Jones should assess whether Dr. Smith's behavior, as he understands it, is unethical or symptomatic of illness. If he believes Dr. Smith to be one of the estimated 5–10 percent of all physicians whose professional performance is impaired by mental or physical illness, Dr. Jones would be acting responsibly in reporting him to one of the special committees set up by hospitals and medical societies to confront and rehabilitate sick doctors. The committee will conduct an investigation to determine whether Dr. Smith's condition interferes with his ability to practice medicine. If it does, they will meet with Dr. Smith to communicate their concern, discuss concrete incidents and the effect on patients, and offer confidential counseling and referrals.

Ideally, the committee will monitor Dr. Smith's rehabilitation and his practice, helping a sick colleague while protecting the public from injury. If Dr. Smith rejects or abandons treatment or continues to jeopardize patient welfare, the committee may refer the case to state disciplinary authorities, which could result in loss of license.

The scenario would be played out differently if Dr. Jones believes that his colleague has deliberately deviated from the profession's code of ethics. This would merit a more punitive approach. Clearly, doctors' decisions about why, how, and when to intervene in a colleague's practice reflect choices among prevailing—and sometimes competing—views of the problem. Indeed, different methods of social control are available, depending upon how the problem is perceived. The range of actions that is open to Dr. Jones highlights professional self-governance as a highly social enterprise, which is shaped by individual and professional notions of what counts as substandard performance, unethical conduct, or medical impairment, and what response is appropriate and effective.

6

The "Student Doctor" and a Wary Patient

Marc D. Basson

Like many medical schools, State Medical College permits its third-year students to rotate through Anesthesiology for a month. During the first week, students follow Anesthesiology residents as they visit patients. Then students are assigned their own patients. After obtaining informed consent, they administer anesthesia under supervision.

James Denton is one such third-year student, rotating through the Smithville VA, an affiliated hospital. His first solo patient is Robert Criswell, a sixty-four-year-old man with metastatic prostate cancer who is scheduled to undergo bilateral orchiectomy (castration) in the morning. Criswell has a history of heavy smoking and poor pulmonary function, so James reasons that a spinal anesthetic would be safer than general anesthesia.

The attending anesthesiologist tentatively agrees to this plan. "You've done lumbar punctures before, haven't you?" the anesthesiologist asks. James says that he has done one spinal tap previously, but had great difficulty with it. He adds that he has seen three others performed. "Well, you've got to learn some time," responds the anesthesiologist. "Don't worry, I'll be with you."

James returns to the ward and finds Mr. Criswell. The residents have advised him to introduce himself as "Doctor" Dencton so as not to frighten the patient unnecessarily. Some of James's fellow students use deliberately ambiguous phrases such as "one of the anesthesiology team that will be taking care of you." James selects a popular alternative, introducing himself as "a student doctor from Anesthesiology."

James tells Mr. Criswell that he would like to use spinal anesthesia and explains the procedure for lumbar puncture. "You should know," he says as he fills in the consent sheet, "that like any other medical procedure a lumbar puncture has risks, including bleeding, infection, paralysis, pain, and perhaps even death. Also, a few people develop severe headaches after such a procedure and we will ask you to lie flat for twenty-four hours afterwards to lessen the chances of this happening."

"Tell me, Doctor," Criswell asks, "have you ever had any of these problems with your patients?" James feels uneasy at being called a doctor and at Criswell's assumption that he has done many lumbar punctures before, but he decides that this is not the time to bring up his inexperience. "No, never, although I have seen one moderately severe spinal headache lasting for three days in a friend's patient," he responds.

"That's OK, I can take a headache," Criswell says as he signs the consent form. "I didn't want to insult you or anything. It's just that I've heard all kinds of stories about those medical students from the university coming over here to practice on the vets and leaving them paralyzed for life."

How should James Denton introduce himself? Is he morally or legally obligated to discuss his inexperience in obtaining an informed consent? Would it make a difference if the patient had never raised the issue of experience?

COMMENTARY

Gerald Dworkin

Considering the frequency with which situations similar to the one described in this case arise in everyday medical practice, it is surprising that the legitimacy of what occurs has not occasioned greater ethical scrutiny. Perhaps this is a specific instance of the generalization that the amount of attention paid to ethical issues is inversely proportional to their frequency in practice. Abortions performed because the life of the mother is threatened by pregnancy account for a miniscule proportion of the total, but occupy a fairly high proportion of the philosophical literature. This case, involving the training of students by allowing them to practice technical procedures on patients under supervision, occurs routinely. Yet the only public discussion I have seen concerned the bizarre case of a salesman from a medical instrumentation company who was allowed to operate on patients—without their knowledge—in order to demonstrate the nature and value of his company's products.

We are not faced here with a moral dilemma. This is not a situation in which there are good reasons of a fairly weighty nature for and against a certain course of action. A patient is being misled as to the qualifications, experience, and competence of his "healer." He thinks that James is a doctor (when he is not). He thinks that James has performed this procedure many times before (when he has not). He thinks that James has fairly wide experience with the possible side effects of the procedures (when he has not). While the violation of informed consent is not as gross as that which occurs very commonly when a surgeon does not tell his patient that the operation will actually be performed by a resident or intern (under the surgeon's supervision), the interference with the patient's ability to make an informed choice is clear. In the absence of exceptions to the principle of informed consent, we must condemn this practice.

By exceptions to the principle of informed consent, I mean factors such as impossibility (the patient is unconscious or an infant), waiver (the patient has waived the right to be informed), external justification (getting the consent of the patient would violate more important rights of others), internal justification (the ends served by the rule would be better served by making an exception).

In this case I do not see that such factors are present, and I conclude therefore that James ought to inform his patient of his status, experience, and qualifications. The patient then could either decide to go ahead or ask for a more experienced physician. The fact that the patient has explicitly raised the issue of experience is only relevant insofar as it offers empirical evidence that this patient is particularly worried about this matter. But it is reasonable to assume that all patients have a concern about their doctor's experience and competence, and would want to know that this is the first time he or she is performing a fairly risky procedure.

This answer to the particular issue does not, however, address the more general concern underlying the practice; namely, that we would all be worse off if surgeons and anesthesiologists could not be trained and training requires "hands on" experience. The solution is not deception, but finding ways to make it attractive for patients to agree to being the subjects of such training. It is reasonable for teaching hospitals to claim that the quality of care they provide is better than that of nonteaching hospitals, and that the "price" for this is that patients agree to being part of the training process. As long as this is done forthrightly, and patients have some degree of choice as to the hospitals they enter, I see no objection. Or perhaps there could be a price differential, depending on whether a doctor performed the operation or merely supervised it. This is common practice for analysts-in-training, who charge their patients a greatly reduced fee.

It is worth noting that the problem of "hands on" training is not confined to the medical profession. Airline pilots, automobile mechanics, sushi chefs, student drivers, hairdressers, psychotherapists—all have to impose risks on others in order to learn their skills. But those who bear the risks ought to be aware that they are doing so and be compensated in some fashion for their cooperation.

COMMENTARY

Eric J. Cassell

The case raises two distinct questions. The first is how the medical student, James Denton, should respond to the patient who questions his qualifications. The second is the more general question of whether medical educators are justified in allowing trainees to have primary responsibility for the care of the sick when more qualified physicians are available.

James Denton is obligated to tell the patient, Robert Criswell, the truth. But that is not the end of the matter, it is merely the beginning. Ethical issues such as truth-telling are too often dealt with as though they stood alone and timeless, like public monuments. These problems achieve their importance because of their place in human relations—of persons to themselves and to others. In medical practice, telling the truth serves something larger than itself. It is, for example, an important aspect of trust, and trust is fundamental in the doctor-patient relationship. But trust is a complex, poorly understood matter and so it is easier to discuss truth-telling in the same oversimplified way that we often discuss other ethical issues like autonomy.

Consider this case again. Robert Criswell has metastatic cancer of the prostate and he is about to have his testicles removed. From this history we do not know much about him, but if he is like most of us, he may be frightened by his situation. He is in a VA hospital where the care is sometimes impersonal and where his need for reassurance and for the information that might reduce his uncertainties may not be met.

Into that setting walks James Denton, third-year student-cum-anesthesiologist, also frightened and unsure. The way this case history is recounted suggests that they are adversaries. On the contrary, they are natural allies (like many, perhaps most, doctors and sick patients) because they need each other. Should Denton be honest? Of course he must tell the truth. But then he must actively set out to win Criswell's trust because both he and the patient need it. He must make it clear that he is a novice, but just because of that he will be more attentive and more concerned about Criswell's well-being than another, more experienced anesthesiologist might be. For this and other reasons (including the fact that information can itself be therapeutic when properly employed) he will carefully explain what is to be done, why it is being done, and what it means to Criswell, answering each of the patient's questions (and getting the correct information when he does not know). He will point out that the attending physician will be watching over them to make sure nothing goes wrong, and that he, James Denton, will visit Criswell while he is in the hospital.

For the rest of his life, if he takes care of patients, James Denton will be talking people into doing things that, while for their benefit, may be fraught with risk and fear. And on many of those occasions he will be pursued by doubts and well aware that others might do things better. That is the nature of medical care. Of course, when trust has been created and nurtured, it must not be betrayed because that is worse than lying.

This case does not describe an isolated instance, although "see one, do one, teach one" is an exaggeration of the problem. It is the strength of American medical education that physicians learn while taking care of patients under the guidance of more experienced teachers. However, the teachers, especially attending physicians, could often give better, more efficient, and less costly care to a particular patient than their trainees. Indeed, the student or house officer may be learning on someone who has been the patient of the teacher for many years. In that case the attending physician further helps the doctor in training by including him or her within the bonds of trust that have developed over those years. How, then, can we justify this method of education? Without this system of supervised learning by doing, teachers themselves would not be well trained and the qualifications of the whole profession would suffer.

What I have touched on so briefly describes a complex system of relationships and bonds that are part of the moral nature of the institution of medicine. Many would be quick to point out the ethical error if James Denton lied to Robert Criswell about his professional status. Those same critics, both inside and outside of the profession, might consider it old-fashioned, "hierarchical," or too conservative to worry about such important moral flaws as the failure to give deference to attending physicians and patients, the failure to protect the bonds of trust between patient and doctor, and the failure to protect both the past and the future of the profession of medicine. But a lie by James Denton threatens only Denton and Criswell, while those other "old-fashioned" flaws endanger the integrity of the profession without which no one would take this case seriously.

7

Proxy Consent for a Medical Gamble

Dennis F. Saver

Norma Walker left her job when six months pregnant. Nine days after the baby was born she experienced severe headache, fever, and a mild reaction to light. The next day, Sunday, she met with her obstetrician in the hospital emergency room. He found no abnormalities and felt strongly that further evaluation by an internist was imperative.

Since Mrs. Walker did not know an internist, she and her husband were worried about finding a physician who would come to the emergency room on a Sunday morning. Dr. Stanley, a physician whom they both knew personally, happened to be in the emergency room at the time, and Mr. Walker asked him to assume care of his wife. Her obstetrician agreed.

Dr. Stanley learned that the Walkers' two-year-old child had recently had viral meningitis, as had several other children and adults living near their home. When reached by phone, their pediatrician confirmed that two children had been proven by lumbar puncture to have aseptic meningitis and had been treated conservatively at home. During the interview the Walkers expressed anger about the impersonal and unpleasant way Mrs. Walker had been treated by hospital personnel in the labor and delivery suite a week earlier. Mr. Walker was especially bitter and was certain she would have had better care at home.

The results of laboratory tests showed that Mrs. Walker probably had a just-beginning viral meningitis (for which no specific treatment is necessary), but may have had a bacterial meningitis (a life-threatening illness requiring treatment with intravenous antibiotics).

The test findings were carefully explained to the Walkers. Dr. Stanley stated that because of the circumstances, the chances of Mrs. Walker having viral meningitis were very high. But the result of the spinal fluid test raised the possibility of bacterial meningitis. The physician argued that, if he or his wife were the patient, he would play it safe and go into the hospital for two days of intravenous antibiotics until the spinal fluid culture was complete.

Mrs. Walker felt too ill to think clearly—she would, she said, do whatever her husband decided. Mr. Walker was determined to be involved in the decision. He was clearly concerned for his wife, but wasn't sure whether "playing it safe" was the best course of action. He appreciated the personal favor of the physician who had agreed to undertake her care on short notice and had given a detailed explanation of the medical evaluation. However, her recent hospitalization had left a bad impression. Also the couple had no insurance. Was the small chance really much of a gamble? Mr. Walker needed time to think and went for a walk.

Upon returning, he announced his decision—to take the gamble. He would take his wife home, fully aware of the risks and of Dr. Stanley's discomfort with his decision. Who ought to have made the decision about treatment in this case? Was Mr. Walker's decision justifiable?

COMMENTARY

Ronald A. Carson

Hospital care is often brusque and inconsiderate, at times even unkind. Patients understandably recoil from such treatment and seek to avoid it. Patients also, increasingly, want to take part in determining the shape of their care. The sophisticated patient expects a full explanation of what ails him or her and wants to contribute to decisions made regarding the course of treatment. The unsophisticated, too, often want to know—not the detail, perhaps, and all the possible options, but certainly the odds and the risks. They, too, often wish to say, and have taken into account, how much discomfort and what degree of suffering they are prepared to undergo for this or that outcome.

While sensitive physicians are trying to be responsive to these sorts of expectations, an important and useful distinction ought not to be sloughed over, namely, the distinction between treatment decisions and decisions about the course of treatment. Treatment decisions are medical decisions in the strict sense, decisions predicated on the special knowledge of the medically trained. Assembling relevant evidence, examining it, and interpreting it is the proper business of physicians and should be left to them. Acting on an interpretation of that evidence to treat a patient in distress is also the physician's responsibility. Difficulties arise in cases such as Mrs. Walker's not in diagnosis or treatment, but on the way from one to the other. It is at this point that the physician must consider the treatment options available and weigh their probable outcomes. It is at this juncture that competent adult patients rightfully become partners with their physicians in the decision-making process.

Course-of-treatment decisions are not medical decisions but life decisions. At issue are the physical, psychological, and social effects this or that treatment is likely to have on this particular patient and those nearest him or her. Gauging those effects does not require medical expertise but rather knowledge of the patient's circumstances "from the inside." Choices about the course a treatment should take (and, indeed, the choice between treatment and no treatment) are most appropriately made by those who stand to bear the consequences of the decision.

The decision required in this case is a medical one. This does not mean that the patient and her husband should be excluded from the discussion. But, knowing the consequences of bacterial meningitis, Dr. Stanley was right in recommending hospitalization for prophylactic treatment until lab results conclusively ruled out a bacterial infection. He had to consider the possible effects of Mrs. Walker not receiving adequate care at home (antibiotics, administered intravenously) and of her being at home with what might turn out to be a contagious disease. True, the evidence for viral meningitis was all but overwhelming, but it was also circumstantial. The presence of those white cells caused Dr. Stanley to hesitate and recommend precautionary treatment.

It is clear that Mr. Walker considered the decision one he had to make (a course-of-treatment decision) and that the physician saw it as a treatment decision. What is not clear is the degree of forcefulness the physician used in recommending hospitalization. If the proper interpretation of symptoms and test results is what is at issue, the recommendation to hospitalize and initiate prophylactic therapy should be insisted upon by the physician. The Walkers may, in the face of that insistence, take it upon themselves to go home, but the physician will not have encouraged that decision by offering them a choice which is not theirs to make.

COMMENTARY

Henry Aranow, Jr.

I have conducted my medical practice on the assumption that competent adults have the right and the responsibility to make final decisions about their own medical care. They may, if they so desire, delegate this responsibility to another competent adult of their choosing.

The inflammation of the covering of the brain designated by the term "meningitis" is almost always accompanied by some inflammation of the adjacent brain substance. This latter, if of sufficient extent and degree, may cause disturbances in thinking. Some patients with meningitis are manifestly mentally incompetent to make a reasoned decision about their treatment options. The case description states, "Mrs. Walker felt too ill to think clearly—she would, she said, do whatever her husband decided." The portion of the history of the patient's illness given in the abstract is very scanty, nor are any of the details of the physical examination performed by Dr. Stanley included. The statement that her obstetrician found no abnormalities seems to refer to abnormalities of her reproductive system, since he felt that further evaluation by an internist was *imperative* [my emphasis]. Such information might have been of value in attempting to evaluate Mrs. Walker's mental competence.

When the decision of a person given the responsibility of making a therapeutic decision on behalf of another differs sharply from that recommended by the physician charged with the patient's care, I believe it is the duty of the physician to present to the patient himself or herself the considerations that led to the recommendations rejected by the patient's delegate. Under such circumstances, the mental competence of the patient is of utmost importance.

The case description leads me to believe that Dr. Stanley felt that Mrs. Walker was competent to delegate the decision-making responsibility to her husband. This competence means to me that, when Mr. Walker's decision differed so strikingly from his own, he should have re-presented his arguments to Mrs. Walker, explaining the bases of his professional recommendations, informing her of the risks inherent in the course chosen by her husband, persuading her to withdraw the delegation of decision-making authority from him, and deciding for herself to accept Dr. Stanley's advice.

In my view, the medical arguments for in-hospital treatment are overwhelming until the test results definitely exclude bacterial meningitis. Bacterial meningitis can be a fulminating illness in which a delay in therapy for even a few hours may lead to death or permanent disability. To permit the mother of two children, who has a central responsibility in their care and upbringing, to run such a risk because of her anger and that of her husband "about the impersonal and unpleasant way she had been treated by hospital personnel in the labor and delivery suite a week earlier" strikes me as, in the highest degree, unwise and irresponsible.

We are asked, "Was the small chance really much of a gamble?" My answer is that for such stakes, "It is an appalling one!"

The wisdom of any medical intervention may be evaluated by computing the cost/benefit ratio to the patient and, less importantly, to her family and to society. With the possibility of the death or serious disability of a young mother in one pan of the balance, against two days of undesired and possibly unnecessary hospitalization in the other, the indicator bangs against the end of the scale in the direction of hospitalization and treatment.

It is clear that I do not believe Mr. Walker's decision was justifiable. The fact that Dr. Stanley was only "accidentally" involved in Mrs. Walker's care raises the possibility in my mind that he might have pushed his recommendations much harder with both the Walkers had he been their "regular" or "personal" physician.

COMMENTARY

Nancy K. Rhoden

Competent adults can, in general, refuse medical treatment even when their refusal is unwise, ignorant, or life-threatening. Such situations are agonizing, but more agonizing, and much more complicated, are situations where third parties refuse treatment for others. In the case at hand, Mr. Walker is making a decision with potentially disastrous consequences for his wife's life and health.

Initially, at least, he has the right to make this decision, since his wife has delegated decision-making power to him. There should be a strong presumption in favor of a proxy's decision when he has recently, and competently, been authorized to decide by the patient herself. But this presumption should not be absolute. Any third-party decision maker has an obligation to promote the patient's best interests and to make a decision which the patient could reasonably have made herself. Decisions by parents or court-appointed guardians which violate this duty can be challenged. Decisions by authorized proxies should be subject to similar scrutiny, to guard against unreasonable decisions or decisions based upon ulterior motives.

In this case, despite the couple's lack of insurance, the facts as presented suggest that Mr. Walker acted from concern for his wife. Obviously, if his motives were suspect, Dr. Stanley should take further action. But the real problem here is not Mr. Walker's motive, but the reasonableness of his decision.

Given the facts at hand, is his decision justifiable? Such decisions can be evaluated in several rather disparate ways. They can be considered in purely medical terms—what is the probable diagnosis, what are the relevant risks of alternative courses of treatment, and so on? By these criteria, Mr. Walker's decision is probably unjustifiable. Competent physicians would likely agree as to the need for hospitalization here, at least for observation, because bacterial meningitis can very quickly become life-threatening.

Mr. Walker's decision, however, should not be evaluated solely on medical grounds. Individuals do not make personal treatment decisions in exactly the same way doctors do: rather, their decisions are necessarily, and properly, influenced by their personal values, needs and preferences. Though proxy decision makers are, correctly, given less leeway to be idiosyncratic, their decisions should not automatically be deemed unjustifiable whenever they differ from medical judgment. Rather, we should ask if the proxy's decision is based on factors which the patient would find relevant and important, and if his weighing of risks is one a reasonable person could make.

Thus it is not inappropriate for Mr. Walker to consider his wife's subjective response to hospitalization, since it is a factor which would probably have influenced her decision, even though it is irrelevant to a purely medical judgment. Nor is it inappropriate for Mr. Walker, in weighing the risks, to take into account that his wife's illness was probably viral. The more unlikely that she has bacterial meningitis, the more reasonable his gamble becomes. Additionally, since one reason for recommending hospitalization is to provide careful observation and ready access to treatment, he can consider how closely he will be able to monitor his wife's condition, and how quickly he could get her to a hospital should changes occur.

Mr. Walker, of course, has an obligation to weigh these factors against the risks of taking her home. To do this, he must be accurately apprised of the risks. From the presentation of facts in this case, it is hard to tell exactly how grave Dr. Stanley believed the risks to be. Although the Walkers were told that bacterial meningitis is a life-threatening illness, we do not know whether they were told that it can progress very rapidly to the critical stage, so that a delay in treatment may be fatal or may cause permanent neurological damage. If Mrs. Walker had been told this, it is less likely that she would have been genuinely uncertain as to what to do: there is no indication that her values are so unusual that she would prefer death in a friendly environment to cure in an impersonal one. If Dr. Stanley feels that he inadvertently characterized the risks of going home as less serious than they are, or that Mr. Walker interpreted them wrongly, he should at least try to re-present the facts to both of them before accepting Mr. Walker's decision. And if Mr. Walker remains steadfast, perhaps Dr. Stanley should also try to get Mrs. Walker to take the responsibility herself.

If, however, Dr. Stanley believes that, in his best medical judgment, his characterization of hospitalization as simply "playing it safe" (rather than medically imperative) does not minimize the risks, then he might be constrained to find Mr. Walker's decision, though far from ideal, justifiable. If this is the case (perhaps because Dr. Stanley feels virtually certain that Mrs. Walker's case is viral, or because the couple live very near the hospital), then he should respect Mr. Walker's decision. He should, however, carefully alert both of them to what changes to look for, and impress upon them the importance of an immediate return to the hospital should such changes occur.

8

Faith Healing for Childhood Leukemia

Within twenty-four hours a ten-month-old boy was transferred from a small local hospital to a university hospital and then to its affiliated cancer center with a presumptive diagnosis of leukemia. Because the diagnosis had not been confirmed by bone marrow examination, information on the type of leukemia—needed for an outline of a specific therapy and a more accurate prognosis—was not available.

When the baby was admitted on a Saturday afternoon, only his mother was present. The child was not acutely ill, and the severe anemia that had concerned the referring physician had been corrected by transfusion before the transfer. The baby seemed much better, according to his mother. However, there were significant signs of tumor. The medical approach currently considered optimal is hydration, medication to counteract excess uric acid, and careful characterization of the leukemia. After that, specific therapy can be offered. The characterization could not begin until after the weekend but some therapy could begin immediately.

This information was explained first to the mother, and a few hours later to the father. After two hours of deliberation, they told the attending physician that they refused therapy. They would, they said, place their faith in God. They had recently seen sight restored to the baby's great-grandmother, when she was taken to a healing service after a debilitating stroke.

They felt that all the cancer center measures would very likely fail and they would then take the child to a faith-healing service. It made more sense to them to refuse the therapy and take the child to the faith-healing service right away. They had prayed for a sign from God to help them make this decision, and took the nurse's failure to start an intravenous infusion on the first attempt as just such a sign.

The physician asked the father why God would allow cancer centers to exist if prayer were a more appropriate mode of exercising parental responsibility. The father replied, "Cancer centers are part of God's plan, so that children of parents who do not believe still have a chance." The parents were then asked whether they could muster a perfect enough faith to mediate the healing. The answer was that such a faith was not necessary—they had a perfect God.

The child was discharged without therapy with a return appointment at the center's clinic, but the family did not keep the appointment.

Did the attending physician take the right course of action by acceding to the parents' desires so easily? Should other staff have been requested to negotiate with the family? Should legal remedies have been sought to ensure treatment for the child? What are the limits of religious freedom and parental authority when a child's medical care is at stake?

COMMENTARY

Baruch Brody

I must confess that I have little sympathy for the parents' decision. Coming from a Jewish theological background, I find their position objectionable on theological grounds. The objection was best put by Rabbis Akiva and Ishmael when they said: "Just as if one does not weed, fertilize, and plow, the trees will not produce, and if fruit is produced but is not watered or fertilized it will not live but die, so with regard to the body. Drugs and medicines are the fertilizer and the physician is the tiller of the soil." It is strange to find people actively intervening through natural means to produce desired results in all areas but matters of life and death, and insisting that in those areas alone man should merely pray and leave himself in the hands of God.

My views about the family decision, and the views of the readers of this case study, are not, however, what is immediately crucial here. That issue is a different one, namely, who has the right to make the decision for the ten-month-old boy. Only if we decide that we as a society, or some agents of ours (the physician, the hospital, the courts), should be making the decision will it be relevant to ask what *we* think should be done for the child.

One other preliminary point. There are those who believe that adults should not be allowed to refuse medical treatment *even for themselves* in such cases. They believe that society, through its agents, should insist upon making the judgment even for an adult patient. The many people who hold this view will certainly not want to allow the parents the authority to decide to refuse treatment for the child. So this case is a difficult one *only* for those, like myself, who think that adult patients can choose for themselves to rely upon faith healing rather than medical treatment. The question then becomes whether they can also make this decision for their child who is incapable of deciding for himself.

What is the extent of parental authority over the child and to what extent should society intervene to override certain parental decisions? I know of no adequate theoretical answer to this question. We can, however, reject as inadequate two often-held but nevertheless crude models. One maintains that making decisions for the child is a right of the parents, and when society or its agents intervene, they violate these parental rights. The other maintains that making a decision for the child is an obligation placed by society upon the parents, and society may intervene whenever it judges it to be in the best interest of the child.

I would like to advocate a third model for the parental role. In this model, parents do have a right to make decisions for their child. At the same time, the child has a right against the parents that the parents not use their capacity and right to make decisions in ways that are harmful to the child. Society's role here is part of its general role to adjudicate between members with conflicting rights. If we adopt this model, what shall we say about this case? All parties involved believe that the continued life of the child is the value to be promoted; the dispute is about the efficacy of different ways of pursuing this value. (This differentiates the present case from Jehovah's Witnesses cases.) Therefore, it seems to me perfectly appropriate for society to say (a) if there is ever a case where the child's right to protection takes precedence, it is where the child's life is at stake; (b) in this conflict, where the dispute is about efficacy, and not values, we can easily decide that medical treatment is likely to be the more efficacious; and (c) we therefore expect our agencies (doctors and hospitals acting with the approval of the courts) to protect the child by insisting upon treatment.

But what about the religious freedom of the parents? Surely, if anything is settled in this area, it is that freedom of action (as opposed to belief) where the rights of others are seriously challenged is not justified merely on the grounds that the action is backed by a religious belief.

COMMENTARY

Jan van Eys

Parents' responsibility for the care of infant children is total. Their absolute authority can be overruled, however, if the state decides that parental decisions are not in the best interest of the child. Such state action is a lengthy process, which stirs wide debate unless the action is based on generally unacceptable behavior by the parents, such as overt physical abuse. In the case of life-threatening illness in a child, the choice of medical care by the parents is based on their perception of the illness. It is frequently argued that an inadequate understanding of the disease may prevent parents from making a valid and reasoned decision. Nevertheless, the state does not intervene a priori in making such decisions.

In this case, involving leukemia in an infant, the parents' perception of the probability of poor outcome was not unreasonable. Chemotherapy is never an easy road to follow and is often more difficult in infants. The outcome does vary with the type of leukemia and a prognosis could not be given. But even in the type of leukemia with the most optimistic prognosis, an optimistic outcome would be statistically less certain in an infant than in a four- or five-year-old.

The judgment that a parent is making a decision in the best interest of the child is usually based on the medical personnel's perception of whether parents are seeking a mode of care that has curing as a goal. The harshest judgments are given to those parents who forego the application of proven or near-proven effective therapy. In this case the parents chose to substitute one mode of treatment with curative intent—chemotherapy—for another—faith healing—thereby creating the dilemma.

There is in the United States a strict separation of church and state. In matters spiritual the parents' decision-making power is even more absolute than in matters physical. Not to feed a child would be considered child abuse; not to give a child spiritual instruction is the business of the parents and not of the state. In addition, although the state makes judgments about what constitutes adequate nutrition, there are very few state judgments about what constitutes adequate spiritual sustenance.

Does separation of church and state imply a separation of church and medicine? Is medicine in fact allied with the state or with the spiritual realm? There is no doubt that the treatment offered the child was wholly biological. However, this does not mean that medical therapy lacks a strong component of faith, even at its most overtly physical, such as in cases of surgery. Clearly medical and spiritual matters are not nearly as separate in the eyes of patients as they are in the eyes of many physicians.

The juxtaposition of faith healing and medicine puts the burden of response squarely on the physician. Does the physician accept the proposition that these are comparable alternatives? As an analogy, Laetrile and classical chemotherapy for cancer are comparable alternatives in the sense that both are attempts to cure the disease. Given such a choice, the decision can be based on recorded past experience. Presumably, an objective decision can then be made about the preferability of conventional chemotherapy over Laetrile.

Obviously the juxtaposition of faith healing and classical medicine does not readily allow an objective evaluation. On the other hand, to reject faith healing a priori as an element of care by the parents would force the physician to confront his or her own belief system. To reject faith healing as an alternative that is outside the system of organized medicine, and thereby to argue that faith healing is not a selection of care but a rejection of medicine, demands an a priori rejection of the concept of faith.

Usually parents use faith healing as a form of support, a "hedging of one's bets." As such it can be ignored, endorsed, or condoned by physicians. In this case the confrontation was stripped of any smokescreen, and the question was presented in its barest form. The parents rejected the concept of classical medicine and faith healing as complementary modes of care: classical medicine, they said, is God's plan for those of little faith.

The fact that an infant is involved in this argument is not as important as the argument itself. Its application to infants recalls the long-standing theological debate over infant baptism. There are arguments that a child should not be baptized until he or she can purposefully make that choice. However, if there is no time to let the child select the alternatives, such debates become irrelevant. The implications inherent in faith healing are clear: the parents feel a responsibility to ensure that their child follow their convictions. No doubt different physicians would have reacted and responded to this challenge differently. The response is clearly dependent on the physician's own deep-seated spiritual beliefs. Any absolute solution would reflect the attitude of the person who proclaims such wisdom, not a fundamental truth about human existence and parental responsibility.

9

Who Speaks for the Patient with the Locked-in Syndrome?

Before his stroke, Mr. B. was an alert and active resident in an intermediate care nursing home. The staff described him as fiercely independent and deeply religious. They routinely try to assess residents' wishes concerning Living Wills and resuscitation measures, but Mr. B. consistently refused to discuss these matters.

His stroke was caused by a clot in the large artery at the base of the brain and was accompanied by paralysis of nearly all voluntary muscles. He could neither speak nor move except for opening and closing his eyes. He was, however, alert and able to understand conversation. He was, in neurological terms, "locked in," aware of himself and his surroundings but unable to communicate effectively with his relatives or the health care team.

Using a simple code of open eyes for "yes" and closed eyes for "no," the staff was able to get answers to simple questions. However, when a question with even minimal emotional content was asked—Do you recognize your niece?—Mr. B. would begin to cry and was unable to give a clear response. Further, his capacity to respond to simple questions waxed and waned.

The diagnosis of brain stem stroke was confirmed by two neurologists who agreed that the prognosis for even minimal recovery of function was near zero. In this situation, long-term survival depends largely upon the vigor with which complications such as pneumonia are treated.

By the fourth hospital day Mr. B.'s condition had stabilized and he was able to breath without ventilator assistance. But he remained "locked in" and unable to speak or move.

How vigorously should the staff press Mr. B. with questions on resuscitation or restoration of the ventilator for treatment of pneumonia? Given the difficulty in communicating, can Mr. B. be considered competent to consent to or to refuse treatment? How might his guardian justify consent to or refusal of vigorous, life-sustaining therapy? Might the attending physician write a Do Not Resuscitate (DNR) order without approval of the patient's guardians?

COMMENTARY

Grant E. Steffen

Is Mr. B. competent to give or withhold consent to treatment? This is the central question, for if it is answered "no," then the answer to the first question—how vigorously the staff should question him—is "not at all." It would be pointless to push Mr. B. for answers only to discard them as the views of an incompetent person.

But probably one must ask such questions in order to *determine* if Mr. B. is competent. Competence to consent to or refuse treatment involves (1) the capacity to understand and reason about choices; (2) the capacity to communicate one's choice; and (3) the possession of a stable set of values and goals upon which to base one's choice. While most questions of competence focus upon the first element, for Mr. B. the second element is the problem.

We are told that Mr. B. can communicate with a simple yes/no code by blinking his eyes but that this strategy fails when questions with emotional content are asked. This, along with his waxing and waning capacity to respond, probably makes Mr. B. incompetent to give or withhold consent. Nevertheless, I feel that an attempt should be made to test his desire and capacity to enter into a dialogue about treatment choices.

One need not ask him directly about DNR orders, but may gently ask if he would like to discuss treatment options. This question should be asked on at least two different occasions. If the answers are both positive and consistent, then Mr. B. is probably competent and discussions about specifics should proceed. Further questioning may well uncover confusion and inconsistency. If these persist, then I would stop the dialogue.

Even then, such a discussion may be of questionable value. A stroke, whether or not it causes loss of speech, may commonly affect the intellect and make any response questionable. So we may not know that even a consistent response is what Mr. B. really means.

Concerning the third element of competence we are told that Mr. B. is deeply religious. While this gives no clue about the content or the stability of his religious beliefs, we may nevertheless assume that Mr. B. does possess that stable set of goals and values. However, to the extent that they involve questions of Living Wills, he has refused to talk about them. Does this past refusal give us an adequate reason not to ask about treatment choices? I do not think so, since we are not told who asked what questions or how the questions were asked in the nursing home. Now Mr. B.'s situation has changed and he should have one more chance at this dialogue.

The last two questions in the case description suggest that in fact Mr. B. was ruled incompetent. Who, then, may speak for Mr. B.? A competent family member such as Mr. B.'s niece, though having no legal status, may give consent to treatment. If the niece is aware of Mr. B.'s wishes, she could give consent on that basis. But there is no record of a Living Will and Mr. B. has refused to talk about such matters. So there seems to be no basis for a substituted judgment.

To determine if the niece is capable of or likely to make decisions in Mr. B.'s best interest, I would want to know if her relationship to her uncle was close and caring, cordial but distant, or one of indifference or hostility. Will she benefit by his death? While the nursing home staff may be able to clarify this relationship, the answers to the questions may remain unclear; if so, the physician should ask the court to name a guardian.

The guardian has the same problem as the niece—to decide what is in Mr. B.'s best interest. If the neurologists are correct in their prognosis of no chance of significant recovery, then I believe that most people in Mr. B.'s predicament would decline vigorous life-sustaining therapy. For the quadraplegic life is restrictive, frustrating, and grim; but there is at least communication and a sharing of memories, feelings, and hopes with one's friends. But for the person who is "locked in," communication is severely restricted and life would offer little more than discomfort, frustration, and despair.

I feel that the quality of Mr. B.'s life is minimal, the burden of his illness intolerable, and that life-sustaining therapy should not be given. This analysis claims neither a logical nor an empirical basis. It is simply my intuition that the difference between the benefits of treatment—prolonged life—and the burden of that life is too great.

The last question is not whether a DNR order is appropriate but rather if it may be written without the guardian's approval. If the attending physician does not think that cardiac or respiratory arrest is imminent, then there is no reason to exclude the guradian from sharing in that decision. If a guardian has not been appointed and if arrest is thought to be imminent, then the physician may write the order with the niece's approval. If the niece refuses to be involved in the discussion or is not available, then the physician may write the order on his own.

Though writing a DNR order should be, whenever possible, a shared decision between the physician and the competent patient, or between the physician and the incompetent patient's family, if this sharing is impossible the physician is not thereby relieved of the duty that exists in all clinical settings—namely, to act in the patient's best interest.

In that classic tale of revenge, *The Count of Monte Cristo*, Alexandre Dumas gives us two examples of locked-in people. Though the hero, Edmund Dantes, was locked in the Chateau D'If for fourteen years, his prison was outside himself. He could still walk and talk and plot his escape. M. Noirtier de Villefort was also locked in, but his prison, like Mr. B.'s, was his body. M. Noirtier could communicate with eye signals and quite effectively influence and sometimes even control his family.

Given the primitive state of medical care in nineteenth century France, I assume that the character of M. Noirtier was not copied from life, but rather constructed from Dumas's superb imagination. I know of no locked-in patient with a long-term survival and a level of function similar to those displayed by Monsieur Noirtier. Mr. B.'s only escape from being locked in (the Monte Cristo syndrome) is death.

COMMENTARY

Cory Franklin

The central issue in this case is whether life-sustaining care should be delivered to this patient. This decision depends primarily on two factors: the ability to ascertain the patient's wishes and the outcome if such care is delivered or withheld. The facts strongly suggest that vigorous, life-sustaining therapy should be applied.

In most situations, the definitive indication not to administer aggressive support (endotracheal intubation, cardiopulmonary resuscitation, intensive care) involves either a prior declaration by the patient to that effect (not present here) or a discussion with the patient where he refuses these measures. To be valid, this type of communication must meet certain standards: the patient must understand the nature of his disease and the proposed therapies. He must further understand the potential consequences of refusing these therapies. Finally, the caregivers must be reasonably confident that the patient is expressing his true wishes, that is, his understanding and refusal are not compromised by pain, fear, anger, depression, or denial.

Mr. B. can only answer yes or no by blinking. His answers to simple questions are unclear. According to the standards, the caregivers cannot render a reliable clinical judgment on Mr. B.'s competence to refuse therapy given the limitations on communication. The problem is simply too complex for yes or no answers.

Mr. B., like other locked-in patients, is conscious, alert, and can understand what is being said to him. To deny him the option of life-sustaining therapy because he cannot communicate is to apply an unfair standard. Similar patients unable to speak or write, such as quadraplegic, ventilator-dependent patients would not (and should not) be denied agressive therapy on this basis. Where doubt exists concerning a patient's wish to be resuscitated, the principle in most cases is "to err on the side of life." Without his prior request, Mr. B. should not have aggressive support withheld simply because his consent cannot be clarified.

When the patient's wishes cannot be ascertained, we must revert to other criteria to determine whether aggressive support is warranted. In this case, the most important issue is the patient's prognosis. Mr. B.'s problem illustrates the axiom that "good facts promote good ethics." The information presented states that, soon after the stroke, two neurologists agreed that Mr. B.'s prognosis for even minimal recovery was poor. This point deserves further scrutiny.

Locked-in state is a relatively new syndrome, first described in the medical literature less than twenty years ago (see F. Plum and J. Posner, *The Diagnosis of Stupor and Coma*, 1966). (Ironically, the condition may have been first mentioned by Alexandre Dumas, describing M. Noirtier de Villefort in *The Count of Monte Cristo* over 100 years ago.) Though the condition was originally considered uniformly fatal, several studies reported in the *Annals of Neurology* and *Transactions of the American Neurological Association* in the last five years have documented patients who have recovered. Many of those who recovered suffered from the same type of cerebrovascular disease as Mr. B. Some patients recovered almost complete function (walking, talking, bowel and bladder control) and were discharged from the hospital.

In several cases, patients' paralysis and loss of speech persisted for three months before recovery began. The largest series of patients with locked-in syndrome described in the literature comprise less than ten patients. This is far too few to permit identification of clinical signs associated with future recovery. As is true with other neurologic disorders, early prediction of the extent of recovery for individual patients is difficult, if not impossible.

Numerous authors and at least one current neurology text (*The Clinical Neurosciences* edited by R. N. Rosenberg, 1983) recommend vigorous medical support early in the course of locked-in syndrome, since potential for significant recovery exists. Measures to prevent pneumonia and other pulmonary complications are considered standard medical care. When these patients require life-sustaining care there is no medical justification for withholding it. For Mr. B., one potential future scenario illustrates this: at some point he may require a tracheotomy to control his lung secretions and avoid asphyxiation. If this were not performed, he might suffocate on his own secretions while conscious, alert, and unable to notify anyone.

Mr. B. may not recover from the locked-in syndrome. Ultimately he may be completely dependent on others and require lifetime institutional care. This situation might last weeks, months, or even years. He may not be completely helpless. Some patients with the syndrome have learned to communicate through Morse Code and computers. (Language interaction with Mr. B. and patients like him presents a challenge to our future computer technology.) The future care problems of these patients must be confronted not only on an individual, but on a societal level. We should be prepared to care for these patients in the same way we care for spinal cord injury victims. Mr. B.'s condition leaves him unable to represent himself, but does not divest him of his right to medical care. His is exactly the type of case where our safeguards for ensuring care must be redoubled. As the question stands, both on the basis of personal autonomy and appropriate medical care, Mr. B. is a candidate for vigorous life-sustaining therapy.

PRIVACY AND CONFIDENTIALITY

10

AIDS and a Duty to Protect

Mr. B., age twenty-eight, reported to the community health center of a large city teaching hospital for counseling after being confidentially informed that his blood test was positive for antibodies to the Human Immunodeficiency Virus (HIV), the virus that causes AIDS. The patient had no symptoms.

Dr. T. informed Mr. B. that although he did not have AIDS, there was between a five and thirty-five percent probability that he would develop the disease within the next five years. He was also told that he could probably infect others through sexual contact, by sharing needles, or by donating blood and blood products. He was counseled not to donate blood, and to engage in "safe sex," that is, sex that does not involve the exchange of bodily fluids such as semen.

Mr. B. then revealed that he was bisexual, and that he believed that he had contracted the infection during one of his homosexual encounters. He also said that he was engaged. Dr. T. advised him to inform his fiancée of his diagnosis. But Mr. B. refused to do so, saying that it would ruin his marriage plans.

Should Dr. T. inform her of his patient's test results, or should he protect the confidentiality of the therapeutic relationship?

COMMENTARY

Morton E. Winston

Dr. T. must weigh his duty to safeguard confidential information against a duty to protect his patient's fiancée, and any children the couple might conceive, from possible harm caused by Mr. B.'s infection.

The American College of Physicans Ethics Manual (1984) states that "the physician shall keep secret all that he knows about the patient and release no information without the patient's consent, unless required by the law or unless resulting harm to others outweighs his duty to his patient." The laws of most states require reporting of cases of sexually transmitted diseases such as syphilis, gonorrhea, and hepatitis B, to public health authorities.

At present, AIDS is a reportable disease in all states. However, only a few states, Colorado and Montana among them, presently require confidential reporting of persons who test positive for antibodies to HIV.

In this case, however, the relevant ethical question is not whether the physician should report the patient as being seropositive to public health authorities, but whether Dr. T. should warn his patient's fiancée that she may be at risk of developing AIDS.

Because the law is presently unclear regarding cases of this kind, physicians are exposed to uncertain legal risks: they may be sued by patients for wrongful disclosure and personal suffering that might result from such disclosure if they breach confidentiality; they may also be sued by their patient's sexual partners if they knowingly fail to protect them from preventable harm or risk of infection from their patient's illness.

In 1976 in the case of *Tarasoff v. Regents of the University of California*, the California Supreme Court ruled that therapists who know or should know that a patient poses a violent threat to an identifiable third party have an obligation to take reasonable steps to protect that person. It also noted that "a doctor is liable to persons infected by his patient if he negligently fails to diagnose a contagious disease, or having diagnosed the illness, fails to warn members of the patient's family."

However, the medical risks involved in the present case are different from those in diseases spread by casual, that is, nonsexual contact. Not all seropositive persons are viremic, that is, known to be producing virus, and some might not be infectious. There is evidence that male-to-female transmission of HIV occurs, but the efficiency of such transmission is unknown, though it may be high in some settings. Finally, the outcome of infection with HIV is not predictable with confidence, and not all infected persons will develop fullblown AIDS. These risks may vary for persons in different age, sex, and other groups, and our medical understanding of this disease is undergoing rapid change. These uncertainties argue strongly against instituting legal requirements mandating contact tracing for persons who have tested seropositive to HIV. The exceptional cases, such as this one, where patients refuse voluntarily to disclose their diagnosis to their sexual partners, are best handled on a case-by-case basis.

But then physicians must weigh carefully their responsibility to protect confidentiality against their duty to protect others who might be placed at risk by their patients' illnesses. While physicians should violate their prima facie obligations to protect confidentiality only with the greatest reluctance, it is morally permissible, and may sometimes be obligatory, for physicians to do so.

The *Tarasoff* decision is often incorrectly interpreted as creating a "duty to warn." In fact, it creates a duty to protect potential victims of violence that can be discharged in various ways. If a physician determines that a patient's illness poses a significant risk to others, he could have him arrested for being a danger to public health, or move to have him civilly committed. In either of these cases, the damage done to the patient's rights and civil liberties would be considerable. In the present case, such extreme measures would be unjustified. In general, the duty to protect should be discharged in the way that is least invasive of the patient's rights while still effectively serving to protect potential victims from harm and significant risk.

Dr. T. could best discharge his duty to protect by persuading Mr. B. to reveal his diagnosis to his fiancée himself, and by offering serologic testing and counseling to her through his patient. Given contemporary sexual mores, it is possible that the patient's fiancée may have already been exposed to the infection; she should still be informed of her risk of exposure, offered testing, and counseling, particularly concerning the risk of infecting any children she might conceive. Since the patient's fiancée is presumably not aware that she is a member of a high-risk group, it is unlikely that she would suspect that she may have been exposed.

If Mr. B. will not agree to voluntary disclosure, Dr. T. must seriously consider revealing the information himself. He should first discuss the case with appropriate legal, public health, and perhaps ethical authorities. If, after such consultation, he determines that the risk to his patient's fiancée is significant, and if all other means of persuading the patient to accept his moral responsibility have failed, then Dr. T. should attempt to contact her, either directly or through public health authorities.

COMMENTARY

Sheldon H. Landesman

The question posed in the case is whether a physician is obligated, that is, has a legal or ethical duty, to inform the sexual partner of an HIV-positive man that she may be at risk of acquiring AIDS through intercourse with him. Such a duty would appear to violate the principle of patient-physician confidentiality.

Medical confidentiality, however, has never been sacrosanct. The physician has always had the *option* of *not* maintaining patient-doctor confidentiality. Confidentiality can be breached when the patient's life is at stake and, in certain clear-cut situations, for society's benefit. The requirement to report communicable diseases and gunshot wounds, as well as suspected cases of child abuse, are clearly violations of confidentiality that are legally mandated and socially sanctioned.

The question can best be answered by looking at the broad societal problems associated with HIV infection. A central aspect in controlling the epidemic is counseling and testing the 1.5 to 2 million infected individuals in the U.S. Mandatory testing of the entire population is a logistically impossible and ethically unacceptable way of reaching infected persons. Encouragement of voluntary, confidential counseling and testing is more acceptable. The expectation is that many, if not most, people who discover they are infected will behave appropriately by informing their partners and practicing safer sex.

Any legally or socially sanctioned act that breaches confidentiality or imposes additional burdens (such as job loss or cancellation of insurance) acts as a disincentive to voluntary testing. Thus if all physicians were legally required to report HIV-positive persons to a health department or to inform sexual partners at risk from the HIV-positive person, no one would come forward for testing. This is especially true if the physician is known to treat many patients with AIDS and HIV infection. The public knowledge that such a physician has violated confidentiality would result (indeed, has resulted in several cases) in a sharp decline of potentially infected persons seeking counseling and testing. Consequently, a growing number of persons would remain ignorant of their infectiousness as would their sex partners.

Furthermore, which sexual partners might the physician inform? The spouse, the current girlfriend, the old boyfriend, the sexual partners not yet identified? As a general rule physicians should not be *legally* required to breach the confidentiality of an HIV-infected person for two reasons: it is ultimately counterproductive to the broader goal of encouraging voluntary testing and is difficult to implement fairly.

The price of such a policy is high. The woman discussed in this case may pay the price; her future infection might have been prevented. For a Dr. T. to sit back and let such a scenario be played out is a painful, difficult thing to do. But his discomfort and the woman's infection may be the cost that society pays if it wishes to implement public health measures to minimize the spread of the virus.

Dr. T. does have room to maneuver. He can strongly urge Mr. B. to inform his fiancée, he can act as an information broker and make himself available to counsel the patient and the partner, or he can work with Mr. B. over weeks or months and gradually move him to a more reasonable position.

If all else fails, Dr. T. must review his own situation: he always has the *option* of informing the fiancée, although he should not do so without telling his patient of his intentions. If the physician is heavily involved with this epidemic; if he counsels, tests and treats many such patients, then violating confidentiality and informing the fiancée may ultimately result in more infected individuals. The breach of confidentiality will undoubtedly discourage others from being counseled and tested. If he does not have an "AIDS practice," it is easier to justify the violation of confidentiality.

The courts are the ultimate arbiter of the presence or absence of a legal duty to protect a sex partner from infection. In the absence of a clear legal mandate, the difficult ethical dilemma is one of balancing long-term societal benefits against short-term benefit to an individual. Although it is a difficult decision, and there may be exceptions to the rule, maintaining the patient's confidentiality ought to be the first principle.

11

When X Rays Show, Must Prison Doctors Tell?

Ken Jones, a twenty-year-old prisoner, was admitted to the prison hospital for evaluation of abnormal liver-function tests and intermittent jaundice. An intravenous heroin user prior to incarceration, he had a history of acute hepatitis B several years earlier.

After gallstones were eliminated as the cause of his liver abnormalities, it was decided that Mr. Jones should see a gastroenterologist. As part of the routine examination prior to the consultation and possible liver biopsy, the admitting physician took X rays of Mr. Jones' abdomen.

Later that day the radiologist notified the admitting physician that the X rays revealed foreign objects in the rectum. One was a half-inch linear metallic article that appeared to be a needle. Another object of low radiographic density had an oval shape.

When sequestered contraband is inadvertently discovered during the course of a routine examination do rules of physician-patient confidentiality apply? If so, how should the admitting physician proceed? Should he or she report the discovery to prison officials? If so, what does the obligation to report such unexpected discoveries mean in seeking informed consent from prisoner-patients? What if the discovered contraband appeared to be a weapon?

COMMENTARY

Kim Marie Thorburn

A predetermined covenant of confidentiality characterizes the physician-patient relationship. Possession of contraband in prison is illegal but the discovery in this case occurred during a routine medical examination. Should the physician report a crime or should confidentiality prevail?

Professional communications between physicians and patients are statutorily protected as confidential. A routine physical examination is part of the confidential communication, like information obtained by taking a medical history and data entered in the patient's health record. Health professionals have an interest in maintaining confidentiality so that patients will feel comfortable in revealing personal but necessary information.

Prisoners do not possess full constitutional rights to privacy but they generally retain rights to privacy when there is a special relationship between communicants, such as the physician-patient relationship. In fact, respect for confidentiality is particularly important in a prison hospital setting where patients feel distrust because physicians are often employed by the incarcerating institution.

Clinical autonomy for health professionals in the prison setting is essential for good medical practice. Physicians working in prisons also retain the privilege of confidential interactions with patients, although the prison authorities may try to pressure doctors to supply information. Even if physicians are employed by the prison, their first responsibility is to their patients. It remains the physicians' decision when to give privileged information to the prison authorities. If physicians yield to prison authorities' demands for information they will lose the trust of patients and diminish their ability to deliver effective health care.

The contraband detected during the routine examination of Mr. Jones has the appearance of drugs and paraphernalia. This finding, like all others during the examination, is privileged information to be treated confidentially. The right to privacy supersedes a duty to report the discovery because there is no imminent threat to others.

In contrast, a weapon harbored by a prisoner represents an imminent threat to other prisoners and to prison staff. Thus, upon discovering a sequestered weapon during the course of a routine examination, the physician has a "duty to warn." According to case law, when the physician believes that a significant threat of harm exists, the duty to warn takes precedence over the patient's right to privacy.

The case raises the issue of where to draw the line between duty to protect the public and duty to protect patients' privacy. While legal guidelines can assist the physician in making the choice, the health professional must rely on a guiding principle of the medical profession: where no danger to others exists, patients come first. Practice in a regulated, bureaucratic institution like a prison does not change the principle.

The possibility of discovering contraband during routine examinations of prisoner-patients reinforces the need for informed consent at several stages. First, prisoner-patients should be evaluated and treated only after they provide informed consent unless they are incompetent. Before an X ray is taken they should be informed that it can demonstrate metal and other foreign bodies, and agree to the procedure.

Second, if a concealed weapon is discovered during a routine examination the prisoner-patient should be informed that the discovery will be reported and given the opportunity to surrender the weapon to authorities before more forcible means are taken to remove it. Mr. Jones is probably harboring drugs and a needle and drug use is quite possibly contributing to his health problem. It is the physician's responsibility to educate him about the potential harm to himself from drug use.

The prison setting often presents health professionals with the need to choose between the duty to protect the public and the duty to protect patients' rights to privacy. The decision must rest with the health professionals.

COMMENTARY

B. Jaye Anno

Under ordinary circumstances, prisoners who are patients have a right to expect that their encounters with health professionals will remain confidential. However, that right is forfeited at the point when the health professional's withholding of information may result in some harm to the patient or to others, such as in this case. The admitting physician cannot simply ignore the presence of possible contraband, especially without knowing what the patient is secreting. The physician's first step is to tell the patient what the X ray revealed and ask him to surrender the objects voluntarily. If the patient refuses, the physician's next step is to notify the appropriate prison authorities so that a body cavity search can be conducted, presumably according to written protocols.

If the patient agrees to surrender the items (or to have the physician remove them), the physician's next step depends upon what the objects turn out to be. If the items are harmless, the physician need not notify the prison authorities. However, a referral for some type of counseling may be indicated.

If, on the other hand, the objects turn out to be a needle and a capsule of drugs, the physician must notify prison officials. The physician's motivation for doing so is not to punish the patient, but rather to prevent Mr. Jones from further harming himself. The patient's history of intravenous drug use and hepatitis suggest that his present liver condition may be a product of continued intravenous drug use. Prison officials should be informed so that they can investigate how Mr. Jones obtained the contraband and institute measures to prevent a recurrence.

In my opinion, the present case has few implications for altering informed consent practices. It would be most unusual for a prisoner not to be informed at the time of admission regarding the institution's policies on contraband. Similarly, health professionals are generally told at the time of employment what their obligations are to report rule infractions. In the present case, it was not suggested that Mr. Jones was unaware of the rules and possible consequences of carrying contraband. Therefore, there was no special obligation for the admitting physician to warn the patient that she or he had a duty to report any contraband found that might be harmful to the patient or to others. In short, while it would not hurt to provide a second warning, the rules governing informed consent would not require it. Obviously, my response would be different if I believed that prisoners were not routinely informed of institutional rules.

In the second scenario—namely, "what if the discovered contraband had the appearance of a sequestered weapon?"—the physician's response is much more clear-cut. She or he must report this immediately to the appropriate authorities. The possible harmful consequences of not reporting the presence of a weapon far outweigh any claim the prisoner may make for privileged information.

For me, then, the prison physician's duty to report versus his or her duty to maintain the patient's confidentiality turns on the issue of which decision has the potential for doing the most harm. Any circumstance that involves the possibility of doing harm to others must be reported immediately. Further, in a prison environment, situations involving the possiblity of harm to self must be reported also. Prisons are charged with maintaining the health and welfare of inmates in their custody. No prison staff member, including health professionals, should fail to act on information that might cause that patient harm.

12

A Duty to Warn, An Uncertain Danger

Ms. L., a twenty-eight-year-old, unmarried woman, is admitted to General Hospital to deliver her first child. In the past, she has been treated for pyromania and schizophrenia (paranoid type), and since the age of eighteen she has spent a total of five and a half years in a state mental hospital or in the

inpatient unit of the local community mental health center in the suburban community where she lives. She has also been arrested for arson on three occasions. Each arrest led to a court referral for psychiatric care.

Mrs. D., the social worker on the Ob-Gyn service at General Hospital, is familiar with Ms. L.'s psychiatric history and arrest record because she was formerly employed by the community mental health center where Ms. L. had been a patient. During a pre-delivery conversation with Ms. L. about her plans, Mrs. D. discovers that Ms. L. has no current residence and spent the previous year drifting from shelter to shelter. Ms. L. informs Mrs. D. that after her baby's birth she is planning to move in temporarily with a local Rabbi and his family, who occasionally share their home with people in dire straits.

Mrs. D. immediately begins to wonder about warning the Rabbi, Rabbi P. about the possible danger to him, his wife, and young children. As a member of Rabbi P.'s congregation, Mrs. D. is aware that, on occasion, he opens his home to transients. She is very concerned about the welfare of Rabbi P.'s family, given Ms. L.'s documented history of arson. The next day, Mrs. D. asks Ms. L. for permission to talk with Rabbi P. about her housing needs and about the difficulties she has experienced over the years. Ms. L. refuses permission for such disclosures.

Is Mrs. D. obliged to warn Rabbi P. about Ms. L. and her history, despite Ms. L.'s refusal to consent? Is it relevant that Mrs. D. came upon the confidential information about Ms. L. serendipitously, as a result of her previous employment in the local community mental health center?

COMMENTARY

Frederic G. Reamer

The commitment to confidentiality in the various health and mental health professions is deep-seated. Codes of ethics routinely cite the professional's obligation to hold in confidence information that a client shares. The Code of Ethics of the National Association of Social Workers—which is pertinent to Mrs. D.'s predicament—is representative: "The social worker should respect the privacy of clients and hold in confidence all information obtained in the course of professional service."

Difficulties arise, of course, when there appear to be good reasons for revealing confidential information against a client's wishes. The circumstances surrounding Ms. L. are typical in this respect, and every profession can produce similar stories. Understandably, confusion exists about the circumstances that warrant a breach of confidentiality, especially when a threat to a third party is involved. Though every professional knows that there must be limits to guarantees of confidentiality, there is no consensus about where the line should be drawn.

Debates about professionals' duty to warn generally address several often conflicting rights and obligations: the client's right to privacy; the professional's duty to protect the client's interests, along with those of the general public; and the professional's right to avoid being held liable. Based on these considerations, a good case can be made that Mrs. D. has a duty to warn Rabbi P. and his family about Ms. L.'s history and, thus, has a right to reveal confidential information against Ms. L.'s wishes. As do many codes of ethics, the NASW code qualifies its principle on confidentiality with a statement that "the social worker should share with others confidences revealed by clients, without their consent, only for compelling professional reasons." Though this code does not define "compelling professional reasons," no doubt most would agree that the genuine threat of arson qualifies (especially since Mrs. D.'s information is based on law enforcement and mental health records, not hearsay).

This position is also supported by case law established by the California Supreme Court's well-known *Tarasoff* decision. *Tarasoff* held that when a therapist determines that a client presents a serious danger of violence to another person, the therapist incurs an obligation to use "reasonable care" to protect the potential victim from harm. This may require the therapist to warn the victim, notify the police, or take whatever other steps "are reasonably necessary under the circumstances." Though Ms. L. has not threatened to harm Rabbi P. and his family, the spirit of *Tarasoff* supports disclosure of confidential information in this case.

Is it relevant that Mrs. D. acquired her knowledge of Ms. L.'s past accidentally, by virtue of her previous employment? No. What matters is that Mrs. D. has become party to confidential information that may need to be revealed in order to protect a third party from serious harm. No victim would be consoled to learn that information about an impending threat was withheld because it was not acquired through ordinary channels. Though we would not want to advocate or condone the use of improper channels, we cannot afford to ignore compelling information that lands in our lap as a result of fortuitous circumstances.

It is not enough merely to conclude that Mrs. D. has a duty to warn. One must also ask what specific information ought to be shared. As a rule of thumb, professionals should reveal as little as possible, while ensuring that a potential victim has sufficient details to be able to react in an informed way. Professionals sometimes reveal more information than is necessary to warn a potential victim adequately. In this case, Mrs. D. should limit her disclosure to information about Ms. L.'s history that appears to pose some genuine risk to Rabbi P. and his family. If Ms. L. does not contact Rabbi P. no confidential information should be disclosed to him. Mrs. D. would do well to have a committee comprised of hospital colleagues and administrators review, critique, and authorize her plan, to protect both Ms. L.'s right to confidentiality and the right of Mrs. D. and the hospital to avoid being held liable.

How likely is it that Ms. L. will harm Rabbi P. and his family? Unfortunately, there is no way of knowing. The ability of mental health professionals to forecast dangerousness in such cases does not have an impressive track record. Our instinct to protect potential victims in these circumstances is a good one, however. Though professionals must take care to avoid gratutitous disclosure of confidential information, we cannot fail to acknowledge, as *Tarasoff* makes clear, that "the protective privilege ends where the public peril begins."

COMMENTARY

Sylvan J. Schaffer

The practitioner in this case faces a difficult choice: whether to preserve a confidence or to protect the safety of a generous cleric and his young children. In trying to resolve this dilemma it is important first to consider the purpose of the confidentiality rule and then to consider when it applies.

In social work, as in the other mental health professions, honoring confidentiality is a fundamental consideration in fostering a trusting relationship with the patient. Without the promise of privacy few people would be willing to trust relative strangers with their innermost thoughts, fears, and secrets. Thus, confidentiality allows the therapeutic relationship to develop and continue. It is difficult, if not impossible, to imagine psychotherapy without the guarantee of privacy.

Recognizing the importance of confidentiality to the psychotherapeutic process, some states have extended the right of privileged communication to mental health professionals. (While there may be some differences between statutes concerning psychiatrists, psychologists, and social workers, for the purposes of this article the professions will be treated as equal.) John H. Wigmore, a legal scholar, has delineated the criteria that warrant the recognition of confidential communications: the communication must originate in confidence; the confidence is vital to maintaining the relationship; the relationship is one that should be encouraged; and the detriment to the relationship through the fear of disclosure is greater than the benefit which would result from disclosure.

However, confidentiality is not absolute. There are circumstances under which a social worker would not be bound to keep a confidence. These include cases in which a patient has introduced his mental condition in a civil proceeding; or a judge has ordered a psychiatric examination and the patient is informed that confidentiality does not exist; or there is imminent physical danger to the patient or to a third party. This case is an example of the third type of exception. That exception provides the mental health professional with the most difficult choice since the standard of "imminent danger" is subjective and difficult to delineate.

The most influential source used by the courts and mental health professionals in dealing with the conflict of danger and the duty to warn is *Tarasoff v. Regents of the University of California*. In that case it was held that a psychotherapist whose client had indicated during a therapy session that he would kill a particular third party had a duty to warn that party. The ruling in *Tarasoff* indicates that, given the circumstances present in that case, a psychotherapist who is engaged in a therapeutic relationship with a patient who has threatened to do physical harm to a particular person has a duty to breach confidentiality and warn the intended victim.

It is not clear that the duty enunciated in *Tarasoff* would apply to this situation as significant differences distinguish the two cases. To begin with, the social worker is not engaged in a psychotherapeutic relationship with the client. This is important for two reasons: first, she does not have the type of detailed, intimate knowledge about Ms. L. that would enable her to make such a difficult judgment concerning her future behavior. Accurate prediction would be difficult even for a psychotherapist who knows a patient intimately; it seems an almost impossible task for a relative stranger. Second, the law generally does not impose an affirmative duty to control the behavior of another person or to warn of a threat. The duty in *Tarasoff* arose from the special relationship between the therapist and patient, which did impose an affirmative duty on the therapist. Mrs. D. did not have such a special relationship with Ms. L. Her familiarity with the patient was based solely on secondhand information. This is not the kind of relationship present in *Tarasoff.*

Second, the nature of the danger is different from that in *Tarasoff*. In *Tarasoff*, the patient made a definite threat against a specific identifiable person. In this case, Ms. L. has indicated no malice toward anyone. We do not know the nature of her arson arrests. Were they for fires in garbage pails? In abandoned buildings? For insurance? Is there any indication that she would do the same to people who were showing her a kindness, with her own newborn baby in the house? Also, to what degree can her past behavior be considered an accurate predictor of future behavior? Had her treatment for schizophrenia and pyromania been effective? In sum, does Ms. L. present a threat to the Rabbi and his family that justifies that breach of confidentiality? What will be the fate of the social worker if she erroneously breaches confidentiality when the patient presents no real danger? Is the social worker liable for malpractice? Defamation of character? Breach of fiduciary duty?

Third, even if there is an element of risk, is the breach of confidentiality necessary in order to warn Rabbi P? In *Tarasoff* the intended victim did not know of the potential risk. The Rabbi in this case had previously hosted transients and could reasonably be expected to have assessed the risk of allowing strangers to stay in his home. Thus he would not be a naive victim dependent solely on the warning of the social worker.

This last point raises the possiblity of a third course of action—neither silence nor breach of confidentiality—an alternative that has its own advantages and perils. The social worker, who is a member of Rabbi P.'s congregation, and is aware of his work with transients through a nonprofessional source, could engage in a general conversation with him about the risks of such an activity without ever referring to her knowledge about a particular patient. In this way she could ensure that the Rabbi is aware of the possible risks posed by strangers, without ever mentioning Ms. L. or divulging any information about her. Admittedly, this alternative treads a fine line between breaching confidentiality and preserving it. Yet it would allow the social worker to alert Rabbi P. without defaming Ms. L. or disclosing confidential information. Given the paucity of guidelines and legal precedents dealing with such cases and the state of the art in predicting the future dangerousness of patients such dilemmas will continue to trouble conscientious mental health professionals.

13

"My Husband Won't Tell the Children!"

Forsythe Archer, a successful scientist with exacting standards and a rigid personality, is being given palliative treatment for cancer. During the course of the relapses and remissions of the disease, Mr. Archer has steadfastly refused to discuss his illness with his two teenage children and has barely discussed it with his wife. He has made her promise to keep it a secret. His treatment program with its ups and downs has caused severe and unpredictable mood swings, which have exacerbated the children's emotional problems.

In an effort to help the children cope with their father's behavior, Mrs. Archer wants to break the promise and tell the children what is happening. However, when she suggests this to him he angrily rebuffs her. Mrs. Archer believes his refusal is causing undue distress and she fears for the emotional health of her children; one daughter in particular has been showing serious tendencies toward self-destructive behavior.

In desperation, she pleads with the family doctor to do whatever he can– even use coercion if necessary– to get her husband to "open up," lest his cancer destroy not only his life, but the life of one or more of his children. What should the physician do?

COMMENTARY

Nancy Neveloff Dubler

The physician-patient bond is forged by combining need and special skills. It is supported by tradition and by the much maligned and oft-disregarded doctrine of confidentiality.

The clear directive to a physician to protect the utterances of the patients—to hold privacy primary—has its roots in three sorts of ethical and legal developments. Ancient oaths contain exhortations to guard confidentiality. Modern state licensing statutes refer to these credos as a measure of ethical conduct and impose penalties for breach of the standard. Finally, the patient's utterance may be privileged, an issue which the patient may raise in a court of law.

Most patients do not consider it necessary to make explicit the implicit though fuzzy protections for their physical and emotional secrets; they assume it and hope that their wishes will be understood. But in this case the patient was quite explicit: he did not want his children told. He would not or could not discuss, consider, or confront the issue. Perhaps he even chose to remain silent out of perversity, anger, disregard, or conscious cruelty. Any of the above are possible; none justify disregarding his specific directive.

There is neither a direct danger to the population, which justifies breach of confidentiality for public health, nor an identifiable action that both threatens another and violates a legal and moral norm, as for example, an instance of child abuse. It may be argued that this behavior was in fact a sort of child abuse, that exclusion and silence will result in developmental disability or adult inability to function.

This assertion has a number of unconvincing aspects. First, child abuse reporting laws represent a required departure from the standard of professional behavior. Second, they challenge the usual prerogatives of adult caregivers in relation to their children. This last is most important. Parents may be charged and held to account for violence that oversteps understood societal limits. Clearly, spanking a two-year-old who runs in the street in front of an oncoming car is not child abuse. It may (or may not) be bad parenting. Beating that same child insensate or burning him with cigarettes to punish the same infraction is child abuse. The excessive and inappropriate physical battering of a child is the sort of action that requires professionals to speak and that shatters the privacy claims of parents.

This case presents no such immediate and recognizable danger. What if this same father—not ill—declared that he loved one of his children most and would thus finance college for that one child; all others could fend for themselves. Is that abuse? Does the physician want to enter the complex emotional web of interfamily relationships over this sort of issue? Is the danger any more quantifiable or direct in the case under discussion?

Many children suffer from the inept emotional responses of their parents. Many are limited in adulthood from bizarre or destructive parenting. Lacking more data, should the physician enter these marshes? Will the Archers' children suffer more than a child who has been "scape-goated," or deprived of a college experience, or forced to enter adulthood with stunted emotional skills? Our belief in parental prerogatives and physician limitations wisely decrees forebearance.

Furthermore, in this case there is another option. These children can be provided with outside counseling and support. Counseling may not make up for the withdrawal and loss of their father, but it may offer comfort and more. In contrast, Mr. Archer may feel lost if his wishes are disregarded. This physician is his support—directing his care, responding to his needs, and honoring his integrity. The failure to honor his clearly stated wishes may leave him feeling abandoned at the moment of greatest need.

Mrs. Archer has a clear problem—the sort of conflict in loyalty that often besets a parent. Parents differ in the skill and creativity with which they handle their children. Children seek to "divide and conquer," to capitalize on the differing approaches. Often a united front supports parenting. Sometimes the divisions must be acknowledged.

In this case the mother must take those measures necessary to protect her child. She must tell the child the truth and seek the professional assistance that is necessary to sustain her daughter through the present medical crisis and the death of a father. But she need not tell Mr. Archer. Withholding this information will require courage and thespian accomplishment but it need not threaten her relationship with her husband. Lying is not always a wrong when it prevents pain and suffering and alleviates danger. This mother may be paralyzed by fear, conflicts of loyalty, lack of courage, or despair. The physician must offer her support, which can permit her to act. As there is another route available to protect the children, the physician need not endanger his relationship to the primary patient—the father.

Physicians in family practice often negotitate intergenerational conflicts involving clashing personality and value systems. They often weigh the risks and benefits of sharing information imparted in confidence. The justifications for breach of confidentiality are narrow: direct and immediate danger with no alternatives. This family's situation does not qualify. This father has explicitly invoked the protections of confidentiality for the time surrounding his death. He is entitled to the physician's full support.

COMMENTARY

Lawrence J. Schneiderman

This case illustrates a potential conflict in duty facing the physician who cares for more than one member of a family. The patient's right to privacy is a powerful ethical warrant that runs from the Hippocratic tradition to the present. Of more recent vintage is a concept arising out of family therapy and family medicine, which views illness as not limited to an isolated person but rather as potentially involving a nexus of persons who are intimately connected. The latter concept logically requires that the physician's treatment decisions must weigh risks and benefits to all the Archer family members and indeed to the family structure itself on which their well-being depends.

A patient's right to privacy mandates that the physician resist any demands by third parties to violate confidentiality in the absence of rare justifiable exceptions. Is Mrs. Archer's claim such an exception? She pleads that Mr. Archer's failure to reveal and discuss his illness with his children is jeopardizing their health. Her claim might be difficult to evaluate and problematic if the physician were not caring for these children as well as for Mr. Archer. But the physician is professionally obligated to all of them.

Obviously, the thoughtful, experienced, sensitive physician will seek to use his or her skills in ways that will resolve the problem without causing conflict. Perhaps gentle persuasion, emotional support, and counseling will persuade Mr. Archer to "open up" and the family will benefit from the new level of intimacy and honesty achieved. But the possibility exists that Mr. Archer will adamantly refuse to alter his personal mode of coping with his illness. What then? Almost certainly the physician with the aforementioned attributes will also use his or her skills to counsel Mrs. Archer on ways in which to deal with this problem at home. After all, they are her children too. She must pursue ways to inform the children about her husband's condition and seek to open communication among them.

Chances are, however, the physician will inevitably be drawn into this process. The children may have questions a mother cannot answer, and will need emotional support beyond that which the mother can provide.

Can the physician, under these circumstances, refuse to recognize the needs of these other patients? Is Mr. Archer's right to privacy so inviolable? In my opinion, no. Admittedly, this view that the father's behavior is part of the illness that is affecting the children puts us on the notorious slippery slope. Would the physician feel entitled to intervene if Mr. Archer had capriciously excluded one child from his will—an act that surely could lead to unpleasant emotional consequences? How forceful should the physician be? Should the physician use threats to get a parent to stop smoking? Substantial evidence documents the adverse health consequences of smoking behavior on children. Lose weight? A shortened life span of the breadwinner has adverse implications for the dependents. Keep up life insurance and health insurance payments? It is notorious that unexpected health diasters have ruined family fortunes and prospects.

Obviously one has to draw a line. Where? One place to begin is that area of health care for which the physician was consulted. Within this circle, the physician must weigh the relative risks and benefits not just to one person but to all the parties to whom a duty is owed. Although the physician is not entitled to challenge privacy rights in matters of wills, life insurance payments, and so on, the physician would regard it as his or her ethical duty to take strong measures to warn and protect the other family members if Mr. Archer were harboring a serious contagious disease. It is not at all farfetched to extend the analogy to emotional disorders. Emotional illness in one family member can have severe impacts on the others.

How to weigh the risks and benefits? If the physician goes so far as to break confidence or attempt to coerce Mr. Archer into doing something he finds unacceptable, the physician puts the therapeutic relationship (and Mr. Archer's well-being) at risk. What would justify such an act? Surely, in my opinion, if the children's self-destructive behavior included threats of suicide. But also if the children's behavior had ominous implications for their futures, such as delinquency, drug use, or school problems.

From the family-oriented perspective, the patient's refusal is a manifestation of dysfunctional coping with his disease, which is not only harming him but harming others as well. The physician's duty is to ameliorate such harm. Thus I believe that in this situation Mr. Archer's wishes with respect to privacy may have lesser weight than the needs of the children for information and communication, benefits that potentially will influence long future lives.

The physician faced with this ethical dilemma cannot confine his or her duty to one person, thereby ignoring the extensiveness and complexity of the medical problem. In my opinion, the physician is forced off the ideological position of protecting privacy to the slippery slope of weighing risks and benefits. The physician's duty is to all the patients under his or her care.

Selected Bibliography

Annas, George J. *The Rights of Hospital Patients: The Basic ACLU Guide to a Hospital Patient's Rights.* New York: Avon Books, 1975.

Benjamin, Martin, and Curtis, Joy. *Ethics in Nursing.* New York: Oxford University Press, 1981.

Bok, Sissela. *Lying: Moral Choice in Public and Private Life.* New York: Pantheon Press, 1978.

Cassell, Eric J. *Talking with Patients.* 2 vols. Cambridge: MIT Press, 1985.

Childress, James F. *Who Should Decide? Paternalism in Health Care.* New York: Oxford University Press, 1982.

Faden, Ruth R., and Beauchamp, Tom L. *A History and Theory of Informed Consent*. New York: Oxford University Press, 1986.

May, William F. *The Physician's Covenant: Images of the Healer in Medical Ethics*. Philadelphia: Westminster, 1983.

Muyskens, James L. *Moral Problems in Nursing: A Philosophical Investigation*. Totowa, NJ: Rowman and Littlefield, 1982.

Pellegrino, Edmund D., and Thomasma, David C. *A Philosophical Basis of Medical Practice: Toward a Philosophy and Ethics of the Healing Profession*. New York: Oxford University Press, 1981.

President's Commission for the Study of Ethical Problems in Medicine and Biomedical and Behavioral Research: *Making Health Care Decisions*, 3 vols. Washington, DC: U.S. Government Printing Office, 1982.

Ramsey, Paul. *The Patient as Person*. New Haven: Yale University Press, 1970.

Veatch, Robert M. *A Theory of Medical Ethics*. New York: Basic Books, 1981.

PART TWO

Reproductive Rights and Technologies

INTRODUCTION

Nothing, it seems, could be more natural than human reproduction. And, in fact, most babies are conceived, brought to term, delivered, and reared in traditional ways. But modern technology—the ability to manipulate conception in previously unthinkable ways and to terminate pregnancy safely and effectively—has altered the moral equation. The question is no longer the scientific one: Can we intervene in reproduction? It is the moral question: Should we intervene?

The first section in Part Two—"Reproductive Rights"—examines questions of the ethics of familial relationships and responsibilities in an era of in vitro fertilization and embryo transfer (the process of fertilizing an egg outside the mother and reimplanting it in her, or another woman's, womb). Along with the technology of conception has come increased knowledge about the developing fetus, including its risk if the pregnant mother uses drugs, alcohol, or cigarettes, to name only a few potentially harmful behaviors. What are her responsibilities to avoid harm to her fetus? Another case raises the question of society's responsibilities to support a wanted child of a single mother on public assistance.

While these cases concern wanted, indeed deeply wanted, babies, the cases in the second section, on "Abortion," concern unwanted offspring. Discussions of abortion are among the most divisive in biomedical ethics. Those who hold to absolute positions on this question are unlikely to be moved by the cases in this section, but those who find plausible moral arguments on both sides of the issue will find these discussions illuminating. What, for example, is the appropriate policy to follow when a fetus is born alive after an abortion? Can a mentally ill woman consent to an abortion? What if she resists the pressures of family and professionals to have an abortion, even though she will never be able to care for the child? What is a hospital's duty toward rape victims when its policies prohibit abortions? And bringing the discussion full circle to technologically assisted reproduction, when a woman has a multiple pregnancy, caused by fertility drugs, is it ethical to perform a selective abortion, reducing the number of fetuses to the desired level? The last case in this section raises the question of what a genetic counselor's role should be.

The cases in this part offer a multi-faceted look at reproduction in a technological era. The ethical questions they raise go to the heart of the human desire to reproduce and to control the terms of that process. With control comes choice, and with choice comes the responsibility to choose wisely.

REPRODUCTIVE RIGHTS

14

When Baby's Mother Is also Grandma—and Sister

David Fassler

Sally Morgan is forty-six years old and has been divorced for ten years. She has one child, a twenty-five-year-old daughter. Recently she married Frank Charlton, a forty-nine-year-old childless widower. They would like to start a family of their own, but she is now infertile.

Mrs. Charlton consults a university in vitro fertilization (IVF) program, where she is told that she is not a suitable candidate for the procedure. However, her husband's sperm could be used to fertilize an egg cell from an anonymous donor. The embryo could then be implanted in a surrogate mother and carried to term.

Since Mrs. Charlton would like her child to be genetically related, her daughter offers to donate the egg cell to be utilized in the in vitro fertilization process. Each of the daughter's cells contains 50 percent of her mother's genetic material; therefore the baby would have one-half of that amount, or 25 percent. In this manner, the child would be genetically related to Mrs. Charlton. Mrs. Charlton would be in the unusual position of being both mother and grandmother to the child; her daughter would be both its mother and sister.

Should the donation be approved?

COMMENTARY

Lori B. Andrews

This case adds a twist to the debate raised by the involvement of third parties in procreation by asking whether a daughter may serve as a gamete donor. Although the advantages and disadvantages of such a situation will differ markedly depending on the particular individuals involved, such an arrangement should be allowed.

The donation would allow Mrs. Charlton and her husband to have a child genetically related to both of them. It may be the only realistic opportunity for her husband to have a child within the marriage since anonymously donated eggs may be scarce and costly (particularly in comparison to donor sperm).

The donation could give the daughter the chance to express her altruism. The prospective child might gain by experiencing greater love and support as well as a more definite identity than if produced by an anonymous donor. And permitting the donation would reinforce the strong moral and legal protection of autonomy regarding decisions about how to create and raise a family.

Some may object to the procedure because it seems unnatural, contrary to traditional notions of family, or may present risks to the parties. In attempting to assess the ethical merit of the donation, professional practices and the law should follow the model used for determining the scientific merit of a new therapy. Under the best of circumstances, a medical innovation is adopted when it is anticipated to be an improvement over the existing treatment modalities and is unlikely to cause risks that outweigh its potential benefits. In this ideal situation, as the procedure is done more frequently, its effects are closely monitored to determine whether it should continue to be used.

All forms of parenting, including traditional reproduction, present potential physical and psychological harm to the participants; yet society is reluctant to interfere with procreative decisions. This is the backdrop against which the donation of an egg from a daughter to a mother must be judged. I do not think that the risks presented by a daughter's gamete donation are sufficiently different in type or greater in magnitude to warrant banning the procedure. Rather, such donations should be allowed and scrutinized for their actual, rather than possible effects.

The potential physical risks to the participants do not appear serious enough to preclude the procedure.

Since many women have undergone laparoscopies and pregnancies, the potential physical harm to the daughter and surrogate is readily quantifiable and can be explained during the informed consent process. When IVF first came into use, the potential physical risks to the child were unknown. Although there are still not enough births to assess whether IVF presents a slightly increased risk of anomalies in offspring (say, 5 percent), it is clear that IVF is generally safe and surely does not present the 25 percent risk of affected offspring that parents with a lethal recessive gene trait run when they choose to have children.

Although most of the human IVF births have involved pregnancies in which the embryo was implanted in the woman who provided the egg, the use of a surrogate should not present additional risks. Indeed, most of the animal IVF studies (showing no increase in anomalies) have involved transfers of the embryos to a surrogate.

Nor do the potential psychological ramifications for the participants seem a sufficient reason to ban the donation. Unlike the unknown risks presented by manipulations of embryos in the early attempts at IVF, the psychological harms can be predicted by analogy to existing situations, such as an adoption or a grandmother raising her daughter's child because of divorce or the daughter's young age.

In this case, three women and one man have an emotional investment in the creation of a child. The physician should discuss with the participants the ways in which the proposed donation arrangement might threaten their emotional well-being. This is in keeping with the approach taken by Great Britain's Warnock Committee and the Victoria, Australia legislation, which require careful counseling when an identifiable egg donor is used.

The discussions should not be a form of licensing for parenting. Since we do not prohibit forty-six-year-old women from conceiving, bearing, and raising children naturally, Mrs. Charlton should not be discouraged because of her age from entering this arrangement. Rather, the interviews should focus on how the participants will handle the unique aspects of this case—the severing of the maternal genetic relationship and the maternal rearing relationship, with the former being provided by the daughter and the latter being provided by the mother.

One of the principal potential hazards lies in the possibility that the daughter could be coerced into donating her egg. In attempting to assure that the daughter has given her voluntary informed consent, the physician should make sure she has thought through the many possible future ramifications of the procedure. How would she feel if she lost her ability to conceive (perhaps as a result of the laparoscopic surgery itself) and her mother's child was her only link to motherhood?

How will the parties deal with the impression, though not the reality, of incest? Currently, stepfather-stepdaughter sexual relationships are considered incestuous and subject to civil penalties in eleven states and criminal penalties in five states. Although fertilizing the daughter's egg with her stepfather's sperm in a petri dish does not violate these laws, the unusual relationship may make the parties uneasy or cause them difficulties in dealing with outsiders who feel they have violated a basic taboo.

The physician should also discuss with the participants whether or not they will tell the child that its sister is the genetic mother. Because of the emotional harm unplanned disclosure can cause the child, the possibility of being candid with the child should at least be raised. It will clearly be stressful for the family unit if the parties do not agree on how to handle this point.

Yet the practitioner's ethical responsibilities do not end with the application of appropriate policies and principles to this particular decision. Since the request for gamete donation between friends or relatives is likely to come up again, there is an ongoing responsibility to better inform the next decision. Just as a new medical procedure is monitored to collect information on the physical risks it presents, physicians and mental health professionals have a responsibility to research the psychological effects of the new reproductive technologies they introduce. The track record of the medical and psychiatric professions in conducting such studies is poor—witness the dearth of well-designed research about the psychological effects on the donor, recipient, recipient's spouse, and child of the century-old technique of artificial insemination by donor. But such studies are especially important where practitioners are helping to conceive a new individual in ways that give birth to new ethical dilemmas.

COMMENTARY

Hans O. Tiefel

A forty-six-year-old mother of a twenty-five-year-old daughter who wants to start parenting all over again, who will not be denied by nature, who will be sixty-two with a husband of sixty-five when the hoped-for child will reach the mature age of fifteen—such a woman must be extraordinarily optimistic about what it means to raise a child. One cannot help but wonder whether a child out of season meant to enhance the marriage may prove extraordinarily taxing to a couple who normally would welcome the visits, and the departures, of grandchildren. Yet such doubts seem condescending since both Mr. and Mrs. Charlton are old enough to know what they are doing. Foolishness need not be immoral. Therefore one should assume that they are willing to pay the price for wanting to start "a family."

But not any child will do. A handicapped child, an abandoned child, a racially mixed child are not mentioned. The offspring must be their own genetically. This genetic connection necessitates the circuitous route of in vitro fertilization and surrogate motherhood. Yet the value of genetic linkage should be questioned when it is pursued in such a complex manner, when it draws other agents into this marriage as contributing agents, and when it raises the possibility of harm to the offspring since sperm deteriorate with aging. Moreover, since genetic percentages seem to matter in this case, 25 percent of the genetic inheritance will come from Mrs. Charlton's divorced husband. One expects that neither Mrs. Charlton nor her husband Frank care much for this genetic interloper. But this unhappy link does offer an opportunity to ascribe any undesirable characteristics of the child-to-be to that man who is well gone but not gone completely.

The role of Mrs. Charlton as both mother and grandmother does not seem troubling; both roles are nurturing and many grandmothers take over the functions of mothers by default. More questionable in this case is the exact meaning of "mother." There are three contenders for that title: the genetic mother (the daughter who contributes the egg), the surrogate, and the social mother (Mrs. Charlton). Whom shall the child call "Mom"?

And if that seems a trivial question, who will be responsible for the care and nurture of the child when it turns out differently than expected? Would Mrs. Charlton still acknowledge the child as hers if it were born with a genetic defect, since her genetic contribution is half that of her daughter? Would she claim to be the real mother if the child were born with a handicap that could be directly attributed to the carelessness of the surrogate mother during pregnancy? Normally mother and child are bound to each other by birth, for better or worse. When these natural ties disappear, bonds of loyalty and care for offspring may also weaken.

More interesting than the combined role of mother and grandmother is the dual status of the daughter and egg donor as both mother and sister. The arrangement assumes that the genetic relationship, which is decisive to the couple, should be disregarded by the daughter. The child-to-be will be half hers, genetically speaking, but this is considered irrelevant once the child is conceived. The parties seem to have contradictory value judgments about genetic derivation.

The surrogate's role is also problematic. Surrogates have been known to become unexpectedly attached to the children they have borne for profit or love. Assuming that the child is carried for love rather than money, would love require her to undergo amniocentesis and, if that showed the presence of defects, an abortion? If she refused abortion out of love for the child-to-be, would the child become hers in every sense, including responsibility for its medical care and upbringing?

And what of the child-to-be itself? It is still too early to tell if in vitro fertilization and embryo transfer pose long-term risks to the child. Even if aspiring parents take that risk (not for themselves but for their offspring), other problems remain. If our self-identity is shaped largely by lineage, if it is important to whom we belong and who belongs to us, then the child may want to relate to all three mothers. The couple cannot expect the child to be indifferent to "the woman who is my flesh and blood" or to "the woman who brought me into the world."

Even naturally born children complain of not being loved enough and of not belonging. Won't triple motherhood create additional tensions and resentment? Will the child not seek refuge from real or imagined grievances with the most sympathetic, and therefore the "real," mother? One might reply that the risks of dispersed kinship ties will not outweigh the good of this child's existence. But that begs the question, since such a value cannot be invoked before the child has come into being.

We live in relationships. But this case reads as if complex begetting were a private matter, as if the issues pertain only to this particular case and as if the wishes of the couple should be decisive. The case reads true enough in times in which morality is reduced to private choice, legality, and consumer satisfaction. But it is also misleading, especially in regard to medical matters. Medical professionals play an indispensable yet deplorably passive role here: Just tell us what you want and we will make it possible. Happily this is counterfactual; no institution is yet quite so accommodating.

Should physicians demur, the couple could claim that its rights have been violated. For rights remain the only powerful and public tool in otherwise privatized ethics. True, no one has a right to interfere with claims to beget children. But such rights remain negative. They establish no corresponding duty on the part of the physician to facilitate reproduction, any more than my right to marry obligates any woman to marry me. Moreover, relying on rights is rather self-centered. Rights cannot guide us in deciding who we should be as spouses or parents or what we owe one another in love.

The loving decision in this case is not what Mrs. Charlton and her husband "would like." It is one that seeks the good of all who are part of these relationships, especially the child-to-be. And the good of this envisioned offspring is obstructed by the risk of harm, by contradictory values about genetic ties, by confusion over who may claim the child and who is responsible for it (and whom the child may claim and be responsible to), and by a need for personal selflessness on the part of the genetic mother that exceeds realistic expectations. In this case moral judgment supports common sense: this foolishness is also immoral.

15

When a Pregnant Woman Endangers Her Fetus

Janet M., in her early twenties, is pregnant for the third time. She has been an insulin-dependent diabetic since the age of twelve but has experienced no major complications of diabetes.

Dr. L. has repeatedly advised her of the risks that uncontrolled diabetes poses to her fetus. Congenital malformations are two to four times more common in infants of mothers whose diabetes is poorly controlled. Furthermore, uncontrolled diabetes can result in the birth of a premature, stillborn fetus.

He admits her at fifteen weeks gestation as an inpatient to treat her diabetes, but she discharges herself against his advice five days later before her diabetes has been satisfactorily controlled. Once home, she ignores pleas from Dr. L. and other physicians to obtain chemstrips or a dextrometer for monitoring blood sugar. In response, she tells them she "has no money" or "forgot."

At twenty-one weeks gestation she is hospitalized for a threatened abortion but quickly announces her intention to leave. Dr. L. decides that her behavior poses a clear risk to the well-being of her fetus. Unless she changes her mind, he says, he will seek a court order to keep her hospitalized.

Is his response justified?

COMMENTARY

Thomas B. Mackenzie and Theodore C. Nagel

Three generic questions can be posed in cases like this one. First, does the physician have an obligation to the fetus to ensure its well-being that cannot be abrogated by the parents? Second, is there sound scientific evidence of a relationship between the specific condition or behavior observed and fetal risk (or damage) to justify concern? And third, is there any way to control the condition that does not significantly endanger the physical health of the mother?

We believe that in order to justify legal action, the answer to all three questions must be yes.

Did this woman's physicians have an obligation to her fetus that superseded her wishes as expressed in her conversation and behavior? In answering this question one must consider two intertwined issues: abortion and viability. Present judicial doctrine clearly subordinates the physician's obligation to the fetus in favor of the woman's right to abort prior to fetal viability. Thus the intention to abort would waive any obligation to protect fetal well-being. But Janet M. gave no indication that this was her intention.

Whether the physician's obligation to the fetus (presuming an intention to carry to term) is the same before as it is after viability is a complex question.

From an ethical point of view that demarcation is not compelling, since fetal conditions that require diagnosis and treatment can be identified prior to viability. Thus the fetus can be a patient independent of the mother in the sense that it is the sole possessor of a disease or condition. It is also clear that maternal behavior during early pregnancy may adversely affect the fetus and result in irreversible injury. Consequently the physician's ethical responsibility to the fetus prior to viability (or prior to the woman's decision to abort) is not different than it is at a later stage of pregnancy.

Whether the physician has a legal obligation prior to viability is less clear. While all American jurisdictions allow a child to recover for prenatal injuries negligently inflicted after viability, only some jurisdictions have abandoned the viability standard. Thus whether a physician could be sued by a child for malpractice regarding care given before viability depends on the state.

At the time when intervention was considered in this case, Janet M.'s fetus was not viable. However, we do not feel that the fetus's nonviability diminished the obligations of her attending physicians. The mother clearly had information about her pregnancy and the potential consequences of uncontrolled diabetes. Her behavior was not a result of ignorance. Her explanations for failing to obtain the equipment that was necessary to control her diabetes were inconsistent and vague. Overall her behavior indicated an unwillingness to manage her diabetes in a manner that minimized the risk to her fetus. Under these circumstances, we believe her physicians had an obligation to the fetus that could not be waived by the mother.

The second question asks whether there is sufficient certainty of a relationship between a recurrent behavior and damage to the fetus. In other words, a physician could not tyrannize the mother by holding her to frivolous or unproven standards in the name of fetal welfare. The answer to this question is yes. A clear relationship has been established between careful management of insulin-dependent diabetes mellitis and reduced incidence of stillbirth, intrauterine deaths, respiratory distress syndrome, macrosomia, and congenital malformations.

The final question asks: Can the threatening condition be reasonably controlled or reversed without significantly endangering the physical health of the mother? If the answer to this question is no, then positive responses to our first two standards would be immaterial. In the case at hand, effective control of diabetes during pregnancy appears well within reach. This may involve close surveillance in the hospital with three to four subcutaneous insulin injections per day. Hospitalization also permits early recognition of emerging complications in the last weeks of pregnancy. Alternatively, patients may monitor their diabetes at home using home blood glucose monitoring, with fetal monitoring done as an outpatient. The latter was offered to Mrs. M. but was not accepted. Thus the answer to the third question is yes.

Since we have answered all three questions in the affirmative, we would support the decision of Janet M.'s physicians to seek enforced hospitalization and treatment to protect and preserve the well-being of the fetus. After noting that protecting the fetus would involve violation of the mother (drawing blood and administering insulin), the court might well decide against the actions urged by the attending physician. Such an outcome would not indicate that her physician was overly zealous. It would reflect the growing capacity of medicine to observe, diagnose, and treat the developing fetus and the consequent conflict between the woman's freedom to control her own body and the potential adverse effects of her behavior on her unborn child.

COMMENTARY

Barbara Katz Rothman

Had this discussion been written twenty-five years ago, it might have read as follows:

> Janet M., a diabetic, refused her DES treatment, prescribed as especially important in the prevention of miscarriage among diabetics. Further, although she was eleven pounds overweight at the time of conception, she refused to limit her weight gain over the course of pregnancy to under thirteen pounds. She compounded the problem by not taking the diuretics prescribed, and twice refused to show up for scheduled x-rays, citing a distrust of medications and radiation. Her irrational refusal to comply with her doctor's advice, plus her unwillingness or inability to limit her weight gain, indicate fetal abuse. Should Dr. L. seek a court order . . . ?

And a potential scenario for twenty-five years from now:

> Mrs. M., suspecting pregnancy, engages the services of an attorney who specializes in family law, especially prenatal agreements. On her initial visit to the fetologist, Mrs. M. and her attorney will be informed of the conditions to which she must adhere throughout the pregnancy, and a second attorney will be appointed to act as fetal guardian. Violations of the prenatal contract will result in the state gaining custody of the fetus: either forcibly removing it to an artificial womb, or putting Mrs. M. in one of the new high-security wings of the maternity hospital for the duration of her pregnancy.

These two scenarios, past and future, illustrate the two major problems I see with an obstetrician calling on the power of the state to control a pregnant woman's behavior in the interests of her fetus. First, obstetrics has too long a history of errors in management for us to be certain that obstetricians always *know* the best interests of the fetus. Each of the procedures cited above, recommended twenty-five years ago, has since been discarded as dangerous. It is too soon to be certain of the standing today's obstetrical practices will come to have in the future.

But even if one had perfect faith in obstetrical knowledge, a second and more serious problem remains: the costs to the civil liberties of pregnant women are too high. We are in danger of creating of pregnant women a second class of citizen, without basic legal rights of bodily integrity and self-determination. Competent adults in this society have the right to refuse medical treatment, even when it is believed to be life-saving. But as reproductive rights attorney Janet Gallagher has warned in a chapter from a forthcoming book, *Biology and Women's Policy,* "The law's concern for human dignity and self-determination can all too readily yield to the recurrent temptations to view and treat pregnant women as vessels." It is wrong to allow obstetrics or the state to subsume the interests and the civil rights of pregnant women to those of the products of conception within them.

The basic ethical question in this case is: What are the obligations of obstetricians toward their patients? Or more precisely, who exactly is the patient of an obstetrician? A long-standing definition of obstetrics is "the branch of medicine concerning the care of women during pregnancy, labor and the puerperium." But that definition may no longer seem appropriate, as obstetricians such as Dr. L. increasingly define themselves as physicians to the fetus. The medical model of pregnancy, as an essentially parasitic and vaguely pathological relationship, encourages the physician to view the fetus and mother as two separate patients, and to see pregnancy as inherently a conflict of interests between the two. Where the fetus is highly valued, the effect is to reduce the woman to what current obstetrical language calls "the maternal environment."

A more appropriate and ultimately more useful perspective is to see the pregnant woman as a biological and social unit. With a more holistic view, Dr. L. might remember that Mrs. M. has controlled her diabetes for over half her life, and through two pregnancies. It may not be a matter of behaving "as she chooses." As a mother of two young children, Mrs. M. may have a variety of compelling reasons preventing her from staying for more than five days in the hospital, from returning for an indefinite period, or even from taking good care of herself at home. As *her* physician, Dr. L. might consider what *her* needs are—social and economic as well as medical—and how he might help her to meet those, rather than calling on the courts to control her.

16

AID and the Single Welfare Mother

Dr. Arnold Franklin, an obstetrician, performs about ten artificial inseminations by donor (AID) a week. His usual practice is to interview single women twice to determine whether they are suitable candidates, medically and psychologically. He also requests that they supply letters from friends, family, relatives, or coworkers attesting to their sense of responsibility and emotional stability. However, he does not ask his single women patients for any detailed financial information.

A year or so ago, a thirty-year-old unmarried woman, Teresa Stevens, came to Dr. Franklin requesting artificial insemination. She said that she was working part-time and intended to stay at her job once the baby was born. She also provided assurances from family and friends that they supported her desire to be a mother. Dr. Franklin decided to go ahead with the procedure, which was successful.

Several months later, to Dr. Franklin's surprise, the press reported that Ms. Stevens was receiving $161 in monthly pregnancy welfare assistance. In addition, she had recently learned that she was eligible for $401 a month from Aid to Families with Dependent Children after her child was born, and intended to file for those benefits. Ms. Stevens admitted that she knew about the pregnancy benefits before she contacted Dr. Franklin, but the doctor never raised the issue with her.

The community reacted indignantly. Some suggested that she should not have been artificially inseminated. Others said the physician should pay the cost of the pregnancy. Dr. Franklin was troubled too. On the one hand, he felt strongly that an unmarried woman "has deep feelings about wanting to become pregnant," and that it is impossible for a man to understand that need. On the other hand, he was deeply concerned about abuses of welfare and "didn't want to deliberately tax the system."

Should the doctor have performed AID in this case? Should single women who want AID be required to supply more detailed information than married women? How can the belief that every woman has a right to have a baby be reconciled with society's right not to have to pay for that choice?

COMMENTARY

Theodora Ooms

Ms. Stevens's story confronts us with our ambivalent feelings about voluntary single parenthood. Her behavior challenges two fundamental assumptions: first, that children are best reared in a two-parent family; and second, that parents' primary function is to provide economic support for their children. These assumptions are gradually being eroded by the unrelenting increase in the number of single parents, although most of this parenthood is "involuntary"—a result of unplanned, out-of-wedlock pregnancies or of separation and divorce. Since some, or even many, single parents are reported to be doing a fine job, Dr. Franklin can now talk about the right of any woman, married or not, to bear and raise a child.

But Ms. Stevens not only wanted to bear a child, she planned to support it with public assistance funds. Her welfare check was a result not of accident or unfortunate circumstance but of a personal choice. This deliberate quality of her indigency triggered the question of whether she was somehow defrauding the public and "deserved" assistance either from Dr. Franklin or public funds.

The concepts of the "deserving" and "undeserving" poor have dominated recent discussions about the main federal welfare program, Aid to Families with Dependent Children (AFDC). This program, enacted in 1935, was originally intended to provide financial support to widows and their children. Since then, the number of recipients has increased enormously. Now 80 percent of the adult recipients are divorced, separated, or never-married women; only 4 percent are widows. As the costs of the program have soared, it has come under increasing attack. The system is accused of supporting and encouraging undesirable or immoral behavior (laziness, cheating, paternal irresponsibility, and promiscuity). The public outcry in some states led to attempts to deny assistance to welfare mothers who have boyfriends (the "man in the house" rule) and illegitimate children. Some people advocated sterilization of welfare mothers.

A series of definitive court rulings in the late sixties defeated these attempts, and public policy assumptions are now quite clear. Eligibility for welfare is determined only by relatively objective criteria such as economic need, marital status (in only twenty-six states is aid given to two-parent needy families), and willingness to work, if able. The degree to which an individual is morally responsible for creating her need is not considered a legitimate factor in determining eligibility.

On ethical grounds, Teresa Stevens cannot be accused of sexual immorality, since she chose an immaculate form of conception. And on both practical and moral grounds it is very difficult to make the distinction between the voluntary ("undeserving") nature of her pregnancy (and consequent public dependency) and the so-called involuntary ("deserving") behavior of other types of welfare mothers. Consider the many teenage mothers with flimsy explanations as to why they did not use birth control, or the mother who seeks a divorce because of unhappiness with her spouse, or the married couple applying for welfare because the husband's wages are too low to pay the medical bills of their five children.

The attitude that wants to deny Ms. Stevens the right to welfare benefits for her child, or condemns her physician for helping her become pregnant, is based on an indefensible double standard: federal assistance to the poor in the form of welfare should be contingent on "good behavior"; but federal assistance to the middle class and wealthy in the form of tax relief, social security, student grants, and so on, should be available with no such strings attached.

Turning to questions of professional ethics, if donor sperm is in short supply, Dr. Franklin must establish priorities, and he should be free to develop his own criteria for accepting applicants (although considerations of income could discriminate against poor women). But if the supply of donor sperm is unlimited, Dr. Franklin may be misguided in his attempts to screen a single woman applicant by a higher standard than he would use for a married couple. Though being a single parent is usually tougher than sharing the job, the present high rate of divorce (approximately one out of three marriages) indicates that he would be wise to screen married couples also to determine their fitness for parenting and the stability of their marriage. Such subjective assessments may lead down a slippery slope: why not apply such criteria to all cases of infertility or indeed to all prospective parents?

Finally, even if Dr. Franklin had full knowledge of Ms. Stevens's intention to seek public support, he should not be held responsible or blamed because his client claims public benefits to which she is clearly entitled. His assistance to her might be compared to that of a lawyer helping a mother of three get divorced and advising her that she may have to go on public assistance to support herself while her children are young. The members of

Dr. Franklin's community should not project onto him and Ms. Stevens their own discomfort with a public policy that declines to sort out the deserving from the undeserving poor.

COMMENTARY

Margaret O'Brien Steinfels

Of the three persons in this case, the interests of one, Baby Stevens, are never cited. The assumption that those interests are congruent with the interests of Ms. Stevens is unwarranted. While Ms. Stevens may not want or have a husband, we can easily imagine Baby Stevens expressing the desire for a father. True, many children in our society have fathers without their mothers having husbands. Unlike Baby Stevens, however, these children have been fathered by a man known to their mother, a person that a child can imagine even if the child has no contact with him. AID babies born to married couples can center their attachment on the adoptive father. AID babies born to single women are left to imagine an anonymous donor who provided sperm for a fee—a stud.

More important, Baby Stevens, like all children, has an interest in a normal family life. The large number of single-parent families notwithstanding, there is no evidence that a single-parent family is better than a two-parent family for a child. In fact, increasing evidence suggests that divorce and single-parenting can be detrimental to a child's well-being. The baby's well-being is further compromised by Ms. Stevens's decision to go on welfare. Placing her desire to be a mother above the psychological, social, and economic needs of her child does not bode well for the rigors of child rearing.

And what of Dr. Franklin's interests? He was not concerned about providing AID to a single woman so long as he could establish her sense of responsibility and emotional stability. Assured by letters and interviews (in which Ms. Stevens apparently misled him), he decided to go ahead. Unfavorable publicity, an indignant community, and an implied threat of suit now lead Dr. Franklin to worry about burdening the welfare system. But neither the community nor Dr. Franklin can keep Ms. Stevens and her baby off welfare, if they are otherwise qualified. Other legal sanctions seem of dubious value. Efforts barring physicians from providing artificial insemination to indigent women would likely violate the constitution and shock another segment of public opinion. An adventuresome district attorney might sue Dr. Franklin and the sperm donor for support payments, but that would discourage physicians from providing AID to all but the most prosperous women—a power of selection most would not want a physician to exercise.

Central to Dr. Franklin's problem, and the community's, is his abandonment of standard medical practice—providing artificial insemination solely to married couples with proven infertility. (Now that Dr. Franklin is in a reflective frame of mind, he ought to scrutinize his acquiescence in the political rhetoric underlying the statement, women have "deep feelings about wanting to become pregnant" that men cannot understand.)

If the medical standard is expanded to include single women, what guidelines, if any, should the profession adopt for identifying "responsible and emotionally stable women"? Should physicians be the judges? Or should men and women who have successfully raised children help establish guidelines? In short, Dr. Franklin would be helped not by new laws or legal sanctions but by reexamining the standards of his practice and by exploring his reason for being guided by the sentiments of the day rather than serious moral reasoning.

The same holds true for Ms. Stevens. Has she adequately reflected on the responsibilities of being a single mother or on the consequences to a child raised under such odd circumstances? Does she believe that the desire to be pregnant will translate into the capacity to be a good mother?

She must also answer a larger question: what claim does she have on the material resources of others to help her raise her child? Her legal right to welfare does not automatically translate into a moral right. AFDC, Medicaid, food stamps, and other support programs are intended to provide for those whose income, through no fault of their own, falls below a set level. According to surveys, most welfare recipients qualify for this aid because they have no other choice. Ms. Stevens has another choice, but prefers to apply for welfare. This penalizes other welfare recipients by giving credence to the view that recipients prefer welfare to work. It penalizes taxpayers whose contributions to the welfare system are based on the premise that there is a level of poverty below which no one should live, not on the premise that individuals who are able to support themselves can choose to live on welfare.

Many people who might prefer four children to the 1.8 national average limit their families because they are not able to support more children. For good reasons, we do not make laws regulating people's decisions about having one child or ten or none. This absence of constraints makes the obligation of individuals to care for and support the children they do bring into the world all the more important.

ABORTION

17

The Unwanted Child: Caring for the Fetus Born Alive after an Abortion

Last spring [1976] the California State Legislature passed a bill specifying that a viable fetus which is live-born following an abortion or attempted abortion is a ward of the state. Furthermore, the bill required that physicians performing abortions must take "all reasonable steps, except extraordinary means, in accordance with good medical practice, to preserve the life and health of the live-born person." However, the bill also specified that it was not to be construed as granting priority to the live-born person over its mother with respect to the provision of livesaving medical treatment.

The bill defined a "viable fetus" as one which is biologically viable, based on the consideration of a minimal number of independently sustained, basic, integrative functions. The viable fetus is able to (1) increase in tissue mass, (2) increase the number, complexity, and coordination of basic physiological functions, and (3) develop into a self-sustaining whole organism independent of any connection with the mother. A "fetus" would be considered a live-born person if, outside the womb, it manifests a sustained heartbeat, umbilical pulsation, spontaneous respiration, and movement of voluntary muscles.

In addition to any criminal or civil liability which may be imposed by law, any violation of the law would constitute unprofessional conduct under the State Medical Practice Act.

In August the bill was amended and sent to Governor Edmund G. Brown Jr. in this form: "The rights to medical treatment of an infant prematurely born alive in the course of an abortion shall be the same as the rights of an infant of similar medical status prematurely born spontaneously." Three of the commentators whose views are presented here (Walters, Nathan, Nathanson) also presented written testimony on the bill.

The bill was signed by the governor in its amended form, as part of the California Health and Safety Code, in September.

[The law is still in effect.]

COMMENTARY

Sissela Bok

We are asked to imagine the following irrational behavior. First, medical personnel and a pregnant woman cooperate in abortive practices usually fatal to an embryo or fetus. But, if by chance the fetus survives their assault, they proceed to do everything in their power to sustain its flickering life. This is what the California assembly bill requires. It allows abortions to proceed, then it declares a live-born product of the abortion to be a ward of the state, and requires what it calls "all reasonable steps" to be taken to preserve its life and health.

Some will conclude that the first activity, the abortion, was wrong from the outset; for them the proof is that a reversal is required when the effort fails. They will argue that consistency demands that all fetuses be treated as patients throughout pregnancy.

Others will argue, on the contrary, that it is right and lawful to perform the abortion, and that what is irrational is to reverse directions in midstream, without carrying the act of abortion to its intended end.

We have then two polarized opinions. But this polarization depends on a blurring of important moral distinctions. We need to ask two questions: what should be done in cases of live-born aborted fetuses? and what social policies can prevent these dilemmas from occurring in the first place?

My premise, in answering these two questions, is that women must be allowed to have early abortion on request. Few will deny that there is a basic need for families and individuals to control their fertility. While I consider contraception, abstinence, and sterilization to be preferable to abortion as birth prevention, it is sometimes too late to use such methods. Many are beginning to forget the inevitability of the choice previously confronting most women who were pregnant against their wishes—the choice between a dangerous, uncertain, and unlawful abortion, and the terrors and burdens and ruined lives which have afflicted so many: maternal weakness or death from childbirth, children for whom no one had the strength or the resources to care adequately, young girls bringing babies to the world without having had a childhood of their own.

Given this premise then, what would I advocate doing if a live-born fetus results from an abortion? First, I think we have to set aside as irrelevant the fact that such births are rare. This fact does not eliminate the moral dilemma which exists whether there is one victim or ten thousand.

Take a very clear case and undoubtedly a very unusual one. Say that a hysterotomy has been performed on a women who mistakenly reports that she is in her sixth month of pregnancy and that an intact four-pound live-born baby emerges from this operation. There can be no question, it seems to me, that in such a case the baby ought to be treated and cared for like any newborn, with the appropriate supportive techniques. If we can agree with respect to this one, admittedly unusual, case, then I believe that we have necessarily concluded that it is not the fact of abortion which should in itself determine the fate of the premature baby.

At this point you may well think that I have landed myself in a contradiction: I believe that abortion can be justified; yet am I not also saying that fetuses *are* to be treated as patients? If so, how can they be aborted in the first place?

The way out of this seeming contradiction is to stress that while a woman does have the right to an abortion in the sense of the termination of her pregnancy, she does not have the right to the death of the fetus. The termination of early pregnancy carries with it, at present, fetal failure to survive. But in later pregnancy, where abortion and death of the fetus do not necessarily go together, it is a fallacy to believe that a right to the first also implies a right to the second. I can maintain, then, without contradiction, that abortion is justified, but that if a live birth should result, it must be protected.

But let us now return to the realities of abortions. If a fetus survives an abortion there will be every reason to fear that it has been severely damaged by the procedure itself and that it will be further damaged by efforts to maintain its life. As a result, any law requiring the maintenance of life in such survivors might result in extraordinary suffering on the part of those who are rescued. The effort to maintain life might well then constitute battery.

In cases of life resulting from abortions, medical personnel should therefore be allowed and expected to exercise the same judgment as they do with prematurely born babies. But they *must* be allowed to make a realistic appraisal of the chances of survival and of quality of life after the abortive procedures, and not be forced by legislation and fear of repercussions into providing care they would never give to similarly burdened prematures. Insofar as it would inspire such fears, the California legislation is unwise.

Now to the second question: what social policies can help individuals to avoid such dilemmas in the first place? For the best way out is obviously not to fall into this tragic predicament in the first place.

In many nations which permit abortion, such dilemmas are largely avoided, for the simple reason that late abortions are prohibited. Abortion on request is permitted in these societies only during the first trimester and later only under very special circumstances.

But in this country, we have no such clear guidelines. As a result, we encounter agonizing dilemmas; and our abortion debate is much inflamed by the thought of viable or nearly viable fetuses subjected to abortion. Why does our society have this special dilemma? The root of the problem lies in one provision of the *Roe v. Wade* decision by the United States Supreme Court, striking down a statute which prohibited abortion: it set no clear time limit in pregnancy after which abortions should no longer be performed. It merely declared that states may, if interested in protecting fetal life after viability, proscribe abortion (except in cases of threat to the life or health of the mother).

This may be all that could be done on constitutional grounds. But it left the abortion situation in the United States extraordinarily open-ended. I believe that we, as a society, must now arrive at a time limit in pregnancy after which most abortions are out of the question. Needless to say, however, such a social choice should not be exercised retroactively so as to punish those having performed abortions lawful at the time.

If such a time limit is set, questions of viability will not come up. Legislation such as California Assembly Bill 2346 will be unnecessary. And much greater social efforts to help individuals cope *before* pregnancy with unwanted fertility will have to be undertaken.

If given a choice between accepting the California assembly bill and rejecting it, therefore, I would definitely reject it. But I would wish to work for improved and careful social policies limiting late abortions. For as stumbling and imprecise as this California legislation is, it does represent an effort to respond to the present failure of our institutions to set such limits.

COMMENTARY

Bernard N. Nathanson

When we first began to do abortions on a large scale following the passage of the 1970 New York statute, the question of the fate of the (accidentally) live-born fetus was an unanswerable argument consistently brought up by antiabortion factions. It was not really a medical dilemma; we reacted by placing these infants in the appropriate nursery facility. But it *was* a moral dilemma, and the proabortion group for the most part simply had no response.

The dimensions of this dilemma were exemplified by the *Edelin* case, which was a profound misunderstanding.* Dr. Edelin regrettably labored under the same misapprehension that a great many obstetricians and proabortion advocates have labored under: that abortion necessarily implies the death of the products of conception. It does not now and it never did. Abortion merely intends to remove the products of conception from the unwilling host. And if one views abortion in that way—namely, that the woman's rights as the unwilling host are respected and that the products of conception are removed—then the fetus's rights (and it *does* have rights regardless of the Supreme Court's meaning within the Fourteenth Amendment) are also respected in that it is removed and cared for in the best manner possible.

Obstetricians and gynecologists are well aware of the increasing number of fetuses which are born alive, because of the increased use of prostaglandins. In order to respect everyone's rights, the fetus should be removed from the uterus and then placed in the appropriate nursery environment. However, two technological advances would be required: (1) a huge leap forward to permit the fetus to be removed from the uterus in such an atraumatic way that its existence would be spared, and that it would not be seriously damaged in the process; and (2) the availability in nurseries of sophisticated life-support systems to maintain even very small fetuses of perhaps six, eight, or ten weeks. I envision a time when this level of technology will be available to us.

However, I hope that there will be a parallel advance: that really efficient birth control means will be available and will be used; the immune sera which are being tested in India are promising. Such an advance would reduce the number of abortions to a manageable number. Instead of a million abortions a year, we would probably perform a thousand, two thousand, or five thousand. With fewer abortions, the few live-born fetuses could be placed in these life-

*The *Edelin* case referred to in the Commentaries is a criminal case unsuccessfully brought by the Commonwealth of Massachusetts against Dr. Edelin as a result of an abortion he performed. Dr. Edelin was charged with manslaughter for allowing the death of the fetus in the process of performing the abortion. The Supreme Judicial Court of Massachusetts, the highest court in the state, directed that Dr. Edelin be acquitted on the ground that there was insufficient evidence of "wanton" or "reckless" conduct by Dr. Edelin.

support systems and raised at the expense of the state with little additional burden to the taxpayer.

I left the abortion arena two years after abortion became legal. As director of a perinatal unit in a hospital affiliated with a medical school, I began to face some perplexing questions which necessarily demanded answers from me not only in terms of patient care but in terms of moral questions. One of them is the question of when to interfere during a labor when the fetus is in distress. The implications for interference with respect to Caesarean section are sharp and clear *medically*, but what about the woman who has a twenty-six week pregnancy which is suddenly in jeopardy during the course of a labor? Do we take heroic measures, that is, do we do a Caesarean section, or do we simply stand by and allow this fetus to expire? What about twenty-four weeks? What about twenty weeks, or fifteen weeks? There are very, very difficult questions to answer in this area.

A similar dilemma is the question of whom and when and how long to resuscitate in the delivery room. Do we spend forty-five minutes with an endotracheal tube on a 400 gram fetus? Do we spend two hours? Ten minutes? These are judgments which regrettably often have to be made on the spot, and there are few guidelines.

The problem is further complicated by the distinction between the state of "fetushood" and the state of infancy. We now have rather interesting, but still crude, methods of monitoring and surveying the fetus, and even of treating it *in utero*. As a result we are coming to consider the fetus as an "intrauterine patient." We are, involuntarily, showing it a certain personhood; we have now been faced with the question of the identity of that intrauterine organism—its rights, its worth, its degree of humanity. We do not have very good guidelines here. And so we are faced in the delivery room, in the operating room, and in the labor room suites with the unpleasant and disagreeable task of triage: whom do we save? whom do we allow to die? It becomes quite as stark as that.

In the California bill certain attempts are made to identify the fetus, to ascertain the degree of its humanity; there are allusions to things like independent activity, increasing complexity of fetal physiology, and so on.

I believe that we have to recognize the humanity of the fetus right from conception, and if we can demythologize the process of birth—view it just as another transition in the life cycle—then we are much more able to identify and respect the fetus. In the framework of abortion, the fetus's rights must be recognized and weighed against the rights of the pregnant female. These rights will become more urgent and more compelling as our technology becomes more sophisticated.

COMMENTARY

David C. Nathan

I have tried to read this legislation in terms of the background in which I have been involved—in the abortion and fetal research issue, and the argument about research on the dying.

I find this statute well-meaning, decent, not particularly self-serving; but I think it derives from two totally unsupported assumptions: first, that in California there are a significant number of viable, midterm fetuses that are aborted and do not receive adequate medical support; and second, that individual California obstetricians cannot be trusted to use their own judgment in the matter of the appropriate application of so-called "reasonable" medical care for aborted fetuses. Almost all obstetricians I know do not abort viable fetuses; if they do produce a viable fetus during an abortion, it is an accident.

Now these assumptions lead to the generalizations which (1) make the aborted fetus a ward of the state, and (2) establish mandatory guidelines for the application of so-called "reasonable medical care," based on a tripartite definition of fetal viability. The first two definitions are totally nonspecific because they would apply to any fetus or even to a newborn. The third definition is one which is nearly impossible to codify within a legal framework. One merely needs to review the testimony at the Edelin trial to see how so-called "experts" disagree on criteria for self-sufficiency, as a result of differences in moral, religious, ethical, and scientific backgrounds.

Hence, if the bill becomes law, obstetricians delivering midterm abortuses would be at the mercy of the local prosecutors who could obtain indictments with relative ease because the disputed facts would require expert testimony before a jury in a courtroom. And that's really the problem—when the state gets into this complex area, judges just can't dismiss cases; there must be a trial with all of the nastiness that follows. Thus the proposed law, perhaps unwittingly, attacks *Roe v. Wade* in a novel fashion. It does not prevent a woman from having an abortion but it threatens her with a brain-damaged infant and her obstetrician with criminal charges. Perhaps the legislators hope that this will discourage abortion without attacking the Supreme Court decision.

The ethical and practical aspects of this bill interest me even more than the legal aspects. The bill forces obstetricians to deliver so-called "reasonable" medical care to all late, first-term and midterm aborted fetuses because the obstetrician cannot be certain that his diagnostic impression of no viability is always correct. Since *Suffolk v. Edelin* occurred in a far less medically litigious state than California, any sensible California obstetrician would incubate and place in an isolette all midtrimester and late first-trimester aborted fetuses. A tiny percentage of such fetuses might survive with the use of ultrasound, most, I suppose, with severe brain damage. To force such an existence on the nonviable fetus, or to protract its living death, is a matter of very serious ethical dispute.

Those who wrote this legislation are rightly concerned about the life and health of the fetus, so one wonders why they wish to sentence all of them to a slow death by strangulation rather than permitting them a mercifully rapid demise. Unless this bill is changed radically to a form that simply urges the obstetrician to use his or her best judgment in an attempt to salvage only those fetuses which can be salvaged, the nightmare of hundreds of isolettes filled with incubated, twitching, demented fetuses will become an actuality.

All because of the physician's understandable desire to protect himself from criminal or professional liability.

The National Commission's report on Research on the Newborn Fetus came to the conclusion that so-called viability research on a fetus that had just been delivered was probably not acceptable. The Department of Health, Education and Welfare did not accept their recommendation and suggested that such research is acceptable if it is for the purpose of extending the life and health of the fetus. This opens up all kinds of Pandora's boxes of very unpleasant research that many of us involved in this field find quite unacceptable.

Aside from that dilemma there is also a practical aspect: financial implications. If there is a significant problem in California, that is, if a large number of viable fetuses are being summarily executed (which I think is clearly not the case), massive costs of medical care in a hopeless situation will be required. Unfortunately, the bill has a peculiar effect; it makes abortion very financially rewarding. The obstetrician can bill not only the mother, but also the fetus, and the hospital can also bill the fetus. I do not understand why the state of California wants to make the process of abortion so financially attractive.

The bill also provides another interesting problem in ethics. Most obstetricians dislike doing abortions; they do it as a necessary service for women with unwanted pregnancies. To force them into a position of further professional and criminal liability in the act of doing something they feel is for the good of their patient is something that we have to consider very carefully.

Finally, I would certainly caution the drafters of this legislation to be very certain that the language clearly distinguishes between aborted fetuses and prematures; their descriptions of what is a fetus and what is a premature are very confused. It seems unlikely that the state wishes to offer ward status to all prematures.

I am afraid that California legislators will find themselves on a slippery slope of their own if they pursue this kind of legislation.

COMMENTARY

LeRoy Walters

There is an ambiguity in the concept of abortion. It may mean "the termination of fetal life," or it may mean "the separation of a fetus from a pregnant woman." In the early stages of pregnancy there is currently no feasible way to effect maternal-fetal separation without terminating the life of the fetus. However, as the gestational age of the fetus increases, particularly beyond the twenty-week mark, the probability of its surviving induced abortion (or spontaneous premature delivery) also increases.

The likelihood of survival following induced abortion also depends on the method of abortion employed. The saline-injection technique raises the salt concentration in the amniotic fluid surrounding the fetus and usually results in the death of the fetus prior to its expulsion from the uterus. In contrast, the hysterotomy technique, which resembles a cesarean section, more frequently produces an infant which shows some signs of life. (This method is often used when a pregnant woman requests tubal sterilization at the time of abortion.) A third technique, the injection of prostaglandins, induces uterine contractions and effects the expulsion of the fetus in a process which, mechanically, simulates childbirth. In its effects on the fetus, this third method is intermediate between the other two: prostaglandins are less toxic to the fetus than concentrated saline solution, but the probability of live delivery following the injection of prostaglandins is probably not as great as following a hysterotomy.

Few reliable statistics exist concerning the frequency of live delivery and infant survival following induced abortion. New York State, where a liberalized abortion law went into effect in July 1970, has compiled the most complete data. In upstate New York between July 1970 and December 1972 there were thirty-eight reported live deliveries following induced abortion. Of these, twenty-seven followed 15,671 abortions by saline injection (live-delivery ratio: 1.7 per 1,000), and nine followed 1,064 hysterotomies (live-delivery ratio: 8.5 per 1,000). Seven of the infants delivered with signs of life expired within an hour of delivery, nineteen between one and four hours, and ten between four and twenty-four hours. Two infants lived more than twenty-four hours; one expired at twenty-seven hours and five minutes; the other survived without evident damage and was discharged into the mother's care (George Stroh and Alan R. Hinman, *American Journal of Obstetrics and Gynecology* 125 (9): 83–90 (September 1, 1976).

Less complete data are available for upstate New York in 1973 and 1974. During 1973 there were seven live deliveries and one survival following 5,751 abortions by saline injection or hysterotomy (live-delivery ratio: 1.2 per 1,000). In 1974, fifteen live deliveries and no survivals followed approximately 5,000 abortions by saline injection, hysterotomy, and the use of prostaglandins (Stroh and Hinman, *op. cit.*). The overall live-delivery ratio for 1974 was 3 per 1,000 abortions; however, the ratio for live delivery following prostaglandin-induced abortions was considerably higher, at least twenty-two per 1,000.

Somewhat more sketchy data are available from New York City for the first eighteen months under the state's liberalized abortion law. Sixty-two live deliveries, including two long-term survivals, were reported following approximately 36,000 abortions by saline injection or hysterotomy (live-delivery ratio: 1.7 per 1,000) (Pakter and Nelson, *Mt. Sinai Journal of Medicine* 39(6): 542, November–December 1972).

These New York figures can be combined with recent statistics from the federal Center for Disease Control (CDC) in Atlanta to compute a tentative national estimate of fetal survival following induced abortion. On the basis of data from seventeen states (CDC, *Abortion Surveillance 1974*), one can project that approximately 6.4 percent, or 49,000, of the nation's 763,000 reported abortions in 1974 were performed by means of saline injection. If the upstate New York live-delivery ratio of 1.7 per 1,000 for 1970–72 held for the nation as a whole in 1974, then the number of live deliveries following saline-injection abortions in 1974 was approximately eighty-four nationwide. Corresponding estimates for hysterotomies are 0.4 percent, 2,896 abortions, and twenty-five live deliveries. Only the most tentative projections can be made on the basis of early statistics concerning prostaglandin-induced abortion. If the initial upstate New York ratio of twenty-two live deliveries per 1,000 prostaglandin-induced abortions is extrapolated to the entire nation, then in 1974 one would have expected eighty-seven live deliveries from 3,950 abortions using prostaglandins. In sum, if these figures and projections are reasonably accurate, it is likely that in 1974 approximately 196 infants were delivered alive after abortion by saline- or prostaglandin-induction or hysterotomy. Of these, as the aggregated data from upstate New York and New York City suggest, perhaps six or seven survived to grow to maturity. In future years these annual nationwide figures may remain relatively constant if the trend toward earlier abortion is balanced by the increasing use of prostaglandins and lower mortality rates among premature infants in general.

As the foregoing statistics indicate, the California state legislature is confronting a problem which involves a small number of infants. Even a maximal treatment program would not be likely to overwhelm the health care system. However, the small number of infants delivered alive following abortion may possess certain human or legal rights which the legislature ought to protect, especially since the members of this class cannot speak for themselves. What principled basis for policymaking can be suggested to the legislature?

Two types of situations can be distinguished, the postabortion and the preabortion situation. Postabortion, I propose that the legislature adopt a formal-equality principle: all newborn infants should be treated equally, without regard to the circumstances of their delivery. The basis for this equality principle is the notion that, subsequent to its disconnection from the mother, the infant possesses independent rights. Two cases will serve to illustrate how the equality principle might work in practice. First, consider the case of a healthy, 2.2-pound infant delivered alive at twenty-four-weeks' gestational age following a hysterotomy. If a hospital's neonatal intensive care unit would normally attempt to save the life of a spontaneously delivered infant of the same health status, age, and weight, then the equality principle would require identical treatment for the hysterotomy survivor. At the opposite extreme, consider the case of a one-pound, twenty-week-old infant delivered alive but with probable brain damage following saline-induced abortion. The formal-equality principle does not specify precisely what treatment should be given to such an infant. It merely requires that this infant receive the same treatment as a similar, spontaneously delivered infant.

The proposed equality principle implicitly rejects two alternative approaches to the treatment of infants that survive abortion. On the one hand, the principle does not recommend compensatory, especially vigorous, or maximal treatment for the survivors of abortion. A simple equality of treatment is sufficient. On the other hand, the principle also implies that, if the mother or both parents request that the surviving infant be allowed to die, this request should be denied if it conflicts with the principle of equal treatment. The independent claims of the infant are thereby recognized.

The preabortion situation raises additional complexities for the legislature. Here the central question is: should the state establish any requirements concerning permissible abortion procedures in the interest of maximizing the probability of infant survival following abortion? Three types of cases can be envisioned, those in which the fetus is clearly viable, clearly previable, and possibly viable. The first type of case is partially covered by existing American law. According to *Roe v. Wade* a legislature may prohibit the abortion of a clearly viable fetus unless abortion is required to preserve the pregnant woman's life or health. But let us suppose that at seven and one-half months of pregnancy immediate termination is medically indicated. Let us suppose, further, that two alternative methods of delivery exist, one of which increases the chances of infant survival but entails higher risk to the pregnant woman, the other of which decreases both the risk to the woman and the probability of infant survival. In my view, the law should not require moral heroism of the pregnant woman in this case by asking her to place her own life at higher risk for the sake of the viable fetus, just as the law should not *require* parents to rescue their children from burning buildings. If the above example is changed, however, to pose a choice between two alternative methods of termination, one of which has a lower risk for *both* pregnant woman and fetus, then the legislature could appropriately decide that the rights of a clearly viable fetus are sufficiently strong to justify requiring use of the safer method (unless other medical contraindications exist).

If the fetus is clearly previable, legislative enactments concerning the method of abortion are meaningless, since there is, by definition, no possibility of affecting the postabortion survival probabilities of the fetus. However, if the fetus is possibly viable, that is, if it is estimated to be between twenty- and twenty-eight-weeks' gestational age, then the choice of abortion method may in fact have a significant impact on its survival probabilities. As in the case of the clearly viable fetus, the legislature would probably not wish to require that a pregnant woman choose a method of abortion which is more dangerous to herself (for example, hysterotomy) merely to maximize the chance of fetal survival. However, if a method of abortion becomes available which demonstrably entails lower risk both to the pregnant woman and the fetus (possibly prostaglandins), then, assuming the general availability of the safer technique, the legislature might wish to require the use of that technique in abortions performed beyond the nineteenth week of gestation (except in cases where use of the technique is medically contraindicated). The dual justification for such a requirement would be the enhancement of maternal health and the protection of fetuses which may have already crossed the viability threshold.

Thus, to return to the ambiguity noted at the beginning of this essay, there may be cases in which abortion means the separation of a fetus from a pregnant woman rather than the termination of fetal life. If a legislature can limit the amount of fetal damage caused by abortion without endangering the life or health of the pregnant woman, then in my view it should do so.

18

When a Mentally Ill Woman Refuses Abortion

Ann Brown is a twenty-seven-year-old woman with a diagnosis of chronic paranoid schizophrenia. She has a history of prolonged institutionalization, with intermittent attempts at independent living. Presently living in a mental hospital, Ann Brown is now twelve weeks pregnant. She has firmly indicated her desire to continue the pregnancy and to keep the child. Abortion, she declares, "is against my principles." The father is unknown.

While Ann's psychiatrist does not consider her capable of responsible parenthood, he does think that she is capable, at times at least, of meaningful moral decisions. Her schizophrenia and medication taken early in pregnancy slightly increase the possibility of fetal defect.

Ann Brown's mother wants her to have an abortion, and has secured legal custody of her daughter in order to effect that result. She feels that the experience of pregnancy and the trauma of labor and delivery will worsen Ann's mental state. Moreover, she herself is unable to care for the child and fears that Ann will suffer further if she is forced to give up the child to strangers.

The hospital attorney has indicated that she will oppose Ann's mother's request for an abortion. She will argue that it cannot be performed without consent.

There is little likelihood that Ann Brown would be allowed to care for her child. However, because of the ambiguity surrounding parental consent, the child would probably be placed in foster care rather than with adoptive parents.

Should the abortion be performed? Who should decide?

COMMENTARY

Mary Mahowald

Among the diverse ethical and legal issues raised by this case, I would like to address two: the moral status of incompetent adults, as well as fetuses; and the relationship between the hospital and the courts.

"Informed consent" is generally viewed as essential to legal and moral justification for medical procedures. There is also general agreement that informed consent entails three factors: competence, understanding and voluntariness. The same factors are present in proxy or substitute consent, which is neither legally nor morally as strong a basis for medical intervention as informed consent. Accordingly, parents' refusal of treatment for their offspring is less binding on practitioners than is their refusal of treatment for themselves. Proxy dissent may be overruled on grounds that it violates the best interests of the person for whom consent is refused.

In securing legal custody of her daughter, Ann Brown's mother has assumed certain rights and responsibilities regarding her, but these do not necessarily imply either Ann's incapability for informed consent or her mother's right to choose abortion for her pregnant daughter. A court judgment would have to be obtained to warrant overriding Ann's refusal of the procedure.

In requesting such an order, Ann's mother could argue that it is in her daughter's best interest to have an abortion, because continuing the pregnancy, experiencing labor and delivery, and probably delivery of the child into another's custody would together entail a burden greater than the abortion. Against that argument stands the fact that Ann has clearly indicated a desire to continue the pregnancy, and that most second-trimester abortions entail the experience of labor and delivery. (Alternatives to labor are available for either childbirth or abortion.) Moreover, the possibility that Ann's sense of "wrongness" about abortion might impose an added psychological burden needs to be considered in evaluating her best interests.

As the psychiatrist apparently recognizes, even legally incompetent individuals may be capable of moral decisions. In addition to mental illness, youth is often a criterion for denying a legal right to choose or refuse medical care. Yet most adolescents, and many younger children, are morally responsible for some of their acts, even as adults may be legally competent while morally incompetent. Moreover, a sophisticated understanding of complicated medical procedures is not requisite to informed consent. The crucial cognitive component of a moral decision is recognition of the cause/effect relationship between election of a procedure and its results. If Ann has a basic understanding of what abortion entails, and what continuation of her pregnancy entails, that cognitive requirement is satisfied.

While ambiguity may remain about whether Ann has made a moral decision in this instance, the moral standing of the fetus tips the scale in favor of respecting her refusal. Moral standing does not imply personhood; it merely means that an individual has some moral claim on others, for example, a prima facie right to, or interest in, continued existence. In this case, the probability that the child will be normal, and live a life that is better than death, argues that the interests of the fetus coincide with Ann's desire to continue the pregnancy.

Nonetheless, since *Roe v. Wade* (1973) there is no legal requirement to consider the interests of a nonviable fetus. Therefore, a legal determination of Ann's competence to dissent or consent to an abortion is crucial. This might be provided through a court decision, based on psychiatric evaluation of Ann's competence.

The possibility that Ann is incompetent both legally and morally suggests an important criticism of the popular "pro-choice" view of abortion. Some women who are pregnant are clearly incapable of autonomous decisions (for example, those who are unconscious or profoundly retarded). Others, particularly minors, are questionably competent. Exclusive emphasis on autonomy undercuts the principles of beneficence and nonmaleficence, which remain applicable in such cases.

COMMENTARY

Virginia Abernethy

There is little question that the hospital attorney would prevail in a court of law and that the abortion would not be performed over her and Ann Brown's objections. But although the case will be decided in Ann's favor, I maintain that this is an absurd outcome based on a fallacious understanding of liberty.

Ann's objection will be honored because abortion is a medical procedure and a competent person has the nearly unqualified right to refuse any unwanted health care intervention. However, this right to refuse apparently does not overwhelm a state interest in protecting *others*, so limited coercion is permitted in issues of immunization or quarantine, or where refusal of blood transfusion endangers a third-trimester fetus. Even when the patient's own life is at issue, if the refusal is "ambivalently" given and the intervention is not major (as in blood transfusion), a patient's refusal may be overridden. Ordinarily, however, a competent person's right to refuse is respected even when the decision appears life-threatening and is "irrational" in terms of others' thinking and values. Legal precedents affirming the person's right not to be touched without personal consent derive both from the common law and from the constitutional guarantee of privacy.

The question thus turns on whether Ann Brown is competent. It is relevant here that competence is presumed and the burden of proof is on those who challenge it; that schizophrenia is not conclusive evidence of incompetence to refuse a medical procedure; that Ann has the capacity to understand the procedure and its meaning to her (that is, abortion means no baby, and no abortion means she will probably deliver); and that the psychiatrist declares "she is capable, at times at least, of meaningful moral decisions." If Ann wanted to have the baby even after being forewarned that, since she was psychiatrically ill and institutionalized, she would never be entrusted with her child, that would constitute telling evidence of her incompetence. But to support the conclusion of incompetency, one might still have to argue that denying those facts because of *hoping for recovery* from schizophrenia is so unrealistic as to be, in itself, grounds for judging a person to be incompetent.

I am unwilling to agree that hoping for recovery is a sign of incompetence. I also doubt that a court of law would find Ann incompetent on the totality of evidence. If she is competent, she can refuse the abortion. End of case.

Unfortunately, this leads to an absurd outcome—so absurd that one must search for an underlying fallacy. The outcome is absurd because Ann Brown does not want the pregnancy and childbirth as ends in themselves; she wants the resulting child. But it is acknowledged by all (except Ann, presumably) that she cannot care for the child, her mother cannot care for the child, and so the child will be taken from her for indefinite foster home placement. No one's good is served: not Ann's and not society's, because society will be burdened with the cost of foster care. All this happens because society will take away Ann's child but cannot prevent or take away Ann's pregnancy.

The fallacy, in my view, is in assuming that Ann has the right to bear a child. This is a wrong-headed belief into which we have muddled because of overemphasis on rights and privileges and neglect of duties and responsibilities.

A well-functioning, stable society matches every right to a responsibility. A "person" in either the philosophic or social sense has both rights and responsibilities. There is a correspondence between them. This suggests that Ann's right to procreate might be compromised by her very limited capacity to be responsible as a parent.

If no one felt obliged to care for the child it would be different; the child would die and Ann's "right" would be nullified. But our society *does* feel obliged; this is not Dickensian England. Since children are thought to create a responsibility, perhaps there should not be a right to procreate by those unable to assume that responsibility.

No right is so broad that, morally, it can extend to harming others. Thus, there is a public right to use water, but not to pollute it. Industry has rights to free conduct of their business, but not to destroy the environment for others. Your right to swing your fist ends where my nose begins. Ann's right to procreate ends where the responsibility to raise her child becomes mine—ours—society's.

Acceptance of the underlying principle would raise questions for others who are arguably deficient as parents: for example, the severely retarded, ambulatory schizophrenics, the socially maladjusted, people who have proven to be "poor parents" in the past and had their children taken from them. Possible extensions of a principle of reciprocal rights and responsibilities are disquieting and raise questions about how due process would develop in order to prevent abuse.

Nevertheless, since the present rules seem seriously flawed I do not withdraw my proposal. Since Ann's pregnancy is leading to a child for which she cannot be responsible, a child for which society will be responsible, her right to privacy does not extend to refusing an abortion. The right to procreate should be limited by the capacity to take responsibility for the result. Ann's right to bring forth ends where my duty to care for her child begins.

19

The Hospital's Duty and Rape Victims

Dr. Maria DeCicco is Chief of Emergency Care at St. Mary's Hospital in a large southern city. She has been put in a difficult situation by the passage of a state Rape Victim's Emergency Treatment Act and recent amendments to the municipal code mandating certain services for rape victims. The state law requires hospitals to collect evidence for the police. Kits are provided for this purpose at no expense to the hospital. Hospitals must also provide, with the patient's consent, minimum treatment including an emergency room examination, counseling, and advice about possible infection or pregnancy.

The city's municipal code specifies the treatment in greater detail and creates the real problem for Dr. DeCicco. The treatment required by the code includes, with the patient's consent, medication against conception and venereal disease. Dr. DeCicco has, as a matter of conscience, always tried to use her medical skills to preserve life. She feels that abortion is morally wrong and went to great lengths to find a position where she could practice medicine without having to provide such services. That is why she joined the staff of St. Mary's. Their policy against abortion was firm and well known. Patients in the community would normally not come to St. Mary's if they were considering abortion.

The new municipal code appears to require that she and her staff provide not only emergency medical services, which she is happy to do, but also medical intervention to interrupt any pregnancy that may result. Although the cells to be destroyed by the "morning after" pill are newly fertilized, to her their destruction is the moral equivalent of an abortion.

Dr. DeCicco recognizes that the ethical issues are a matter of substantial controversy. She is not seeking to impose moral judgments on anyone else. She only wants to practice medicine as her conscience dictates, yet the new state and municipal mandates seem to require her to participate in what she believes is a morally objectionable practice in order to protect the rights of the rape victim.

She has talked with the administrator of the hospital. He strongly agrees that the hospital should not be forced to provide medical intervention to stop any potential pregnancy. He proposes that they ask the municipal authorities for an exemption from the requirement if they would pledge to provide counseling to rape victims coming to their emergency room including information to the effect that the hospital does not provide any services that could lead to an interruption of any possible pregnancy. This would leave the patient free to seek such service elsewhere.

Dr. DeCicco is not satisfied with the suggestion because she objects to being put in a position where she would have to counsel patients or refer patients to services where the end result was possibly going to be an interruption of a pregnancy. She is beginning to feel that she can no longer practice what she considers responsible medicine without violating the law. Should society provide some escape for Dr. DeCicco? If not, should she violate a law that she objects to so strongly?

COMMENTARY

J. David Bleich

Much of the current debate concerning abortion practices is clouded by a failure to distinguish between the legal and moral issues involved. *Roe v. Wade*, the Supreme Court decision governing abortion statutes, established a "right to privacy" insofar as performance of abortions is concerned and serves to prevent governmental authorities from prohibiting such procedures. There is absolutely nothing in that decision that *requires* a physician to perform an abortion. The physician retains freedom of conscience and freedom of religious practice either to perform or not to perform an abortion. The physician, no less than the mother, enjoys a constitutional "right to privacy." Any municipal ordinance *mandating* that the physician destroy a fetus upon the demand of the mother would probably be held unconstitutional by the courts.

A municipal ordinance requiring that a rape victim be informed of the medical options available to her and be provided with information concerning availability of abortion services is an entirely different matter both legally and morally. Legally, failure to provide such information, even in the absence of a legal requirement to do so, may constitute malpractice. As such, the rape victim may have a cause of action to recover damages from the physician. That, however, is a civil matter upon which the legality of the municipal ordinance has no bearing. Morally there is a conflict between the patient's moral autonomy, which can be exercised only if she has an informed awareness of the viable options available to her, and the physician's conscientious objection to providing information which, from his or her moral vantage point, can be used only in an immoral manner.

There may be a way to escape from between the horns of this dilemma. Although, by virtue of the tenets of her faith, Dr. DeCicco cannot refer patients to another medical institution for interruption of pregnancy she may well be able to provide information with regard to the options available. While I am certainly not qualified to pass upon matters of canon law, it would appear that merely providing information constitutes no more than "remote material assistance" to an immoral act which, from the vantage point of Catholic morality, is justified when "serious cause" exists for doing so. Loss of one's profession is recognized as constituting not merely "serious cause" but "grave cause."

Moreover, the prospect of St. Mary's Hospital being forced to close its emergency care department—with all that such a step would imply in terms of availability of treatment in life-threatening situations—is certainly "proportionate reason" for rendering what is no more than "remote material assistance." Whether civil authorities have a moral (or legal) right to require even remote assistance to an act perceived as immoral by some citizens is an entirely different question.

More significantly, the ethical problem posed in this case study may be more apparent than real. Assuredly, if such is her conviction, the physician, as a moral agent, is obligated not only to refrain from destroying the fetus but also to urge her patient not to seek an abortion elsewhere. Surely, any intelligent person living in our society should consider it not only likely but also highly probable that the rape victim will leave the emergency room of St. Mary's and proceed to seek aid in terminating her pregnancy elsewhere. Under such circumstances, it would be no more than proper for the physician to present the moral case mitigating against such a course of action. In the very act of offering moral counsel—which the physician should feel morally compelled to do even in the absence of a legal requirement—the physician will have provided the legally required information.

But let us assume that there is no way for the physician to provide this information without violating her moral principles. Such convictions deserve the respect of both society and the law. Any attempt to compel compliance with a law perceived by a responsible segment of society to be inconsistent with the moral code to which it subscribes, regardless of the goal which such a law seeks to further, is an attack upon morality itself. Violation of conscience very quickly leads to a breakdown of conscience—and surely there are few goals, if any, whose benefits outweigh the societal benefits of preservation of a sense of moral conscience.

Instead of tampering with Dr. DeCicco's conscience the municipal authorities would be better advised to embark upon a public information program designed to provide all citizens with pertinent information regarding available health care facilities and the policies adhered to by the various medical institutions in the community. They would also do well to provide information in an objective, dispassionate manner with regard to the moral perspective upon which the policies of such institutions are grounded. Indeed, it would be wise—and fair—to require St. Mary's Hospital to post a notice in a conspicuous place in the emergency room which would inform patients of the hospital's policy with regard to services leading to termination of pregnancy.

Should a conflict between law and morality remain, there is no question that Dr. DeCicco's duty to conscience is such that she cannot act in a manner which the law prescribes. The only options available to her are civil disobedience or abandonment of the practice of medicine. Under the circumstances I believe disobedience of the law would be morally defensible. One must remember that, for Dr. DeCicco, feticide is indistinguishable from homicide. Who would be unsympathetic to disobedience of a legal requirement to counsel homicide?

Indeed, the constitutionality of an ordinance requiring a physician to provide such information is open to question. Enforcement of such a requirement under these circumstances would require the demonstration of a "compelling state interest." It is not at all certain that such an interest exists. I would therefore urge Dr. DeCicco to pursue the matter in the courts. It may readily be argued that she has a moral obligation to do so. Historically, the courts have been extremely reluctant to permit the law to tamper with religious or moral convictions. May they have the good judicial sense to refuse to do so in this case as well.

COMMENTARY

Carol A. Tauer

Dr. DeCicco believes that the law requires her to participate in a morally objectionable practice in order to protect the rights of the rape victim. The rape victim's rights have already been gravely violated by an invasion of her body about which she had no choice. After the rape, it is essential that her right to choose be restored to her, that she be given the opportunity to decide how she will deal with the actual and potential consequences of the rape and with the weighty moral issues involved.

Beyond emergency care, the rape victim's primary right at this time is self-determination. But in order to exercise this right, she needs information about the options that are open to her. This information is standard scientific and medical knowledge. It is well-known to those who are educated and advantaged in our society. By providing the information to all rape victims, a doctor or hospital is simply equalizing opportunity, the opportunity of all rape victims to make an informed choice.

Dr. DeCicco is not being asked to convince the victim to take the "morning-after" pill. In providing information, she is in the position of a teacher who must clearly outline the scientific aspects of biomedical procedures that raise ethical questions. It is appropriate for either the teacher or the doctor to express her own moral or value judgment. But she cannot make this judgment for others. And in depriving the rape victim of information, the doctor is attempting to prevent the victim from making a particular choice, thus depriving her of moral freedom.

Although the hospital and doctor ought to provide the information the law requires, if they have serious moral objections to prescribing the "morning-after" pill, this should not be required of them. The hospital has a clearly stated position against abortion, and it regards intervention in the period between conception and implantation to be morally equivalent to abortion. In taking this position, the hospital has the support of the Ethical and Religious Directives for Catholic Health Facilities issued by the National Conference of Catholic Bishops. It should therefore be possible for the hospital to obtain an exemption from the specific requirement of providing the "morning-after" pill.

If Dr. DeCicco cannot bring herself to give the information and counseling required by the law and approved by the administrator, she should ask to be removed from her present position and assigned elsewhere in the hospital.

Beyond these immediate decisions, however, both Dr. DeCicco and the administrator should recognize that they may be wrong in their moral evaluation of the "morning-after" pill. For at least ten years, numerous Catholic theologians have been questioning the inviolability of the embryo during the first two or three weeks after fertilization. They respect it as nascent human life, but believe that it does not require all the protections given to an individual human being. For a serious reason, for example, the prevention of pregnancy due to rape, the early embryo could be deprived of the environment it would need for continued development. Dr. DeCicco and the administrator have the obligation to become familiar with this theological literature in order to inform their own moral judgments.

Another point for them to consider is the phrase "morally equivalent." In what sense is use of the "morning-after" pill morally equivalent to a sixth-month abortion? We may say that the energy crisis is the moral equivalent of war, and that chain smoking is the moral equivalent of suicide. Such expressions are at least partly figurative, and to take them literally leads to moral confusion. Catholic adolescents of my generation experienced this confusion on being taught that any deliberate sexual arousal was morally equivalent to premarital sexual intercourse. Sorting actions into large, all-encompassing categories is not a good way of making moral judgments. *Is* taking the "morning-after" pill in case of rape, truly as great an evil as obtaining an abortion at six months? To say *yes* seems to indicate a rigid adherence to set rules and categories without regard for the morally relevant distinction that obtains.

If Dr. DeCicco and the hospital recognize that there is a moral distinction, that even if both acts are evil, one is a lesser evil than the other, then they ought to be interested in preventing the greater evil. Almost any woman who becomes pregnant after a rape will at least consider the possibility of having an abortion. Unless she is sexually ignorant, she will be thinking about the possibility of pregnancy and abortion when she is in the hospital emergency room. Dr. DeCicco claims that she does not want to be part of any practice where the end result might be an abortion. But in not allowing the patient to choose the "morning-after" pill, the doctor is limiting the patient's options so that the end result may well be a direct abortion. If the patient does not want to go through with a pregnancy, the doctor ought to counsel the least evil way of terminating pregnancy, and the more immediate the intervention, the better: physically, psychologically, and morally.

20

Selective Termination of Pregnancy

Ms. Q. is a thirty-year-old woman who is pregnant for the first time, having spent several years in a local infertility program. She had been treated previously with clomiphene citrate, a fertility drug that increases the incidence of multiple births among those who subsequently become pregnant from 1 percent to 8 percent. Dr. G., the physician who prescribed the drug, had indicated to the patient that its use involved "some risk of multiple gestation."

At nine weeks gestation, ultrasound reveals the presence of triplets. After discussion with her husband, Ms. Q. asks Dr. G. to terminate two of the fetuses. She says she really wants to have a child and "be a good mother," but doesn't feel capable of caring for more than one child at a time. Even though all three fetuses appear healthy, her preference is to abort all rather than have triplets.

A technique similar to amniocentesis (in which the uterine cavity is entered) has been used to terminate selectively a defective fetus, when a serious fetal anomaly, such as Down's syndrome, occurs in a multiple gestation. This technique could be used to terminate two of the triplets, but it entails an incremental risk of miscarriage. Legally, Dr. G. could: (1) terminate the pregnancy through a standard method of abortion; (2) selectively terminate the gestation of two of the triplets; (3) refuse to terminate the pregnancy, with transfer of care to a physician who is willing to do so. Should Dr. G. acquiesce in Ms. Q.'s request? Is this request morally valid?

COMMENTARY

Angela R. Holder

The central question in this case is "What are the limits of a physician's duty to do what the patient wants?" No physician is legally obliged to provide treatment he or she deems unwise, dangerous, or not indicated simply because a patient wants it. Dr. Q. is no more required to abort one, some, or all of

Ms. Q.'s fetuses than a physician is to give human growth hormone to a normal-sized child whose parents want a basketball star. The legal doctrine of informed consent means that a patient has the right to choose among reasonable medical alternatives; it does not mean that the physician must perform the chosen procedure if he or she thinks it is ill-advised. In case of necessary medical care, the physician may have a duty to refer the patient to someone who will comply with the patient's requests, but the condition of "necessary" would not apply to Ms. Q.'s situation.

Under normal circumstances, Ms. Q. would have no trouble finding a physician who would perform a standard abortion, and, at this stage in the pregnancy, she has every legal right to decide to have one. (Since family finances have apparently presented no impediment to several years of infertility treatment, presumably she can afford this procedure.)

However, the procedure for selective abortion presents about a 45 percent risk of loss of all fetuses. There is also a risk that triplets will be sufficiently premature to have serious difficulties—many are born at thirty weeks' gestation. While some obstetricians might be willing to abort one fetus with a severe disorder, not many would agree to undertake a procedure still in its developmental stage only because a woman decided she was incapable of being a good mother to three children.

Ms. Q. had been in the infertility program for several years. That experience surely should have presented opportunity for adequate counseling about the possibility of multiple births, since they cannot be predicted or prevented when fertility drugs are used, and what such a possibility would mean in terms of expenditure of energy and finances. In advance of her pregnancy, Ms. Q. should have been able to think through for herself whether she could cope with this eventually. Did she really want a baby, or was she in this program to satisfy the desires of other people—her husband, for example, or her parents who wanted a grandchild? Does she have any idea how much energy *one* baby requires? Several years of treatment should have provided Ms. Q. with better counseling, rather than leaving her in this dilemma, since it was a reasonably foreseeable result of doing what she wanted to do.

Dr. G. should attempt to mobilize family and child care resources (including her husband, who presumably can learn to change diapers as well as she can) and facilitate contacts with mothers of triplets to find out how they cope with three children the same age. Perhaps Ms. Q. will discover that the situation is not as difficult as she assumes and continue the pregnancy.

As Oscar Wilde wrote, "In this world, there are only two tragedies. One is not getting what one wants, and the other is getting it."

COMMENTARY

Mary Sue Henifin

Unlike the "old woman who lived in a shoe, she had so many children she didn't know what to do," Ms. Q. has requested an available medical intervention as a solution. The question of whether Dr. G. should acquiesce in her request for partial termination of her multiple pregnancy is one that tests the limits of a physician's obligation to respect patient autonomy.

Self-determination and autonomy apply to a patient's "negative" right to refuse as well as her "positive" right to choose among beneficial procedures, yet these principles do not guarantee the right to demand nonbeneficial or harmful treatment. Before providing a requested treatment, the physician should determine whether the patient can define a recognizable problem that medical treatment may benefit. If a requested treatment is beneficial, it should be among the options offered to the patient.

In this case, triplet pregnancy presents many recognizable problems to which partial termination is one solution. Once a benefit can be identified, the pregnant woman is in the best position to weigh the alternatives. Each woman brings her own ethical principles to decisions about her pregnancy based on her own life circumstances.

In an ideal relationship, physician and patient share their mutual knowledge and perspectives until they arrive at an agreed upon course of treatment *prior* to commencing therapy. In the case of inducing ovulation with clomaphene citrate, the discussion should include the eightfold increase in the risks of multiple gestation and accompanying maternal and fetal complications, not merely the vague warning provided by Dr. G. that there is "some risk."

What information does Ms. Q. need to make an autonomous decision? First, the physician must present those options that can provide benefit and discuss their risks. Three options could benefit Ms. Q.: carrying the fetuses to term, complete abortion, or partial termination. A triplet pregnancy is by definition high risk, with stillbirth rates three times higher than for singleton pregnancy and perinatal mortality rates almost twenty times higher. Multiple gestation increases the strain on the pregnant woman's circulatory, renal, and endocrine systems, and she is more likely to suffer from hypertension, anemia, respiratory distress, preeclampsia, placenta previa, and placenta abrupta.

The fetuses are also at increased risk. The majority of multiple births are preterm; and intrauterine growth retardation is the rule, caused by placental insufficiency and crowding. Labor and delivery are particularly risky. Moreover, children born of multiple gestation have higher rates of congenital disabilities and developmental problems after birth.

Finally, multiple gestation severely disrupts the life of the pregnant woman and her family. Bedrest is usually prescribed beginning in the third trimester, and lengthy hospital stays may be required for both mother and newborns. Depression and, in rare cases, suicide have been reported to accompany multiple births as families try to cope with the caretaking, social, and economic pressures. Although support groups exist, such as The Triplet Connection in California and Central New Jersey Mothers of Multiples, reproductive choice may be circumscribed by inadequate access to medical coverage, housing, child care, and other necessities.

Once risks have been identified, the physician should avoid paternalism and respect the patient's evaluation of her own unique circumstances. Just as it would be unethical for Dr. G. to pressure Ms. Q. to abort because of the *known* risks of multiple gestation, it would be wrong to try and pressure her to forgo partial termination because of alternative risks. Ms. Q.'s constitutionally protected right to privacy, including the right to make procreative decisions, supports her right to weigh the available options and their outcomes in selecting a course of treatment. Even when more accurate data are available on the relative risks of multiple gestation, abortion, and partial termination, privacy and procreative liberty must extend to protect the pregnant woman's choices. Dr. G. should either respect Ms. Q.'s decision or transfer her care to a competent physician who is willing to do so.

Ms. Q.'s case illustrates how the development of new reproductive techniques leads to technological imperatives: If a technology exists it will be used. The critical focus is usually on the morality of "consumer demand." A more direct approach would examine the moral responsibility of researchers who develop and promote new reproductive technologies like selective termination.

21

Risk Taking and a Minor Birth Defect

Linda Robinson, a twenty-eight-year-old actress, is eight weeks pregnant. Her five-year marriage to a magazine photographer has been strained by their dual career demands and their indecision over whether to have a child. During one particularly difficult period, when her husband had just gone away on assignment and Mrs. Robinson failed to get a part in a play, she became very anxious and started taking about 20 mg of Valium every day. She continued taking the drug in that dosage for about a month, although once she took 35 mg. Then she discovered that she was pregnant and stopped taking the drug. Her obstetrician referred her to a genetic counseling clinic to evaluate the potential effects of the drug on her child.

Dr. Andrews, the genetic counselor, told Mrs. Robinson that the only reported effect of Valium on pregnancy was a three- to fourfold increase of cleft lip and/or palate. Since the normal risk is only one in a thousand, the risk to her baby was only three to four in a thousand, in Dr. Andrews's words, "very small compared to other possible birth defects." Furthermore, he pointed out, cleft lip or palate can be corrected quite easily surgically. He found nothing else in her history (or in as much of her husband's as she could tell him) that would indicate she was at particular risk for bearing a child with any other kind of birth defect.

Mrs. Robinson seemed somewhat upset by the thought of a birth defect that might mar her child's appearance, but said she wanted time to think about this information. She confided to Dr. Andrews that she had just been offered a part in a television series and that her husband would be returning from his trip that week. She would, she said, discuss the situation with him.

The following week Mrs. Robinson returned for a follow-up visit. She said that the risk of a cleft palate was too high, and that she would have an abortion. Dr. Andrews felt that she was not being completely open about her reasons, and that she was ambivalent about her decision. She hinted, but did not directly ask for his advice.

What should the genetic counselor's role be? Should it be to explore the other possible reasons for her decision—her career, her marriage, her concern with physical appearance? Should it be to restate more forcefully the information that the risk was small and the defect, if it occurred, remediable? Or should it be to accept the client's decision on her own terms, on the grounds that she had been given full information and was free to make any choice she liked?

COMMENTARY

Robert Redmon

The questions raised by this case and by countless others that occur in genetic clinics around the world can be viewed as a debate between those who believe in "directive" counseling—emphasizing a particular decision that the counselor believes is preferable—and those who state that the role of the counselor is simply to supply information, so that their patients/clients can apply their own values to make an appropriate judgment, the "nondirective" model. Indeed those who hold the nondirective view do so as a matter of moral principle, since to do otherwise seems to them to violate client autonomy or to impose value structures that may be foreign to the individual.

The active, directive view is often chosen by genetic counselors who view the individual as a patient, not a client. They believe that they must assume some responsibility for the outcome of their contacts with the patient, and thus some responsibility for the patient's behavior and decisions. As one genetic counselor put it, "It is neither right nor desirable to evade a personal commitment when it is desired and might be of help. It is in the nature of the doctor-patient relationship that the doctor assumes at least some responsibility for the patient, influences his decisions and, therefore, must answer for them as well" (W.F.F. Vogel, *Genetic Counseling*, Springer-Verlag, 1969, p. 97).

The nondirective view toward genetic counseling, on the other hand, is expressed in a 1975 statement from the Ad Hoc Committee on Genetic Counseling. The Committee held that the task of counseling is to "communicate" with "clients" (not patients) so that they "comprehend the medical facts," "understand the options," are able to "choose the course of action which seems appropriate to them in view of their risk and their family goals" and can "make the best possible adjustment to the disorder." The task is not to influence the client, but simply to inform her. To do otherwise would be to infringe upon the client's autonomy.

The assumption underlying this directive/nondirective debate is that informing someone or communicating with her is a matter of implanting some thought, imprint, ideas, or whatever, in the subject's mind. How she assimilates, judges, and reacts to the information is a separate matter. The directive counselor says that he has not finished his job until the patient reacts in a certain way, and the nondirective one claims that getting the right ideas in the client's mind is enough.

Informing someone is not simply saying something. It is saying something that has a desired effect. And the effect is not merely in the mind. If A says to B, "It is raining," and B does not rush outside to put up the top of his beloved sports car, then A has not *informed* B that it is raining (B did not hear A, B does not understand English, etc.). To inform someone, to communicate, is to say something that results in actions (or the disposition to act) of a certain sort, which includes being able to cite reasons for those actions.

To return to Mrs. Robinson and Dr. Andrews: Dr. Andrews seems to have failed to inform Mrs. Robinson because Mrs. Robinson's actions are not appropriate. The abortion decision is not the problem. The problem is that she has stated the wrong reason for the abortion. If she did not want to burden a shaky marriage with a baby or if she did not want to interrupt her career at this point or if the fear of other defects was cited as a reason, this would have let Dr. Andrews know that he had succeeded in giving information. But citing fear of a 3/1000 risk (of a minor defect, at that) and ignoring a 6/100 risk (the statistical average) of other problems is irrational and shows a failure to comprehend.

The statement by the Ad Hoc Committee on the goal of counseling must be supplemented by an adequate view as to what constitutes communication, information giving, and so on. The counselor's values must govern his judgment as to whether information has been given. He must decide which effects are more serious (a value judgment) as well as the probabilities of their occurrence. And he must determine if the response is appropriate to these facts, to be sure the client has been informed. If the nondirective approach is best, then the counselor must allow for a wide range of responses. But a wide range does not include every response. It is Dr. Andrews's responsibility to explore the reasons behind Mrs. Robinson's decision; to try to elicit a rational response.

Which brings up my final point: the counselor must be quite clear about his own values. In order to tell if someone is responding irrationally, we must have criteria for rationality. At least two of the major components of rationality are (1) an appropriate set of beliefs about reality, including probabilities and reasoning processes and (2) an appropriate value structure which, for example, places a higher value on the life of a human than of a mouse, or which places a greater dysvalue on Down's syndrome than on a cleft palate. We all require such structures in order to communicate, and the counselor must be aware of his own and those of his clients.

COMMENTARY

Joyce Bermel

Twenty-eight. Married five years. A difficult time in a woman's life. Mrs. Robinson is going through the anxieties of many young women today, caught between her desires for a career and the disturbing realization that if she is going to have a family she had better start soon.

In her case the decision is even harder than it might be for, say, a woman who is a lawyer or a doctor with an established practice. Her career has its ups and downs. It obviously won't pay for a housekeeper. Once the baby is born she may have to cut back on going to auditions, and that in turn could mean fewer jobs and less money.

Her husband, who's wrapped up in his own career, probably won't be much help. He's away on assignment often. It was during one of his trips, while her own career was going poorly, that Mrs. Robinson started taking Valium. Her physician might have done better to refer her to a marriage counselor or a psychologist than to a genetic counselor.

But Dr. Andrews was called in. He thought the information he gave Mrs. Robinson would reassure her. The only birth defect known to be associated with Valium is a three- to fourfold increase in cleft lip or palate, which is "corrected quite easily surgically." The likelihood of the baby having that or any other birth defect is, in his estimation, small. To a genetic counselor that is splendid news. Compared with many of the clients Dr. Andrews sees—women who run the risk of having babies born with Down's syndrome or spina bifida—Mrs. Robinson is wonderfully lucky. Her decision to have an abortion must seem irrational. It goes against the best scientific information.

But what does a baby represent to Mrs. Robinson? Perhaps she sees it as a chance to hold her strained marriage together, a mistake many women persist in. Perhaps she hopes her husband will stay closer to home once he is a father, and take photos of their beautiful child. As an actress, she may put a premium on looks and so may her photographer husband. A baby born with a physical blemish does not fit into the picture. And a child who requires surgery may heap more problems on this already rocky marriage. What, then, should the genetic counselor do?

First, he must recognize that, whatever her reasons, Mrs. Robinson has a legal right to an abortion. It does not matter whether Dr. Andrews regards appearance as sufficient cause; it does not matter whether other reasons are at work. Mrs. Robinson does not have to justify her decision to anyone. With that firmly in mind, Dr. Andrews has several options.

He can simply quote the statistical data and consider his job done. But a mechanical presentation of facts is a poor approach under any circumstances. It adds ammunition to the frequent charge that medicine has become depersonalized, and it ignores the counselor's role as advisor. Many genetic counselors see value-neutrality as a mark of professionalism, but carried to extremes it makes a mockery of the consulting process.

Or, Dr. Andrews can press Mrs. Robinson to make one decision or the other, based on medical information. In this instance, since he believes that the risk of the defect is small and the condition is remediable, he will probably advise her not to abort. But, given the complex circumstances of Mrs. Robinson's life, this advice might not be doing her—or the unwanted baby—a service.

There is another path that Dr. Andrews can take to help Mrs. Robinson clarify her own thinking. He can raise the question of whether Mrs. Robinson is using the scientific data as a smokescreen. He can suggest that other matters seem to be troubling her. Since he has not been trained as a psychologist or psychiatrist he may find himself on slippery territory. And, of course, he may be wrong. Still, he owes it to Mrs. Robinson—and to the baby in formation—to at least raise the possibility, and to suggest that Mrs. Robinson discuss her doubts with him, her husband, or her physician.

It bothers me that Mr. Robinson did not join his wife on the follow-up visit to Dr. Andrews. The counselor should have suggested—even requested—that they appear together to consult about a matter of such importance to them both. While the ultimate decision about whether to have the baby is Mrs. Robinson's, obviously her husband's feelings influence her, or she would not have deferred her decision until his return. She needs to know how her husband feels about bringing up this or any other child, and a three-way consultation might be a good place to start.

Abortion is not an action to undertake lightly. But then neither is motherhood. Mrs. Robinson made her decision to abort shortly after she had been offered a television role. The tradeoff may appear ridiculous to some, but the choice between having a career and caring for children has not yet been resolved in our society.

Selected Bibliography

Part II: Reproductive Rights and Technologies

Andrews, Lori B. *New Conceptions: A Consumer's Guide to the Newest Infertility Treatments.* New York: St. Martin's Press, 1984.

Bayles, Michael D. *Reproductive Ethics.* Englewood Cliffs, NJ: Prentice-Hall, 1984.

Callahan, Sidney, and Callahan, Daniel. *Abortion: Understanding Differences.* New York: Plenum Press, 1984.

Elias, Sherman, and Annas, George J. *Reproductive Genetics and the Law.* Chicago: Year Book Medical Publishers, Inc., 1987.

Kass, Leon R. *Toward a More Natural Science: Biology and Human Affairs.* New York: Free Press, 1985.

McCormick, Richard A. *How Brave a New World? Dilemmas in Bioethics.* New York: Doubleday and Co., Inc., 1981.

Noonan, John T., Jr., ed. *The Morality of Abortion.* Cambridge: Harvard University Press, 1970.

Rothman, Barbara Katz. *The Tentative Pregnancy: Prenatal Diagnosis and the Future of Motherhood.* New York: Viking, 1986.

Thomson, Judith Jarvis. "A Defense of Abortion." *Philosophy and Public Affairs* 1, no. 1 (Fall 1971): 47–66.

Walters, LeRoy. "Human In Vitro Fertilization: A Review of the Ethical Literature." *Hastings Center Report* 9 (August 1979): 23–43.

Warnock, Mary. *A Question of Life: The Warnnock Report on Human Fertilisation and Embryology.* Oxford: Basil Blackwell, 1985.

Wolf, Susan. "Enforcing Surrogate Motherhood Agreements: The Trouble with Specific Performance." *New York Law School Human Rights Annual* Vol. IV, Part 2 (Spring 1987): 375–412.

PART THREE

Death and Dying

INTRODUCTION

Part Two examined the ethical dilemmas at the beginning of life; Part Three turns to the equally vexing questions at its end. Concerns about the appropriate use of life-sustaining technology mark the beginning of the modern era of biomedical ethics. In previous eras doctors could do little to stave off the inevitable death of a patient. Today, however, highly sophisticated machinery—the best-known example being the mechanical ventilator, which breathes for a person unable to do so on his or her own—creates the possibility of a whole range of interventions. Some of these may be life- saving, others only temporarily life-prolonging. Moreover, these technologies carry risks and burdens. Should doctors (and patients) use all the available technology, all the time? Or are there limits? And inevitably one confronts the quintessential procedural question in biomedical ethics: Who decides?

The cases in the first section— "Decisions about Death"—pose these questions in varied ways. They concern decisions about stopping cardiopulmonary resuscitation on the basis of a secondhand report that the patient would refuse if conscious, about informing patients' families of hospital "coding" procedures, about the right of a physician to refuse to operate on a woman who insists on an advance directive prohibiting certain forms of life-sustaining treatment, and about the duty to treat a patient who has attempted suicide.

A second section—"Refusal of Life-Sustaining Treatment and Euthanasia"—addresses the range of situations in which patients, or their proxies, decide that the continuation of treatment is not in the patient's best interests. While the legal right to refuse treatment has been well established, the moral questions are still unresolved. Should a burn patient, who wants to stop the excruciatingly painful treatment that will keep him alive, be treated against his wishes? Should the wishes of an AIDS patient who refuses treatment that would alleviate his current illness but not offer cure be honored? Should a woman totally dependent on life-support technology be allowed to refuse feeding tubes, and thus bring about her own death? Should family have a role in such decisions?

All ethical theories value life. But other values—autonomy, personhood, privacy—are also important. These cases open up the vast array of highly personal decisions that will, at some point, confront us as individuals and as members of society. What individuals choose to do in these life-and-death situations will affect not only their lives but also our collective sense of the dignity of persons.

DECISIONS ABOUT DEATH

22

A Cardiac Arrest and a Second-Hand Report

Mr. R., sixty-five years old, is brought into the emergency room by ambulance. The emergency room staff determines that he suffered a heart attack and was not breathing for an unknown period of time before he was revived by paramedics. After initial evaluation, Dr. A., the family physician, tells Mrs. R. that her husband's condition is serious and that he may have suffered irreversible brain damage. Before he leaves for his office, Dr. A. also says that he is ordering a neurological consultation and that he wants to monitor the situation for the next seventy-two hours.

In the waiting room Mrs. R. encounters Ms. C., the chaplain's intern assigned to the emergency room. Over coffee, Mrs. R. confides to Ms. C. that she and her husband had talked about the possibility of such an event and that both wished that "nothing extraordinary should be done to keep them alive." Ms. C. also learns that Mrs. R. had not given this information to Dr. A.; she makes a mental note to do so. Meanwhile other families occupy her attention.

Approximately one hour later a "code blue" is called. Mr. R. has suffered a cardiac arrest. By the time Ms. C. responds to the code, the code team has begun work. Ms. C. relates the substance of her conversation with Mrs. R. to the nursing supervisor who passes it on to the resident in charge of the code team. The resident is furious with the nurse for interrupting his efforts by reporting "gossip."

The supervisor pages Dr. A., who responds immediately from his office. She communicates the substance of the conversation between Ms. C. and Mrs. R., the fact that Mr. R. has coded, and that the code team is now working on him. The chaplain's report rings true to Dr. A. He has had a longstanding relationship with the family and feels that he "knows" what they would want, even without a direct conversation.

By now the resident has come to the phone. He is angry that Dr. A. is even considering the secondhand report. He tells Dr. A. that Mr. R. can be resuscitated, although his prognosis would still be uncertain.

Dr. A. orders the resident to stop the code, and tells him that he will call Mrs. R. and inform her that her husband has died. The resident hangs up the phone and heads toward Mr. R.'s room. Just then a nurse comes into the hallway, shouting, "He's starting to come back!" The resident turns toward Ms. C. and asks angrily, "What am I supposed to do now?"

COMMENTARY

Stephen E. Lammers and Alan W. Childs

What does the resident see as the problem? Is he troubled about obeying his superior's orders, which he perceives as flawed? Is he angry at the chaplain's intern for meddling in a matter that was not her business? Does he feel confused about the exact meaning of Mrs. R.'s wishes concerning what should be done for her husband? Is there some conflict in his own mind about what is best for the patient?

The resident's conflict can be understood on at least two levels: who should decide? and what should be decided? Under a patient-centered, collective decision model, the competent and informed patient's consistent expression of wishes should almost always determine what is to be done. Unfortunately, Mr. R. is not competent to convey his wishes, so we must rely upon others. However, certain precautions are in order.

First, we must be sure about the information we are receiving. Does the information indicate the wishes of the individual making the decision rather than the patient's actual desires? Are people confusing the best interests of the patient with the patient's wishes? People may have to base their decisions upon the patient's best interests but they should not confuse this judgment with the patient's expression of what he wanted done.

Second, to whom was the information conveyed and under what circumstances? In this case the physician should have contacted the spouse immediately in order to determine what might be done for her husband while the code continued. Dr. A.'s error was to assume that the previous expression of wishes was definitive. Perhaps he presumed too much about his relationship with the Rs. What he owed the patient and his spouse is direct communication. The resident is correct in being cautious about the information.

But the problem does not end here. The resident owes Ms. C., the chaplain's intern, more respect than he showed. Simply because information comes "secondhand" does not lessen its value. At the very least it should be checked. Problems such as these arise too often in hospitals, not simply because of earlier failures to communicate, but because patients often communicate only bits and pieces of relevant information at a time to a variety of individuals. The whole picture may be known to no one or known by persons who have lesser status and reponsibility in the hospital hierarchy. Ways of sharing information must be developed and used. Here the question also involved acting upon information given to an auxiliary member of a health care team. Instead of being treated as a person with valuable information to contribute, the chaplain's intern is regarded as a meddler.

This is not to say that the chaplain's intern is immune to criticism. Given the collective model of health care, the responsibility of health care personnel to communicate with one another expeditiously becomes more important. How much better it would have been if Ms. C. had made sure immediately that Dr. A. learned of her conversation with Mrs. R. If that had happened, and assuming Dr. A. acted responsibly, a conversation could have begun between the primary decision makers, the spouse, and the family physician, and the confusion for everyone involved in caring for Mr. R. could have been minimized or avoided.

Problems like this will continue to arise in medicine unless and until new ways of acting become second nature for medical care personnel. Given that crises with cardiac patients are not uncommon, Dr. A. should have taken the initiative at the time of Mr. R.'s admission and talked to his spouse about the possibility of cardiac arrest. If such a conversation had produced a satisfactory result, Dr. A. could have charted the appropriate orders and the problem would never have arisen. Physicians should always initiate conversations on coding when the condition of the patient warrants it. While such discussions often are avoided to spare families pain or anxiety, they may be more painful at a later, more critical time.

Now we may suggest an answer for the resident. For two reasons, he should continue the code. First, more information is needed about the spouse's wishes. Second, with respect to what should be decided, medicine is not a neutral practice; it is oriented toward the good of patients, and the presumption is that this includes the good of their life. Given appropriate communication with the spouse, that presumption could have been defeated. Otherwise it dictates action in favor of life. Only if we proceed in that fashion can we feel confident that if the patient dies, nothing wrong has been done.

The family physician acted too quickly, and thus wrongly, in ordering the code stopped; the resident should not compound the problem by obeying the order. In a climate where the old medical model of "always battle death to the end" is being challenged not only by a more sensitive understanding of the limits of medical power but also by pragmatic financial considerations, one must not abandon the presumption in favor of preserving life unless the patient's or spouse's wishes are clearly known.

COMMENTARY

Mitchel H. Mernick

In certain instances it is appropriate to withhold life support. Medical progress and technological advances have made it easy for physicians to delay the exact moment of death. However, we are still faced with terminal, irreversible disease for which resuscitative efforts do no more than prolong the dying process and the agony of our patients and their families.

When a competent adult has a progressive, irreversible illness the physician should take the initiative in raising the subject of resuscitation in the event of a cardiopulmonary arrest so as not to subject that patient to unnecessary and futile resuscitative efforts. If a patient is incompetent, the family should be sought to offer what they understand to be the presumed or prestated wishes of the patient regarding terminal care. This case study underscores the importance of accurate documentation regarding Do Not Resuscitate (DNR) orders. The decision not to resuscitate cannot be left to word of mouth or intuition.

The emergency room staff has encountered Mr. R. for the first time. The family physician, Dr. A., on initial evaluation suspects that there may have been irreversible brain damage. To confirm his diagnosis, he orders a neurologic consultation and decides to observe for seventy-two hours to see how much, if any, neurologic function will return. Dr. A. makes no attempt to discuss the patient's desire for resuscitation even though he suspects that the neurologic process may be irreversible. Of course, without knowing how long the patient was lacking oxygen it is difficult to offer an accurate prognosis. This uncertainty may have dissuaded Dr. A. from discussing resuscitation at the outset with Mrs. R.

Everyone should be aware of the alternative approaches that can be followed in the event of serious incurable illness. Mr. and Mrs. R. had discussed these issues. Unfortunately, Mrs. R. had neglected to inform Dr. A. of their feelings. Ideally the family physician should know a patient's wishes in the event of cardiac arrest. Patients are often unable to communicate their wishes once a catastrophic event occurs. A written statement indicating an individual's preference in the event of a cardiac arrest can help prevent misunderstandings.

It became evident to Ms. C. that the patient had, while competent, clearly expressed the wish that "nothing extraordinary should be done to keep (him) alive" in the case of "such an event." I am interpreting as extraordinary measures mechanical ventilation and cardiopulmonary resuscitation, both of which are part of a code blue. We do not know why Mr. R. made this decision. (Did he suffer from a chronic, progressive illness?) Regardless of the reason, Mrs. R. clearly states her husband's wish to Ms. C. The intern at this point might have suggested that Mrs. R. immediately page Dr. A. or alternatively that Mrs. R. make this known directly to the emergency room physicians.

It is routine practice that any patient in a hospital suffering a cardiac arrest will be resuscitated. Some hospitals provide a mechanism by which a physician may write a DNR order. In Mr. R.'s case none had been written and the resuscitative effort was started. We are given no indication that the resident in charge of the code team had any knowledge of Mr. R.'s past or present medical history. The furor of the resuscitative effort usually does not allow time for acquiring this information. The resident was following emergency room protocol and fulfilling his obligation in resuscitating a patient for whom no DNR order had been written. When the nursing supervisor conveys the information that she received from the chaplain's intern, the resident cannot be expected to stop the team's efforts at resuscitation. There is no documentation that Mr. R. actually wished not to be resuscitated.

When Dr. A. is contacted by the nursing supervisor he states that he "knows" what Mr. and Mrs. R. would want, even without direct conversation. Studies have shown that doctors who rely on intuition often make incorrect assumptions regarding their patients' true desires. Had Dr. A. discussed resuscitation with Mrs. R. when they met in the emergency room he could have documented their discussion as well as the possibility of irreversible brain damage and written a DNR order. With proper communication and documentation the resident and code team would not have started resuscitation procedures. Once they were in effect and the patient was responding, to stop them would mean actively removing medications and machinery that were keeping Mr. R. alive. This is an unreasonable order for Dr. A. to have issued to the medical resident.

The medical resident should have known what to do when Mr. R. was "starting to come back." To ask the chaplain's intern "What am I supposed to do now?" was inappropriate. Ms. C. was in no position to make what at that point was a medical decision. The resident should have continued efforts to stabilize the patient.

23

Does "Doing Everything" Include CPR?

Fred Walker, ninety years old and retired since 1955, was admitted to a community hospital with bronchial pneumonia, advanced pulmonary edema, urinary tract infection, and anemia. Mr. Walker responded to treatment initially but then his condition worsened. Mrs. Walker asked the attending physician to do "everything possible" for her husband and assured him that they were able to pay for the costs of treatment not covered by Medicare.

On the morning of the fourteenth day in the hospital, Mr. Walker's physician visited him and found his condition unchanged. Although he was not improving, Mr. Walker was alert and asked, "Am I all right, doctor?" Fifteen minutes later a nurse entered the room and found that Mr. Walker was not breathing and that all vital signs were absent. She summoned the doctor, who immediately decided not to attempt to resuscitate Mr. Walker. The cause of death was recorded as ventricular fibrillation.

According to hospital officials it is the institution's policy to make an all-out effort to revive all unresponsive patients. Like other hospitals, this one has a "code"—usually a series of numbers or a color—for summoning staff members with portable defibrillators and other resuscitation equipment to the bedside of a patient in cardiac arrest. "Code Blue"—as it is called at this hospital—is known only to insiders and can thus be called without alarming other patients and visitors. But physicians may also issue "no code" orders. That is, in certain circumstances they may direct staff not to resuscitate a patient should cardiac arrest occur. Patients, however, are usually not told about coding. "It would make already anxious patients and relatives even more fearful," one official explained. "They don't need to know about it. They will be coded anyway. People should assume whatever care is needed is going to be given."

Mr. Walker's physician and the hospital officials maintained that Mr. Walker was coded, but both conceded that "code blue" was not called. Mr. Walker's physician argued, "Doing 'everything' for a patient in my mind does not include cardiopulmonary resuscitation (CPR). In Mr. Walker's case it might mean doing nothing." According to the physician, Mr. Walker was not sent to the intensive care unit (ICU) for two reasons. There was a shortage of beds in the unit and Mr. Walker "didn't seem like he belonged there" because he was not acutely ill. "When it comes to resuscitating, it's reasonable for a man in his fifties or sixties, but criminal to try to resuscitate in [Mr. Walker's] age group to prolong life a week at the most, given his condition. I don't see any sense in calling code blue with a ninety-year-old man who has no future to look forward to. That's doing him a disservice and increasing his hospital costs."

Mrs. Walker disagrees. Upon being informed that no emergency measures were taken in her husband's case, Mrs. Walker said that that decision was against her wishes. "Doing everything," she says, "is the difference between life and death. The doctor was playing God when he decided he should not try to save my husband. You're not playing God when you've tried everything and exhausted all methods. All I wanted was for them to try. My husband knew how to love and be loved. That was his quality of life. That suited him and it suited me."

Should patients and their families be informed about coding policies? Did Mr. Walker's doctor act ethically in going against Mrs. Walker's wishes?

COMMENTARY

Ronald A. Carson

The routine introduction of life-prolonging technologies into medical care raises questions about the morality of extending life at all costs. Physicians are aware, as perhaps never before, of the centrality of values in clinical judgment and of the need to acknowledge and resolve conflicts in values that arise in medical practice. This is, in the main, a laudable development. But it may, on occasion, have unfortunate consequences, as in this case.

There is no reason not to assume good faith on the part of Mr. Walker's physician. My impression is that he was benevolently motivated when, upon being summoned by the nurse, he decided not to attempt to resuscitate Mr. Walker. Considerations of social worth may have entered into his decision. A young or middle-aged person would almost certainly have been resuscitated in similar circumstances, even in view of the possibility that irreversible brain damage had been sustained. Whether such considerations should enter a decision in cases like these can be debated. What is clear, however, is that to act contrary to the expressed wishes of a competent adult who was speaking on her husband's behalf, is to act immorally.

The physician's reasons for not putting Mr. Walker in an ICU prior to the final acute incident do not bear up under close scrutiny. Three reasons are mentioned. The first—that "doing everything" might mean "doing nothing"—is patently absurd. The second—that Mr. Walker was not acutely ill—is difficult to assess on the basis of the information given but, at the least, this assertion is inconsistent with the claim that, following an initial rally, Mr. Walker's condition worsened. The third reason—that it would have been "criminal" to try to resuscitate Mr. Walker—is the most confused.

The physician cites several factors in support of this last claim: the patient's age, his physical condition, the quality of his life, and hospital costs. But Mr. Walker's advanced age did not make him less worthy of care. His debilitated condition was of central importance in selecting a course of treatment but is not in itself sufficient to justify withholding treatment. Judgments about the quality of Mr. Walker's life were, as Mrs. Walker said, his (and hers) to make. Hospital costs, while inevitably entering into decisions of this sort, appear not to be at issue here since the Walkers were able to pay for services. (Conceivably, Mrs. Walker had an exaggerated notion of what could reasonably be done for her husband, as evidenced by her desire that the doctor "exhaust all methods," but that merely indicates the deep disparity between her expectations and those of the physician.)

There is irony (and perhaps some mean-spiritedness) in the hospital official's statement that entering patients should not be bothered with the details of resuscitation policy but should assume that they will be well cared for and coded if necessary. Mrs. Walker made that assumption. To say that her husband was coded but that the code was not called is a fine distinction—or a mincing of words. Mr. Walker was a victim of reverse moral discrimination motivated, I presume, by the wish not to prolong the dying of a very sick old man. The old man, however, wanted to live and expected to be treated and apparently his wife was not made aware that he was dying. A decision to resuscitate might have prolonged his life, or at least spared his wife unnecessary anguish.

COMMENTARY

Mark Siegler

Should health professionals perform CPR on every patient who is about to die in a hospital? This approach—equal CPR for all regardless of medical condition or patient preference—is indefensible, counterintuitive, and unethical, and would signal the ultimate transformation of medicine from an art based upon clinical discretion into an unthinking, unfeeling bureaucratic system.

Preserving or prolonging life is one, perhaps even a central goal of medicine. But it it not the only goal. In the case of the terminally ill, many physicians and patients often prefer alternative, attainable goals such as the relief of symptoms and the preservation of function. Which particular goals are preferred from a medical encounter (a value matter) should be determined jointly by the physician and the patient, but it is important to note that preferences and desires will be constrained by the medical-scientific realities (a factual matter) of what can be achieved. If dying without being accorded the full ritual of a CPR effort is regarded as the ultimate horror (the twentieth-century equivalent of the morbid nineteenth-century fear of being buried alive, as in Poe's *The Cask of Amontillado*), health professionals might have an obligation to explore any chance, however remote, of saving patients from such a fate. But I believe the existence of a medical technique does not and should not mandate its use in every case, nor should it necessarily generate a presumption favoring its use.

CPR is a relatively new emergency medical technique, developed originally to prevent sudden and unexpected death in the life-threatening situation of cardiac arrest. The standards for CPR issued by a 1980 national conference support this view (*JAMA* 1980: 244:453). It is the physician's responsibility to decide which patients can possibly be treated with which medical techniques, and it is the joint responsibility of the physician and patient to decide which should be so treated. CPR decisions should be examined in this context. For example, I believe that CPR is often not indicated in patients for whom vigorous intensive therapy has not been successful. It is unlikely that a final *pro forma* pounding on the chest or administration of one or several electrical shocks will reverse their progressive downhill course. Even if CPR is temporarily successful, such patients rarely regain consciousness and usually suffer a second arrest.

The principal ethical grounds for making a decision not to resuscitate a patient should be the sound medical judgment that the patient's death from the primary disease is imminent and that further treatment for the primary disease is futile. Although the medical details in this case are sketchy, the principal factor in the physician's decision not to perform CPR seemed to be Mr. Walker's deteriorating clinical condition. After Mr. Walker died, the physician invoked many reasons (some extraneous and some downright inappropriate) to defend his decision not to perform CPR, but this seems to be his central point: "When it comes to resuscitating, it's reasonable for a man in his fifties or sixties, but criminal to try to resuscitate in that age group *to prolong life a week at most, given his condition*" (italics added).

If Mr. Walker's chances for survival were poor prior to the arrest, they were infinitesimal afterwards. I am not aware of a single case report of a successful resuscitation in a patient such as Mr. Walker (i.e., unwitnessed arrest in a ninety-year-old person with multiple serious underlying medical problems).

A second and independent reason to decide not to resuscitate a patient would be if this were the stated preference of an autonomous, self-determining, competent adult. Unfortunately, we know very little about Mr. Walker's wishes or whether, in the face of serious illness, he retained the capacity to process information and to make choices concerning his care.

We know considerably more about Mrs. Walker's wishes. Her motto was: "Do everything!" The question arises: how much legal and ethical weight should be placed on the statements of the angry widow or on her preferences before her husband died? Family members have no legal authority to make decisions on behalf of patients unable to make decisions for themselves, unless such family members have been granted guardianship powers by a judge or by a legislative statute (only three states—Maine, Idaho, and North Carolina—have such a statute). However, the statements of family members may be ethically important for two reasons. First, they may (but do not necessarily) reflect the personal preferences of the patient who is unable to express them. Second, the common practice of turning to family members acknowledges that we exist in communities of concern and that those who care most about us ought to have a special moral authority to assist in making decisions about us when we are no longer able to do so for ourselves. I sense that Mrs. Walker's statements, however, reflect her personal wishes and preferences and not necessarily her husband's. Further, she appeared to be ignorant of medicine's limitations and nourished unrealistic expectations regarding CPR.

Perhaps the physician could be faulted for not having raised the issue of CPR directly or tangentially with Mr. or Mrs. Walker when he first believed the patient's condition was deteriorating and was likely to terminate in a cardiac arrest. Presumably, he could have used the occasion to gently inform them of the prognosis and instruct them on medicine's limitations (including, but not restricted to, CPR technology).

On reflection, however, *perhaps* the physician acted rightly in not raising this matter with Mr. Walker (even if Mr. Walker were competent). If the physician knew (within limits of uncertainty that characterize all medical knowledge) that CPR offered Mr. Walker no possible benefit, the patient's preferences would not have been germane.

Our CPR policies are enmeshed in rules, regulations, and procedures that minimize discretion and maximize bureaucratic bumbling. Some believe that placing the burden for such decisions on patients by invoking autonomy and self-determination will resolve the matter, but let me assure such legalists that the resolution will exist only on paper and not on hospital wards. This arena demands clinical discretion, a discerning judgment reached by the patient and physician after due consideration of all the patient's life (and death) circumstances.

In Mr. Walker's case, the decision not to resuscitate was made by his personal physician who came to his bedside immediately upon being summoned, and discovered that his patient was pulseless and without respiration and might have been so for a period of up to fifteen minutes. In these circumstances, who would have been in a better position to decide on whether to resuscitate? Surely not a code team, or the nurse, or Mr. Walker, or Mr. Walker's wife! The physician acted in the best traditions of equity—with reasonableness and responsiveness—in reaching a judgment based upon discretion not to resuscitate.

24

Surgical Risks and Advance Directives

Mrs. P. is a seventy-six-year-old woman with osteoporosis and a failed left hip prosthesis. In addition, she has severe chronic asthmatic bronchitis. The management of her lung disease has been hampered by her allergy to theophylline, which is one of the mainstays of treatment. As a result, she has had increasing difficulty walking and confinement to a wheelchair is imminent.

When surgery to replace the prosthesis was recommended, Mrs. P. expressed concern about the possibility of ending up after the operation dependent on a ventilator, possibly comatose. She feared that her resources would be depleted for medical expenses. Little or nothing would be left to pass on to her children.

She was willing to have an operation only if she could prepare a legal document that, in the event of prolonged ventilator dependence, would require her physician to remove her from the ventilator after a specified time (for example, two weeks). Should the surgeon agree to be bound by Mrs. P.'s instructions, or should he refuse her request even if doing so means that she will not have the surgery that might prevent increasing disability?

COMMENTARY

Daniel H. Lederer

In agreeing to surgery, a patient, while hoping for a favorable outcome, must accept the risk of a spectrum of adverse effects. These can range from a lack of benefit at one end to permanent disability or death at the other. The surgeon must also accept an element of risk, for the price he pays for failure may include an unhappy, angry patient; colleagues to whom he must explain major complications or death; and, possibly, malpractice litigation with its personal and professional penalties.

In this case the patient is unwilling to accept the risk of an unlikely but possible event, specifically that she may become dependent on a ventilator after surgery. Her attempted solution is to prepare a legally binding document that requires the surgeon to discontinue the treatment after a specified interval. Were the surgeon to accept such an agreement, the patient presumably would be willing to proceed with the operation. But such an agreement does not eliminate the risk; rather, it transfers it to the surgeon, who in accepting it may be placing himself in legal jeopardy. Of course, the patient's signed document may protect the surgeon should the issue come to court, but it cannot prevent the initiation of legal action by those who might interpret the surgeon's actions as collusion in suicide.

Beyond the legal considerations, such an agreement undermines basic principles that should guide every doctor-patient encounter. The first is the dictum of nonmaleficence, *primum non nocere*. With this patient, the risk of prolonged respiratory failure requiring mechanical support of breathing is low, but should it occur, one cannot predict *in advance* the point at which the likelihood of reversibility will seem unacceptably small to either the surgeon or the patient. In other words, a judgment regarding a patient's potential for recovery requires an assessment at that point, not days or weeks ahead.

Nor can one be sure what the patient would have wanted. If Mrs. P. does become ventilator-dependent, it will still be difficult to know whether she would have followed her own directive once a hypothetical scenario becomes reality. In this case, to discontinue ventilator support when the patient's respiratory failure may still be reversible must be considered a harmful act.

The importance of the principle of reverence for life is perhaps self-evident. Although a physician is not required to prolong life at all costs regardless of circumstances, it is the physician's obligation to try to preserve life as long as such efforts, in his or her judgment, are in the patient's best interests. Many factors, including the emotional and financial costs to the patient as well as the patient's projected quality of life, must be considered. For the surgeon to agree to accept a document as a substitute for this delicate judgment is potentially to convert his role from protector to executioner.

The agreement proposed by the patient disregards a third principle, more subtle but equally important, that of mutual trust. It implies that the patient does not trust the surgeon to determine appropriately when treatment is no longer beneficial and then to act accordingly. And the surgeon, by agreeing to the document, contributes to an atmosphere of mistrust by saying, again by implication, that the patient or her family cannot be trusted to make a reasonable judgment regarding prolongation of treatment during the postoperative period. The presence of mutual trust *per se* does not guarantee a successful outcome of surgery, nor does its absence preclude such a result, but without a sense of mutual trust a patient would be ill-advised to embark on any dangerous diagnostic or therapeutic procedure.

For all these reasons the surgeon should refuse the patient's request. This refusal will not be without consequences. The patient will be deprived of an operation that would probably have been successful and the surgeon must wonder whether he has been needlessly rigid and authoritarian in denying the patient some control over her own treatment. But respect for patient autonomy has limits. Although from her own perspective the patient may only be asking to exercise her autonomy, in this case she is asking too much.

COMMENTARY

Dan W. Brock

It is now widely accepted that a competent patient is morally entitled to refuse any medical treatment, including life-sustaining treatment, that he or she judges to be unduly burdensome. Why then should the surgeon be reluctant to make an agreement with Mrs. P. that ventilator treatment will not be continued beyond a specified time?

One reason may be that the surgeon, like many physicians, is reluctant to be bound even by a patient's competent request due to fear of legal liability (criminal or civil) for stopping life-sustaining treatment. Court decisions and advance-directive legislation around the country, however, increasingly support the legal permissibility of physicians carrying out patients' decisions to stop life support. Such fears could also be allayed if hospitals and other health care institutions develop clear policies for making and carrying out decisions to withdraw life-sustaining treatments.

The surgeon's concern in this case may not be legal, but moral. Many physicians believe that although it is morally permissible for patients to decide not to initiate life-sustaining treatment, it is not morally permissible to stop it once it has begun, or at least that stopping it is a graver matter requiring weightier reasons to be justified. While still common, this view is increasingly rejected, quite correctly I believe, by physicians, patients, and their families.

What should ultimately be determinative of whether any form of life-sustaining treatment is initiated *or* continued is the competent, informed, and voluntary decision of the patient.

Even if there is no important moral difference between not starting and stopping life support, physicians and others who must make or carry out such decisions commonly *feel* more responsible for the patient's death when forms of life support such as mechanical ventilation are stopped. As a result, they often find it psychologically harder to stop life support than not to start it.

The most obvious bad effect of the reluctance to stop life support once begun is overtreatment. The case of Mrs. P., however, dramatically illustrates another bad effect. For fear of indefinitely continuing, patients and others may be reluctant or unwilling to accept any treatment. That can result in denying patients treatment that may prove beneficial— either life support itself or other beneficial treatment, such as replacement of the hip prosthesis, without which Mrs. P. is doomed to live disabled.

This is a case in which physicians should be much more willing to agree to—indeed to recommend—time-limited trials of various forms of life support. Such an agreement would allay Mrs. P.'s fears and might reduce or eliminate the uncertainty about whether, and to what extent, the treatment will prove beneficial.

One final issue that this case raises is whether agreeing to be bound by the patient's instructions would unduly infringe on the surgeon's responsibility to exercise his professional judgment. Physicians are not obliged to act in ways that would violate their own moral or professional integrity just because their patients want them to do so. Nonetheless, physicians should be flexible regarding the alternative treatments they are willing to offer. In Mrs. P.'s case she seeks an agreement with her physician only that treatment will not be *imposed* on her in circumstances in which she does not wish to have it.

The surgeon may be concerned that the agreement Mrs. P. seeks could commit him later to stopping life-sustaining treatment when he judges that doing so is not in the patient's best interests. It would be reasonable, even desirable, for the surgeon to seek an agreement that puts not only a time limit on the use of mechanical ventilation, but that also, or even instead, specifies in some detail the circumstances in which life-sustaining treatment will be withdrawn.

Since one of Mrs. P.'s fears is being left on a respirator indefinitely in a comatose state, it could be made a part of the agreement that respirator treatment will be withdrawn if she has suffered an irreversible lose of consciousness and is in a persistent vegetative state. If she so desired, the agreement might further stipulate that other forms of life support such as nutrition and hydration will be discontinued in those circumstances. The agreement should insure both that the physician's expertise and the patient's values are brought to bear on decisions. Mrs. P.'s desire for such an agreement need not be seen as displaying a lack of trust in the surgeon, but only a desire to insure that her own values will guide later decisions.

This is a case in which an advance directive from the patient is appropriate about her care, and/or about who will act as her surrogate decisionmaker should she be incompetent to decide for herself. A number of states, like my own Rhode Island, have enacted legislation to enable persons to appoint a so-called Durable Power of Attorney for Health Care. Encouraging advance planning by patients about their health care is desirable public policy and squarely within medicine's long tradition of serving patients' well-being.

25

Nurturing a Defective Newborn

Baby Girl S. was born at a small community hospital, four weeks prematurely, after an uncomplicated pregnancy. At birth the baby breathed spontaneously, but shortly thereafter had an apneic episode in which respiration stopped, and oxygen was required. She also had unusual face and hands and showed little spontaneous motor activity. For these reasons she was transferred to a neonatal intensive care unit. Physical examination showed findings consistent with trisomy 18, a serious genetic defect. The infant continued to have occasional episodes of apnea which over the next twenty-four hours became sufficiently severe so that respirator assistance was considered. A heart murmur was noted and signs of early heart failure (normally treated with a variety of medications) became evident.

Mr. and Mrs. S. came to the center thirty-six hours after the birth, having been told that Baby S. had multiple birth defects. They met with the pediatrician and geneticist caring for the baby. The infant's primary problem was explained (a chromosomal "accident" resulting in extra genetic material in all of the infant's cells, with diverse manifestations), the immediate difficulties outlined (short periods where the infant "forgot" to breathe, and a heart defect which was probably an opening between the major artery to the body and the large artery to the lungs, with resultant heart failure), the child's abnormal features described (small size, unusual facial features, and deformed hands), and the long-term outlook explored (profound retardation with very high probability of death within the first year).

Within the next day or two decisions will need to be made:

1. Should resuscitative efforts be continued when the baby "forgets" to breathe?
2. Should a respirator be used if that becomes necessary to maintain the baby's life?
3. Should medication to control the potentially life-threatening heart failure be instituted?
4. Should other routine care be given?

Before these decisions are made, should the parents see the baby? Should the physician encourage or discourage them in touching and holding the baby?

COMMENTARY

Richard M. Pauli

Questions about resuscitation, medication, and allowing to die seem appropriate questions to ask in the case of Baby S. This baby has, with any treatment, a very limited life expectancy; should it survive, it has very little likelihood of evidencing even the most minimal level of "personhood" (that is, affective interaction with other persons). Since the parents should have primary responsibility for deciding about Baby S., they must be given accurate information about diagnosis and prognosis as well as predictions about the results of alternative courses of action. But another way of "knowing" about their baby is to see and touch her. This information, like the other pieces of data, must be made available to them by others. Therefore the attitude of the physician-counselor about nurturing will inevitably influence their own decision.

The physician-counselor may already have decided what medical care decisions are "preferred." Based on this judgment, he could opt for or against the parents seeing and touching the baby depending on which action he viewed as being most likely to result in accord with his "preferred" decision. That, of course, would be paternalism and deceit. But even if the physician-knows-best strategy is rejected, one is left with a difficult question. Does nurturing or non-nurturing, in itself, determine what decision the parents will make about resuscitation and medical support?

One could posit that all parents who first held and touched their infant would be *unable* to *ever* allow it to die. I don't think this is true for most parents. For example, decisions about adult incompetents are often made by family with a nurturing commitment of many years duration, and this is held to be the best way of "assuring loving solicitude for the patient" (the Quinlan case is a good example).

On the other hand, the horror of physical deformity might be anticipated to produce the opposite effect. The loving care evidenced by families with surviving but severely defective children indicates that this need not be an inevitable consequence.

The tension for the physician-counselor in the case of Baby S. is the conflict between an active and compassionate concern to minimize the suffering (through overwhelming guilt) of the parents, and the more passive responsibility to allow them to act autonomously. The physician's goal of minimizing parental suffering may be misplaced. Given the opportunity to nurture their defective child, parents will need to be supported through the guilt and grieving following a decision to withhold care, just as a family who elects to treat such a baby will require personal and community support. But attempts to allay their suffering by discouraging or refusing to let them see their baby is to engage in another form of paternal deception.

An informed decision requires accurate information, which we may assume the parents received in the case described. Does a knowledgeable decision require more than accurate information? Perhaps a well-considered choice *requires* experiential nurturing and a special kind of caring.

I think this other way of "knowing" is beneficial in making truly informed decisions, is a parental right, and is the best safeguard against arbitrary or frivolous decisions. The physician-counselor's role, then, is to encourage independence and autonomy. He should allow the parents themselves to decide whether to touch and hold the baby, but should encourage them to do so. Our aim should not be easy choices, but real ones.

COMMENTARY

Eric J. Cassell

The birth of this child is a tragedy. No matter what decision is made, or whether the child lives or dies, sorrow and suffering will follow. Therefore, there are two immediate problems: first, to make a decision about treatment and second, to minimize pain and suffering, because such relief is a necessary and legitimate object of medicine.

There are two alternative decisions to be made about her care. Either the infant should be permitted to die from the complications of her genetic defect and given care that will comfort her and relieve her suffering; or she should be kept alive until, beyond the limits of technological rescue, she ultimately dies, usually, we are told, within a year. If she is to be kept alive, the tools to be used—respirators, cardiac drugs, resuscitation—are merely technical details.

The case offers four alternative treatment levels, suggesting some ambivalence in the medical staff. Physicians may say, for example, "I believe she should be kept alive, but only if resuscitation for apnea is sufficient," or "only if therapy for heart failure is sufficient." This ambivalence makes the baby's failure to survive beyond a certain level of technological support the factor that determines outcome. Such decisions merely extend the wheel of fortune from conception into the neonatal intensive care unit and seemingly remove human agency—an understandable strategy, but an illusion nonetheless.

The parents have two choices. Either life is to be saved at all costs, or the decision to treat the baby is based on the infant's individual characteristics. If the parents believe life must be preserved at all costs, then their decision to treat is obvious. We would all sympathize with them and should do what is necessary to minimize their pain whether the infant survives or dies.

But if the decision is to be made on the basis of what the infant will become—her quality of life, her ultimate length of survival, economics, their ideas about parenthood, the effect on siblings or other family members, and future childbearing—then clear thinking and as much information as possible will be necessary. Clear thinking is the ability to weigh the evidence and the sets of competing needs and feelings as objectively as possible—to sort out wishes and desires from the facts of this infant's existence now and in the future.

This kind of thinking may be difficult for the mother who has given birth, just three days earlier, to a child that probably bitterly disappoints her nine months of dreams and wishes. Clear thinking will be made even harder by the inevitable feelings of guilt that accompany such a birth. The mother will wonder whether she did something to bring on the defects. Indeed, it is often easier to accept blame and guilt than to accept one's helplessness in the face of a capricious fate.

Now we come to the more pernicious question. Should the parents be encouraged to nurture the child—to touch her and to hold her—before making their decision?

If their decision is to save her life at all costs, what harm could come from *not* nurturing? The child will not lack such attention in the intensive care unit where nurses will hold and fondle her without the aversion that the inexperienced first feel with a defective child. What good would come from the physician *encouraging* the parents to hold and touch the infant before making the decision? They could ask to do so if they wished.

If the decision is to be based on a careful weighing of the baby's individual characteristics and the therapeutic possibilities, I cannot conceive how nurturing would clarify the mother's painful thinking or provide her with more "information." If the child lives there will be time enough for nurturance.

And if the child dies? Recent research confirms what even the most primitive people know: the bonding of parent and child occurs through the mother's nurturance and the child's response. If an infant is adopted at birth and after a period the biological mother wants the child returned, we feel sympathy for the adopting parents. Why? Because nurturing experience has formed a bond between the parents and their adopted child, so that the loss of the child is not merely the loss of a desirable object, but the loss of a loved one.

Why do pediatricians sometimes *want* the parents with newborns like Baby S. to nurture the child? Does the physician wish to teach them, starting here, how to be good parents? Or is there possibly something punitive in encouraging the parent to touch and hold? Does the staff share the magical beliefs on which the parents' feelings of guilt are based? Nurturing this infant will not change her defects or the conditions upon which a decision must be based. But nurturance and the establishment of a bond may make a decision to save the life a selfish one based on the parents' unwillingness to lose a loved one. Furthermore, nurturance will only add to the parents' suffering after her death. Is either a selfish decision or further suffering desirable?

26

A Suicide Attempt and Emergency Room Ethics

Michael Jellinek

After the car that he is driving at high speed hits a telephone pole, Mr. D. is brought to the hospital emergency room in serious condition. The physicians who examine him recommend surgery to repair a major internal hemorrhage. But the sixty-eight-year-old man refuses, saying that he wants to be "left alone to die." The physicians also learn that three weeks earlier Mr. D. was diagnosed as having carcinoma of the tongue. He has refused surgery for the lesion and has asked his own physician not to tell his wife that he has a fatal disease.

The hospital physicians believe that Mr. D. will die without surgery for the hemorrhage, and they call a psychiatric resident to evaluate the patient. Dr. M. interviews Mr. D. and finds him coherent, rational, and alert. Mr. D.

describes himself as a man who values independence. He feels he has had a good professional life as an engineer, and a good personal life with his wife and two children. He expresses some sadness at his situation, but says, "I have had a good full life and now it's over."

Dr. M. suggests, and Mr. D. does not deny, that the automobile accident was a deliberate suicide attempt. What should Dr. M. recommend? That the patient's treatment refusal for immediate surgery be accepted as the act of a rational person? That the refusal not be honored, and a court order sought on the grounds that a presumed suicide attempt is per se evidence of mental illness?

COMMENTARY

Richard B. Brandt

The prevailing law governing the requirement of consent for surgery was stated by Justice Cardozo in 1914: "Every human being of adult years and sound mind has a right to determine what shall be done with his own body; and a surgeon who performs an operation without his patient's consent commits an assault. . . . This is true except in cases of emergency, where the patient is unconscious. . . ." (*Schloendorff v. Society of New York Hospital,* 211 N.Y. 125, 129, 105 N.E. 92, 93).

There may, however, be exceptions if the patient's decision conflicts with overriding "state interests" in the preservation of life, the protection of the interests of innocent third parties, and the prevention of suicide. A refusal to accept treatment may not be suicide, since the patient himself does not set into operation a chain of causes leading to his death; but in this case the patient did (it appears) produce the injury for which surgery is contemplated. It is also unclear whether there could be a state interest in prolonging his life, in view of his disease, although another person's killing him would clearly be murder.

Further, some psychologists might claim that his sudden death in these circumstances could be psychologically damaging to his children, so there is a question about the impact on innocent third parties. Both the physician and court might wonder whether he had given careful thought to this potential damage. So it is not self-evident that a court would refuse to issue an order requiring the surgery. However, the specific question raised about this case is a limited one: whether the requirement of consent fails because the patient is not of sound mind.

In this case it would be sound legal practice, and seemingly morally unobjectionable and perhaps morally desirable, for the physician to seek a court order for surgery. The court order would provide a decision on some of these issues, and in any event it would clear the doctor and hospital of responsibility should questions arise later about failure to treat the patient.

Ought the physician/court to decide that a person's having made a suicide attempt is sufficient reason to judge him of unsound mind? Is a suicide attempt evidence of irrationality?

Let us consider some senses in which a person might show himself to be irrational:

1. If his objective is *manifestly* to *injure* himself, irrationality might be presumed (other things being equal, for example, if he is not attempting to help others by self-injury); but it is not manifestly a self-injury to attempt to shorten life in order to avoid the pain of death from tongue cancer. Evidently the present patient has decided that such action would not be self-injury.

2. A person is not rational if he fails to see the connection of means and ends, and refuses to take the means that are essential for his ends. The present patient is not in that condition; he sees precisely the consequences of his actions, and is acting so as to realize his end.

3. A person might be said to be irrational if his end is one he would not pursue if he knew, or anyway visualized clearly, what kind of thing his objective would be if realized. The patient appears not to be in this position. Tongue cancer is normally terminal, at least when not treated (it is so assumed in the description of the case), and a death from this cause is highly unpleasant to the patient and family.

4. A person might be said to be irrational if his end is one he would not pursue if he were not drunk, or seriously disoriented mentally, or in a highly emotional frame of mind. There is no evidence that the patient is in one of these conditions.

A judgment, then, that the patient is incompetent must rest on a conclusion about (1) that it is self-injury to shorten one's life in order to escape pain. It might be argued that the courts should try to prolong life no matter what. But courts have recently been more explicit in affirming what already seems to be public opinion: some treatment refusals are acceptable. (It is unlikely that any rational person would prefer to live fifteen minutes longer, in order to be burned to death, rather than shorten his life by taking a cyanide capsule, except on grounds of some moral conviction.)

Otherwise conservative philosophers such as Philippa Foot hold that life is not worth living in a situation of extreme senility or of intense pain ("Euthanasia," 6 *Philosophy and Public Affairs,* 1977, 85–112). It is true that courts have generally tried to avoid qualitative judgments of this sort. In the present case, however, the patient himself has made a qualitative judgment after careful deliberation to the effect that the kind of life that lies ahead of him, if his life is prolonged, is not what he wants. If the court declares him incompetent, it is, in effect, substituting for his view its own about what kind of life is worth living.

The moral issue might be put in broader terms: would society be better off in the long run if physicians and courts did what is in their power to do, require people to undergo a painful termination of their lives when they do not wish to and when there is no evidence of irrationality beyond the very fact that they have made a decision not to live longer? It is not easy to see what would be the gain. On the contrary, there is the loss of needless suffering by the patient, not to mention his family: and the individual is deprived of assurance that he is in control of his own destiny in matters of most importance to him and which affect others only in an incidental way.

COMMENTARY

Robert E. Litman

Dr. M., the psychiatric resident, should take action as follows:

1. He should notify Mrs. D., the patient's wife, and his children of the emergency. They should be interviewed by telephone and asked to come to the hospital;

2. Dr. M. should get in touch with a senior staff psychiatrist, preferably the chief of the service, and request an immediate consultation;

3. Dr. M. should initiate the legal process for a court order authorizing surgery.

If the patient demands his release from the hospital, the psychiatrist should be prepared to place him on a "hold" order for observation for mental disorder, because he is a danger to himself and to others. Another such suicide attempt might result in injury to a pedestrian.

Meanwhile, there should be a surgical consultation. If the surgeons find the patient's condition immediately life-threatening, then there is no time available for further persuasive efforts to obtain Mr. D.'s cooperation, nor sufficient time to obtain a court order. Given these emergency circumstances, the surgeons should proceed, trusting in the group consensus as a substitute for the consent of the patient, the family, and the court.

The hospital has an ethical and legal obligation to prevent further damage to Mr. D.'s life and health, and the patient has no ethical or moral right to demand that the emergency room doctors cooperate in his suicide efforts. By placing himself in the position of requiring emergency medical help to save his life, Mr. D. has forfeited his autonomy for the time being. In the emergency room, the doctors are properly immersed in, and bound by, the ethic of saving lives; and these physicians, together with the other emergency personnel, simply do not have the time or the training to challenge this ethic in order to make exceptions for individual cases.

This is true in general for suicide attempters, and it is true in particular for Mr. D. The scant data we have strongly suggests that Mr. D.'s recent behavior has not been rational. I would not be inclined to accept his statement, "I have had a good full life and now it's over," as a rational self-evaluation in the given context; but instead, I would suspect that the statement probably represents a delusion of hopelessness, the direct result of depressive mental illness. It is quite likely that the physicians will learn from the patient's wife that there was a noticeable change in the patient's attitude several months ago, a change possibly connected with one of life's important transitions, for example, forced retirement from his job. And his refusal to allow treatment for carcinoma of the tongue because it is a "fatal disease" is another sign of his irrational hopelessness.

Clinical experience suggests that with appropriate psychiatric treatment, including a combination of antidepressive drugs and psychotherapy, the patient will feel much more hopeful in a month.

We can expect that within a month or two, this patient will have regained his full autonomy. At that point, if he chose to commit suicide, he might still do so, choosing, I hope, a method with less potential danger to other persons. Suicide is fairly common in the United States. In California, 2 percent of all deaths are by suicide. A person who is rational and relatively unambivalent about committing suicide can usually find a decisive and effective method for ending his life. Mr. D., on the other hand, chose a suicide method that is unusual, even bizarre, suggesting a great deal of ambivalence on his part. Given this degree of ambivalence, quite typical of suicidal persons, and the excellent treatment for depression that is now available, it is reasonable to expect that the hospital personnel take appropriate action to preserve Mr. D. from further harm.

In principle, however, paternalistic action by physicians should be limited to emergencies, exceptional situations, and situations in which the use of authority is justified by the extreme difference in outcome that can be predicted from action versus inaction. For example, if a person has cut his or her wrists, and refuses remedial surgery, and the person's life is not in danger, I do not think that the surgeons are justified in immediately performing the reparative surgery on the grounds that a presumed suicide attempt is per se evidence of mental illness.

In summary, how Dr. M. should proceed depends on how acute the emergency is (i.e., how many hours will elapse before the threat to the patient's life becomes irreversible). If Dr. M. has time, he is urged to consult with the family and with other more senior psychiatrists and to use whatever time is available to persuade the patient to accept treatment, and failing this, to obtain court approval for emergency treatment. If there is no time, then doctors must proceed to remedial surgery with confidence in their own emergency room ethics. Although the patient's autonomy and self-determination is an important ethical value, Mr. D. has sacrificed his autonomy temporarily by placing himself in life-jeopardy in the emergency room, an eventuality which could reasonably have been predicted when he drove his car into a pole. If it turns out that there is no treatable mental illness, he will, at a later date, regain his autonomy and his capability of disposing of his life as he chooses.

REFUSAL OF LIFE-SUSTAINING TREATMENT AND EUTHANASIA

27

A Demand to Die

Two months after being discharged from three years of military service as a jet pilot, the world of Donald C. exploded in a flash of burning gas. He was then twenty-six years old, unmarried, and a college graduate. An athlete in high school, he loved sports and the outdoors. Rodeos were his special interest, and he performed in them with skill. Upon leaving the military in May, 1973, Donald joined his father's successful real estate business. The two of them had always had a close and warm relationship. On July 25, 1973, they were together, appraising farm land. Without realizing it, they parked their car near a large propane gas transmission line; the line was leaking. Later, when they started their automobile, the ignition of the motor set off a severe and unexpected explosion. Donald, his father, and the surrounding countryside were enveloped in fire. The father died on the way to the hospital, and Donald was admitted in a critical but conscious state. He sustained second- and third-degree burns over sixty-eight percent of his body—mostly third-degree burns. Both eyes were blinded by corneal damage, his ears were mostly destroyed, and he sustained severe burns to his face, upper extremities, body, and legs.

During the next nine months, Donald underwent repeated skin grafting, enucleation of his right eye, and amputation of the distal parts of the fingers on both hands. The left eye was surgically closed in order to protect it from the danger of infection; the cornea was badly scarred and the retina was partially detached. His hands, deformed by contractures, were useless, unsightly stubs. When admitted to the University of Texas Medical Branch Hosptials in April, 1974, the patient had many infected areas on his body and legs. He had to be bathed daily in the Hubbard tank to control infection.

From the day of the accident onward, Donald persistently stated that he did not want to live. Nonetheless, he had continued to accept treatment. Two days after admission to the University hospital, however, he refused to give permission for further corrective surgery on his hands. He became adamant in his insistence that he be allowed to leave the hospital and return home to die—a certain consequence of leaving since only daily tanking could prevent overwhelming infection. The tankings were continued despite his protests. His mother, a thoughtful and courageous woman, was frantic; his surgeons were frustrated and perplexed.

Although calm and rational most of the time, the patient had frequent periods of childlike rage, fear, and tearfulness. He engaged his mother by the hour in arguments regarding his demand to leave the hospital—which, of course, he was physically incapable of doing unless she agreed to take him home by ambulance.

At this juncture, Dr. Robert B. White was asked to see the patient as a psychiatric consultant. Prior to seeing the patient he was given the impression that Donald was irrationally depressed and probably needed to be declared mentally incompetent so that a legal guardian could be appointed to give the necessary permission for further surgery and other treatments. The patient's mother was understandably in favor of his remaining in the hospital. She was deeply concerned about her son's welfare, and the prospect of taking him home to die from pus-covered sores on his body was more than she could bear. She was a deeply religious woman and was also concerned lest her son die without re-accepting the church which he had left some time prior to his burns.

Donald was the eldest of three children. By his family's account, he was an active, assertive, and determined person, who since childhood had tended to set his own course in life. What or whom he liked, he stuck to with loyalty and persistence; what or whom he disliked, he opposed with tenacity. His mother stated, "He always wanted to do things for himself and in his own way." Dr. White soon concluded that the mother's summary was apt. In the course of the first few interviews it was apparent that Donald was a very stubborn and determined man; he was also bright, articulate, logical, and coherent—not by any criterion mentally incompetent. He summarized his position with the statement, "I do not want to go on as a blind and crippled person." Arguments that surgery could restore some degree of useful function to his hands, and perhaps some useful vision to his remaining eye, were of no avail. His determination to leave the hospital was unshakable, and he demanded to see his attorney in order to obtain his release by court order if necessary.

COMMENTARY

Robert B. White

Donald's wish seemed in great measure logical and rational; as my psychiatric duties brought me to know him well, I could not escape the thought that if I were in his position I would feel as he did. I asked two other psychiatric colleagues to see the patient, and they came to the same conclusion. *Should his demand to die be respected?* I found myself in sympathy with his wish to put an end to his pathetic plight. On the other hand, the burden on his mother would be unthinkable if he left the hospital, and none of us who were responsible for his care could bring ourselves to say, "You're discharged; go home and die."

Another question occurred to me as I watched this blind, maimed, and totally helpless man defy and baffle everyone: could his adamant stand be the only way available for him to regain his independence after such a prolonged period of helplessness and total dependence?

Consequently, I decided to assist him in the one area where he did want help—obtaining legal assistance. He obviously had the right to legal recourse, and I told him I would help him obtain it. I also told him that I and the other doctors involved could not accede immediately to his demand to leave; we could not particiate in his suicide. Furthermore, he was, I said, in no condition to leave unless his mother took him home, and that was an unfair burden to place on her. I urged him to have the surgery; then, when he was able to be up and about, he could take his own life if he wished without forcing others to arrange his death.

But Donald remained adamant, and the patient, his attorney, and I had several conferences. Finally, the attorney reluctantly agreed to represent the patient in court. The patient and I agreed that if the court ruled that he had the right to refuse further treatment, the life-sustaining daily trips to the Hubbard tank and all other life-sustaining treatment would be stopped. If he wished, he could remain in the hospital in order to be kept as free of pain as possible until he died.

Had Donald been burned a few years ago, before our increasingly exquisite medical and surgical technology became available, none of the moral, humanitarian, medical, or legal questions his case raised would have had time to occur; he would simply have died. But Donald lived, and never lost his courage or tenacity. He has imposed upon us the responsibility to explore the questions he has asked. On one occasion Donald put the matter very bluntly: "What gives a physician the right to keep alive a patient who wants to die?"

As we increase our ability to sustain life in a wrecked body we must find ways to assess the wishes of the person in that body as accurately as we assess the viability of his organs. We can no longer blindly hold to our instinctive tendency to regard death as an adversary to be defeated at any price. Nor must we accept immediately and at face value a patient's demand to be allowed to die. That demand may often be his only way to assert his will in the face of our unyielding determination to defeat death. The problem is relatively simple when brain death has occurred or when a patient refuses surgery for cancer. But what of the patient who has entered willingly on a prolonged and difficult course of treatment, and then, at the point at which he will obviously survive if the treatment is continued, decides that he does not want further treatment because he cannot tolerate the kind of future life that his injuries or illness will impose upon him?

The outcome of Donald's case does not resolve these questions but it should add to the depth of our reflections. Having won his point, having asserted his will, having thus found a way to counteract his months of total helplessness, Donald suddenly agreed to continue the treatment and to have the surgery on his hands. He remained in the hospital for five more months until medically ready to return home. In the six months since he left, Donald has regained a considerable measure of self-sufficiency. Although still blind, he will soon have surgery on his eye, and it is hoped some degree of useful vision will be restored. He feeds himself, can walk as far as half a mile, and has become an enthusiastic operator of a citizens' band radio. When I told him of my wish to publish this case report, he agreed, and stated that he had been thinking of writing a paper about his remarkable experiences.

COMMENTARY

H. Tristram Engelhardt, Jr.

This case raises a fundamental moral issue: how can one treat another person as free while still looking out for his best interests (even over his objections)? The issue is one of the bounds and legitimacy of paternalism. Paternalistic interventions are fairly commonplace in society: motorcyclists are required to wear helmets, no one may sell himself into slavery, and so forth. In such cases society chooses to intervene to maintain the moral agency of individuals so that their agency will not be terminated in death or in slavery. Society chooses in the purported best interest (i.e., to preserve the condition of self-determination itself—freedom) of the would-be reckless motorcyclist or slave. Or, in the paradigmatic case of paternalism, the choice by parents for their children is justifiable in that at a future time as adults, the children will say that their parents chose in their best interests (as opposed to the parents simply using their children for their own interests). That is, the paternalism involved in surrogate consent can be justified if the individual himself cannot choose, and one chooses in that individual's best interest so that if that person were (or is in the future) able to choose, he or she would (will) agree with the choice that has been made in his or her behalf.

Thus, one can justify treating a burned patient when first admitted even if that person protested: one might argue that the individual was not able to choose freely because of the pain and serious impact of the circumstances, and that by treating initially one gave the individual a reasonable chance to choose freely in the future. One would interpret the patient to be temporarily incompetent and have someone decide in his behalf. But once that initial time has passed, and once the patient is reasonably able to choose, should one respect a patient's request to refuse life-saving therapy even if one has good reason to believe that later the patient might change his or her mind? This is the problem that this case presents.

Yet, what are the alternatives which are morally open: (1) to compel treatment, (2) at once to cease treatment, or (3) to try to convince the patient to persist, but if the patient does not agree, then to stop therapy. Simply to compel treatment is not to acknowledge the patient as a free agent (i.e., to vitiate the concept of *consent* itself), and simply to stop therapy at once may abandon the patient to the exigencies of unjustified despair. The third alternative recognizes the two values to be preserved in this situation: the freedom of the patient and the physician's commitment to preserve the life of persons.

But in the end, individuals, when able, must be allowed to decide their own destiny, even that of death. When the patient decides that the future quality of life open to him is not worth the investment of pain and suffering to attain that future quality of life, that is a decision proper to the patient. Such is the case *even if* one had good reasons to believe that once the patient attained that future state he would be content to live; one would have unjustifiably forced an investment of pain that was not agreed to. Of course, there are no easy answers. Physicians should not abandon patients when momentarily pain overwhelms them; physicians should seek to gain consent for therapy.

But when the patient who is able to give free consent does not, the moral issue is over. A society that will allow persons to climb dangerous mountains or do daredevil stunts with cars has no consistent grounds for paternalistic intervention here. Further, unlike the case of the motorcyclist or the would-be slave, in this case one would force unchosen pain and suffering on another in the name of his best interests, but in circumstances where his best interests are far from clear. That is, even if such paternalistic intervention may be justifiable in some cases (an issue which is different from the paternalism of surrogate decisionmaking, and which I will not contest at this point), it is dubious here, for the patient's choice is not a capricious risking of the basis of free action, but a deliberate choice to avoid considerable hardship. Further, it is a uniquely intimate choice concerning the quality of life: the amount of pain which is worth suffering for a goal. Moreover, it is, unlike the would-be slave's choice, a choice which affirms freedom on a substantial point—the quality of one's life.

In short, one must be willing, as a price for recognizing the freedom of others, to live with the consequences of that freedom: some persons will make choices that they would regret were they to live longer. But humans are not only free beings, but temporal beings, and the freedom that is actual is that of the present. Competent adults should be allowed to make tragic decisions, if nowhere else, at least concerning what quality of life justifies the pain and suffering of continued living. It is not medicine's responsibility to prevent tragedies by denying freedom, for that would be the greater tragedy.

28

Family Wishes and Patient Autonomy

Ralph Watkins, a seventy-five-year-old married man, was admitted to the intensive care unit of a university hospital in acute respiratory distress. He was anxious but fully alert and gasping for help. A retired laborer, Mr. Watkins had been suffering from a chronic pulmonary disease for the past fifteen years. For the past five years he had become progressively debilitated. Prior to admission he had been confined to his home and depended on his wife for the most basic of care: without her assistance he could not dress or feed himself. He had been a fiercely independent man and still enjoyed ordering people around. His wife and married son were totally devoted to him.

The diagnosis was bilateral pneumonia, and Mr. Watkins was given antibiotics and put on a mechanical respirator with supplemental oxygen. Within two weeks the pneumonia was largely cleared and Sarah Radburn, his physician, began attempts to wean him from the respirator. Unfortunately, he had become "respirator-dependent" as a result of a combination of poor nutrition, possible new damage to his lungs, weakened respiratory muscles, and fear of breathing on his own. Despite a slow, cautious approach with much reassurance, the weaning attempts repeatedly failed. Mr. Watkins, short of breath and terrified, would demand to be placed back on the respirator.

Dr. Radburn rated the ultimate chance for successful weaning as "maybe 20 percent." The patient became more and more discouraged with his lack of progress and the frequent painful medical procedures (constant intravenous feeding, frequent needle punctures for arterial blood gases, suctioning, and so on). After three weeks of unsuccessful efforts, Mr. Watkins refused to cooperate with further attempts at weaning. His wife and son became concerned that he had given up the "will to live." They begged the medical staff to "do something to save him." Although he had become less communicative, he remained alert and aware and, in the opinion of the staff, was fully competent. He told Dr. Radburn he wanted the respirator disconnected. "I want to die," he said.

What is the physician's responsibility in this case? Should the physician honor the patient's request? If we assume the patient is legally competent to make medical decisions, on what basis, if any, can the physician refuse or postpone acting on the request to stop life support? How much weight should be given the family's wish to "save" the patient?

COMMENTARY

Stuart J. Youngner and David L. Jackson

This case illustrates the often confusing and conflicting responsibilities that confront physicians in today's modern, high-technology medical environment. To preserve life, relieve suffering, do no harm, and respect the autonomy of this alert, competent man is no simple task. If Mr. Watkins were comatose or delirious, he could be declared incompetent and the family or a court-appointed guardian would make the decision. Confronted with the realities in this case, however, one could "solve" the problem most simply by taking one of two courses—both of which, we feel, are wrong.

First, one could insist that Dr. Radburn's primary responsibility is to try for the 20 percent chance of saving his life. After all, the patient placed himself in her care, and she can dismiss his wish "to die" as irrational, although not incompetent, and press on. This course is unacceptable because it violates the patient's autonomy. It also ignores the great degree of suffering and the small chance of regaining a "meaningful" life.

Equally simplistic, and in our view unacceptable, would be to respond to his expressed wish to die by immediately disconnecting the respirator, while piously proclaiming respect for patient autonomy.

It is noteworthy that both these courses (relentlessly pursuing treatment or rigidly following the patient's request) allow the physician to avoid a time-consuming and potentially painful dialogue with the patient and family. We suggest that before the respirator is disconnected and the irrevocable decision made to let the patient die, the physician must evaluate with the patient and family the following:

1. Does the wish "to die" represent a temporary depression in reaction to pain or a sleepless night? If the depression passes or is adequately treated, the patient may well retract the wish to die. Of course, depression may be a realistic and consistent response to a situation of great suffering and little hope.

2. The patient's request may be a reaction of fear based on misperception or misinformation. Before stopping treatment the physician should identify any fears underlying a refusal of treatment and explore their source with the patient. Fear may be appropriate to many situations, and a reasonable basis for refusing treatment.

3. In similar intensive care units, we have seen several cases in which patients have exhibited true ambivalence about stopping treatment. If adequate dialogue is not established, the physician may hear only that side of the ambivalence with which he or she agrees. Acting on such half-truths is hardly honoring the principle of patient autonomy.

4. A patient's request to have treatment stopped may be a symbolic attempt to regain control in a situation in which he has none. A critically ill, machine-dependent patient has little autonomy in the most mundane and basic aspects of his life such as sleeping, elimination, eating, and privacy. He is totally at the mercy of others. The request for termination of treatment may be a desperate effort by a helpless patient to get the attention of his family and caregivers and to assert his independence. Thoughtful investigation may discover alternative measures that restore the patient's sense of autonomy and with it a revival of the wish to pursue life vigorously.

5. An apparent clash between the wishes of the family and patient may identify underlying problems of communication between them. The physician must clarify with the family the meaning of their cry "to save" the patient. Are they acting out of guilt? Can they distinguish their own needs from those of the patient? A meeting with patient and family together may be the only means of clarifying the apparent disagreement. If the issue cannot be resolved the patient must have the ultimate input to the decision-making process. The physician's contract is with him and ultimately it is his fate being decided.

The possible interventions and evaluations we have suggested will postpone acting on a patient's request to stop treatment. In doing so we could be accused of "paternalism" and violating the patient's autonomy. However, as Eric Cassell (*Hastings Center Report,* December 1977, pp. 16–19) has pointed out, a sick person is not simply a well person with an illness appended. Life-threatening illness, dependence on machines, and the ensuing physical and psychological regression make the concept of autonomy much more difficult to apply. By postponing an irreversible decision until important issues can be clarified, physicians may not be violating the true autonomy of their patients. Reflex acquiescence to patients' wishes that treatment be stopped may be a way for physicians to avoid close dialogue with fellow beings in their hour of greatest need. If the dialogue is completed and the patient's wish to die remains, there is almost always time to withdraw life supports.

COMMENTARY

William Ruddick

In order to sharpen a single issue I shall assume that the courts, the hospital's regulations, and the physicians' professional and moral principles do allow patients in such circumstances to refuse life-saving treatment. Nevertheless in this case as sketched, Dr. Radburn should first explore the conflicting requests.

Her first responsibility is to make sure that the patient's request expresses an informed, autonomous, and resolute desire to die and is not merely a show of "fierce independence."

Suppose that various inquiries convince the physician, staff, and consultants that the patient means what he says for reasons appropriate to his age, condition, character, and other circumstances. His pain is tolerable, but his increasing and irreversible debilitation and dependence are not. Even ordering people around has ceased to relieve his "burdensome" life. Despite his family's pleas, he wants to die—even if he can still be weaned from the respirator.

His wife and son want him kept alive, even if he cannot be weaned. They realize they have no legal means to prevent the physician's termination of treatment, but if the physician refuses the patient's request, they trust that he will be too weak to enlist legal aid (or to turn off his own respirator). For reasons of affection, shame, and "philosophy of life and death," they prefer his forced survival to his death by what they perceive as suicide.

These elaborations simplify the case:

1. The probability of weaning becomes irrelevant: the patient wants to die, even if weaned; his family wants him kept alive, even if respirator-dependent.

2. The direct conflict of their desires shows that the patient is not influenced by self-serving family suggestion or fear that he has become a resented burden.

3. Free of all other opposition to terminating treatment, the physician must base any refusal or further delay solely on the family's desire.

What then are the physician's professional and more general moral responsibilities? Should the family's desire, or considerations of their welfare, deter her from "honoring the patient's request"? I think not. The family is not her patient, nor the patient's proxies. Nor does his decision or welfare depend on their own. A physician often has a derivative responsibility for the welfare of family members who can provide a patient with hope, courage, nursing or financial aid, or legally required representation. But she has no such derivative professional responsibility for the family's welfare here. Indeed, to the extent that she shares her patient's belief that he would be "better off dead" or would die better now than later, she must oppose those who would forcibly continue treatment. A family's welfare does not compete with, let alone overrule, a patient's welfare in a physician's deliberations.

Though not professionally responsible *for* the family, Dr. Radburn is nonetheless responsible *to* them in at least two ways. Given their concern and past care for the patient, they are owed a thoughtful account of the decision to terminate treatment. Whether or not they are employing her, the physician must answer to them for the proposed course of action. Moreover, benevolence requires her to try to reconcile the family to her decision. If their religious principles cannot be interpreted to permit termination, she may only be able to prepare them for the patient's death. Even if the patient is being selfish in his distress, the physician should take concern for those he is (excusably?) ignoring and harming. And even if he is acting "within his rights," benevolence requires the physician to moderate the avoidable suffering produced. The demands of virtue cannot block the exercise of rights (otherwise rights would lose their force), but they can delimit the manner in which others facilitate the exercise of those rights.

In summary, the physician has two grounds for delaying, but none (as the case is elaborated) for denying the patient's request. Time is needed for: (1) making sure that the patient's request expresses a deliberate, resolute desire; and (2) trying to lessen the suffering of the family whose plea she professionally should reject but morally must respond to with compassionate attention. The first delay involves a paternalistic defense of a patient against undue influence by haste, pain, drugs, or others whose desires and welfare are not an integral part of the patient's own concerns. (This "subject paternalism" appeals to a patient's *characteristic* desires, not to his or her "best interests.") The second delay is justified by the coordination of rights with virtues that limit the manner of their exercise, especially with regard to the cooperation of the physician and the suffering of the family. Like any right to life, any right to die must be located in a context of virtues, as well as of other rights. Contrary to current slogans, people do not die alone.

29

"If I Have AIDS, Then Let Me Die Now!"

Dr. Lois Dorsey, a psychiatry resident, was paged by an intern from the Medical Intensive Care Unit (MICU) for an emergency psychiatric consultation. Gary Davidson, a twenty-eight-year-old gay man, had been hospitalized eleven days before for a first episode of *Pneumocystis carinii* pneumonia (PCP). One week earlier he had been told that the presumptive diagnosis for his illness was Acquired Immunodeficiency Syndrome (AIDS).

On the day Dr. Dorsey was called, the medical team discussed with Mr. Davidson the need for a Swann-Ganz catheter, which would be inserted in his pulmonary artery. Mr. Davidson refused permission for placement of the catheter, and requested that medical treatment be stopped. "Take the tubes away and let me die with dignity," he declared.

The medical team discussed in detail with Mr. Davidson, his lover, and his parents and sister his clinical status and prognosis; Mr. Davidson had, they believed, a 50 percent chance of surviving the current illness. However, people with AIDS rarely survive more than two years and Mr. Davidson could expect several bouts of severe illness during his remaining lifespan. They also pointed out that rapid advances were being made in understanding the pathophysiology of AIDS and offered the prospect for a future treatment as a result of current research efforts.

With the support of his lover and family, Mr. Davidson continued to insist on cessation of treatment, citing as his reasons "quality of life" and the "right to die with dignity." In the presence of witnesses he signed a living will and statement of competency. The legal formalities were carried out; however, for "legal reasons" and "completeness," before complying with the patient's request, the medical team was waiting for a psychiatric assessment.

Dr. Dorsey reviewed Mr. Davidson's records and interviewed him. Mr. Davidson reaffirmed his belief that quality of life was more important than quantity of life and that he wished to die with dignity. He admitted that he was feeling pain, fear, loss of control, extreme discomfort on the respirator, and sleeplessness. He added that he was distressed by his inability to eat (on the respirator). When Dr. Dorsey asked how he might feel should he recover from the pneumonia, the patient noted that he knew he had AIDS and that he would die within one or two years. Therefore, he said, he did not deserve to take up a bed in the hospital and continue to receive medical treatment that could better benefit another patient.

The patient had no psychiatric history and had never attempted suicide. He had never had any personal experience with death or dying among family or friends. He could not speak because of the respirator tubes but he communicated by writing notes and nodding his head. He was alert, not disoriented, wrote clearly and logically, and initiated his own statements and topics for the interview. He was not tearful but appeared anxious. In his own eyes he did not want to commit suicide but wanted to be allowed to die.

Dr. Dorsey concluded that the patient showed no evidence of confusion, psychosis, or delusional thinking, but that he did show symptoms consistent with depression, probably secondary to his underlying medical condition.

Mr. Davidson, then, was legally competent, understood the consequences of his decision to refuse treatment, and had the support of those closest to him. Yet, because of his age and depression, the availability of treatment for his current illness, and the possibility that some treatment for AIDS may become available within the next few years, Dr. Dorsey hesitated. Should Mr. Davidson's treatment be stopped as he wished?

COMMENTARY

Sophia Vinogradov and Joe E. Thornton

Dr. Dorsey's conflicting feelings summarize the essentials of the dilemma. On the one hand, her impulse is to evaluate and treat the underlying disease: on the other, she wishes to promote Mr. Davidson's autonomy and sense of control. Hence her hesitation. She agrees that a legally competent patient has the right to refuse treatment, and yet she wonders: when does the patient's right to refuse treatment encroach on the physician's responsibility to work in the patient's best interest? Or to do no harm? When does the physician have the right to impose treatment on competent patients?

Mr. Davidson was suffering from the discomfort of difficult breathing, from the pain of a respirator tube, and the effects of having been drugged and deprived of sleep for over a week—all reversible physical states. He was suffering from this extreme physical duress when his physicians sought his permission to inflict more pain by inserting a Swann-Ganz catheter.

His primary physical illness also led to secondary psychosocial effects of depression, isolation, loss of self-esteem, and altered body image–all reversible mental states. But patients may initially pass through stages of denial or despair and reject medical treatment that later they may be willing to accept. It is here, then, that the physician must seize the prerogative and help the patient adapt to his or her illness before permitting an irreversible or impulsive decision regarding treatment.

The notion of thoughtful decision making, of the reversible vs. the irreversible, of preparedness vs. impulsiveness, is the touchstone of this case. Refusal of treatment here implied cessation of life support therapy followed by immediate and certain death. Faced with a treatable illness that is imminently life-threatening, the physician must obey the injunction to "do no harm." At least in the interim while longer term strategies are being devised, she must work to support life and encourage thoughtful decision making. In the presence of reversible physical or mental states the physician has the right to impose treatment on competent patients in order to prevent irreversible decisions.

It is also possible that Mr. Davidson was being influenced by subtle external pressures. In a period of scarce resources, a vulnerable and distressed patient who is labeled as nonproductive or deviant by society may feel that he does not deserve life-sustaining medical treatment. If Dr. Dorsey recognizes those external pressures, she should resist them by imposing treatment on her initially unwilling patient.

We may appear to be saying "the ends" (life) "justify the means" (violating a person's free will). We are not. We are arguing for "informed refusal." Just as a person under physical or psychological duress cannot give informed consent, neither can a person under physical or psychological duress give informed refusal. As Dr. Randall Weingarten has pointed out to us, physicians have the right to impose treatment on competent patients when the patient is not capable of giving informed refusal.

Far from being antithetical to the right of a patient to decide his own fate, these conditions complement that prerogative. If Mr. Davidson is to make a truly informed decision regarding his illness, health, future treatment, and perhaps ultimately his death, that decision must be made under circumstances that are as free as possible from psychological and physical duress.

It is thus Dr. Dorsey's right to buy Mr. Davidson a little time, to allow him to recover from his initial sense of hopelessness and shock. Even more, she has a duty to permit Mr. Davidson to adapt to his altered circumstances, and to guide and comfort him through the fear and pain of invasive procedures and diagnostic uncertainty. Only then will he be fully free to accept or refuse treatment, free to say . . . "Let me die with dignity."

COMMENTARY

by A-J Rock Levinson

Gary Davidson is a competent, rational adult and hence cannot be subjected to invasive medical procedures without his consent. That is a basic human right and the law of the land. Dr. Dorsey has found that Mr. Davidson knows the nature of his condition(s), has been informed of his options, and is aware of the consequences of his decision. He is "alert, not disoriented, clear and logical in his thinking."

Dr. Dorsey's reasons for hesitating are good ones: Mr. Davidson is depressed, has a potential life of several months even if no new developments are discovered for reversal of AIDS, and has a fifty-fifty chance of surviving his immediate life-threatening condition. However, none of these is reason enough to impose her perception of his situation upon his own perception of that situation.

Time is the crucial element. If Mr. Davidson's death is imminent, Dr. Dorsey could declare the patient incompetent—thus setting into motion the legal process for overriding his decision or declaring him "competent" and able to refuse the procedure. But if a court declares Gary Davidson to be "incompetent," from whom would the medical team get the required consent for the procedure? Those closest to him—therefore the ones best qualified to make a substituted judgment—have already declared their support for Mr. Davidson's decision. Why would a judge be better able to make such a personal decision?

If there is time for further consultation, Dr. Dorsey should talk with the parents, sister, and lover independently to try to elicit the rationale behind what appears to be their too facile acquiescence to Gary Davidson's demand to be allowed to die. Is the family reacting to new knowledge of his homosexuality? Are they all afraid that Mr. Davidson's recovery from this crisis will create for them the burden and threat of caring for an AIDS victim? If his family and lover knew more about AIDS, the evidence about transmission, and the training and supports available to help them care for him, would they try to change his mind?

Dr. Dorsey should also explore with Mr. Davidson his own feelings of abandonment, guilt, fear, shame, loss, despair, and anger. So far, he has had only a discussion of his clinical status and prognosis and an earnest but transparent prediction that research efforts might extend his life-expectancy beyond two years. If he could be reassured of his parents', sister's, lover's, medical team's, and society's wish to have him survive—even for a short time—perhaps his assessment of his situation would be different.

If time does not permit, however, Mr. Davidson must be considered the best judge of his own situation and treatment must be stopped. To do otherwise would exemplify the ultimate in medical paternalism and could have serious legal consequences.

This case raises other, more general questions:

Why was Dr. Dorsey not asked to consult with the patient and family as soon as AIDS was diagnosed? A suicidal reaction to such information is predictable and earlier psychiatric intervention might well have prevented the crisis.

If Gary Davidson had consented to the insertion of the catheter, would there have been "legal reasons" for "competence" to be assessed? Would Dr. Dorsey have been asked to evaluate his psychological condition or was she asked to intervene solely because his decision was contrary to the medical team's evaluation of his needs? (At a time when society—and even the medical profession—is discussing the abandonment of the psychiatric defense for violent crime, it is ironic that the psychiatrist is called in when we want to "preserve" the life of someone who has made an "informed," "competent" decision to relinquish it.)

Who is Dr. Dorsey's client? Is she serving Mr. Davidson's best interest (in which case she will work with him and his family and support whatever conclusion he reaches), or is she serving the medical team who want her to provide "completeness"?

If Mr. Davidson were in his seventies, suffering from terminal cancer but facing a procedure that might (or might not) provide a few more months of life, would the medical team respond differently?

All these questions need to be thoroughly examined by any medical team assessing a situation of this kind. However, their conclusions should not affect the outcome in this or any other case. Decisions made by an informed, competent adult must be respected.

COMMENTARY

Michael L. Callen

Choosing death can, under some circumstances, clearly be a rational decision that ought to be honored. Less clear are the criteria by which an individual can be judged sufficiently competent to make such a momentous decision. The facts presented convince me that Mr. Davidson is almost certainly competent to decide to refuse life-sustaining treatments. I would argue, however, that before affirming Mr. Davidson's competence, Dr. Dorsey has an ethical obligation to test his apparent resolve.

While Mr. Davidson may truly prefer to die, it is also possible that he has taken his dramatic position to see if his lover, family, and/or friends will attempt to dissuade him. Surprisingly, neither Mr. Davidson's lover nor his parents or sister disagrees with his decision. It would be useful and appropriate for Dr. Dorsey to interview each privately to ensure that support for Mr. Davidson's decision is indeed unanimous and genuine.

Should Dr. Dorsey discover that one or more of Mr. Davidson's significant others have misgivings about this decision, she should encourage that individual to share those misgivings with him. The intent here is not to badger Mr. Davidson, but to confirm that he is committed to his position. If the individual is hesitant or unwilling to share his or her misgivings with Mr. Davidson, Dr. Dorsey might offer to discuss their concerns with Mr. Davidson in a general sense—without mentioning which of his significant others expressed misgivings. Obviously, Dr. Dorsey would have to proceed very cautiously.

Dr. Dorsey would also be justified in testing the validity of Mr. Davidson's stated altruism. Mr. Davidson's statement that he does not "deserve to take up a bed in the hospital and continue to receive medical treatment that could better benefit another patient" is worthy of more careful exploration. "Deserve" is a loaded word; many gay men who develop AIDS harbor feelings of guilt about sexual promiscuity and its obvious connection to the development of AIDS in gay men. It would be tragic if such inappropriate "guilt" were playing any role in Mr. Davidson's decision to refuse life-sustaining treatment. Dr. Dorsey could point out the erroneousness of Mr. Davidson's belief that a decision to accept treatment would mean that others would have to be denied a hospital bed or care.

However, assuming that (1) Mr. Davidson's significant others do genuinely and unanimously support his decision; or (2) doubts expessed by his segnificant others do not persuade Mr. Davidson to change his decision; and (3) Dr. Dorsey has concluded that inappropriate "guilt" and/or altruistic misconceptions are not determining Mr. Davidson's decision, then only one additional test remains.

I believe that Dr. Dorsey *herself* has a professional and, indeed, an ethical obligation to encourage Mr. Davidson to reconsider. She should begin by challenging the presumption that everyone dies from AIDS. It is more appropriate to discuss mortality rates in terms of specific opportunistic infections. Although PCP accounts for a large portion of AIDS fatalities, some individuals have survived discrete bouts of PCP and remained free of further life-threatening illnesses for a year or more. Since Mr. Davidson has expressed a preference for "quality of life" rather than "quantity," he should be informed that many who have survived these periods of illness spend whatever time they have left living life quite fully. Some travel to places they always wanted to visit; others begin or finish pet projects; some resolve differences with enemies; and most spend precious time with loved ones.

AIDS is another "closet." Realization of one's gayness can initiate confusion, anxiety, and a sense of isolation; a diagnosis of AIDS can create similar feelings. It is Dr. Dorsey's duty to alert Mr. Davidson to methods and resources for dealing with such feelngs.

There have been some innovative responses to the stigma, misinformation, and emotional upheaval that often attend a diagnosis of AIDS. Persons with AIDS in various cities have formed their own support groups and I would strongly encourage mental health care providers to investigate these unique resources.

At a minimum, Dr. Dorsey should tell Mr. Davidson that support groups exist which include people with AIDS who have experienced the crisis he is facing. It could be extremely useful if Dr. Dorsey could arrange for Mr. Davidson to meet face to face with someone with AIDS who has had PCP and *accepted* life-sustaining treatments. In this regard, plans are underway to create a toll-free number so that people with AIDS can contact others diagnosed with AIDS during periods of crisis. Attempts will be made to match those with common opportunistic diseases.

The importance of such supportive networking cannot be overstated. I have personally experienced—and witnessed in others—how this process of sharing common experiences can radically alter initial perceptions of helplessness and hopelessness.

If Mr. Davidson declines to speak with another person with AIDS who has had a similar experience or if he objects to the idea of support networking, then I believe Dr. Dorsey should sign the necessary forms. If every reasonable effort made to test Mr. Davidson's resolve has failed to change his mind, I believe that his choice of "death with dignity" should be respected.

30

"No Feeding Tubes for Me!"

Pauline Randall, a sixty-five-year-old married woman with three adult children, has been suffering from amyotrophic lateral sclerosis (ALS) for several years. Her neurological condition has deteriorated so that she can no longer control any voluntary muscles. Confined to bed in a nursing home in a small midwestern American city and breathing with the aid of a respirator, she communicates through the electronic monitor that responds to eyelid blinks. She can "write" words and brief sentences in this way.

Mrs. Randall understands that her condition cannot be treated and that it will inevitably lead to her death. But she has been an active participant in her health care and has been determined to continue functioning as long as possible.

Her physician, Dr. Samuels, believes that she is not receiving adequate nutrition and that the time has come to insert a nasogastric feeding tube. When he proposes this procedure to her, she blinks quickly, "No more!" He asks, "Do you understand that you will die slowly of starvation if we do not insert this feeding tube?" "Yes," she blinks, "No more."

When Mrs. Randall's family, which has been close and supportive throughout her illness, learns of her opposition, they have divided opinions. Her husband believes that her wishes should be respected, but two of their three children are convinced that her life should be prolonged. The nursing staff believes that she should not be made to suffer any longer.

There is no question that Mrs. Randall is legally competent, that is, that she understands the procedure being proposed and the consequences of refusal. Should her refusal of the feeding tube be honored, even though it will lead to her death?

COMMENTARY

Richard H. Nicholson

In 1860, the English poet, Arthur Clough, wrote "The Latest Decalogue," only one couplet of which is usually remembered nowadays:

> Thou shalt not kill; but needst not strive
> Officiously to keep alive.

Today those lines are often quoted in the United Kingdom as summing up a proper attitude to terminal care. Repeated used out of context, however—

starting with Bernard Shaw in "The Doctor's Dilemma"—has hidden the lines' origin in parody. Clough's poem went on:

Do not adultery commit;
Advantage rarely comes of it;
Thou shalt not steal; an idle feat,
When it's so lucrative to cheat.

Such an error is not untypical of the deceptions and misunderstandings that surround the care of patients with terminal, or inevitably fatal, illnesses. Mrs. Randall understands that her neurological deterioration will lead inevitably to death; yet one wonders whether Dr. Samuels has accepted that she is a dying patient. After all, at a slightly earlier stage of her illness, he acted in a way that would almost never happen in the United Kingdom. He started to aid her breathing with a respirator.

Since she can no longer control any voluntary muscles, such respiratory assistance, to be effective, would almost certainly be intermittent positive pressure respiration (IPPR), probably administered via tracheostomy. The normal way in which ALS patients die, when not attached to a ventilator, is by suddenly, and usually unexpectedly, stopping breathing; at autopsy it is uncommon to find any reason why death happened at that particular point. Artificial respiration is likely to prevent this mode of death, and was therefore a major intervention in Mrs. Randall's dying.

Cynics might suggest that the only reason why a patient like Mrs. Randall would not be artificially ventilated in the United Kingdom is that the National Health Service cannot afford enough ventilators. In fact for many years U.K. doctors have assessed the value of such interventions in terms of the probable quality of life as well as the probable quantity. In the 1936 House of Lords debate on the Voluntary Euthanasia (Legalisation) Bill, Lord Dawson, the royal physician recently revealed to have eased King George V's passing with morphine and cocaine, said:

> If one goes back fifty years . . . it was an accepted tradition that it was the duty of the medical man to continue the struggle for life right up to the end. With time that has changed. There has gradually crept into medical opinion, as there has crept into lay opinion, the feeling that one should make the act of dying more gentle and more peaceful even if it does involve curtailment of the length of life.
>
> When you pass . . . to lives which are burdened by incurable disease, and where the gap between that stage of illness and death becomes wider, it may be fully admitted that the difficulty is greater, yet when the patient is carrying a great load of suffering, our first thoughts should be the assuagement of pain even if it does involve the shortening of life.

Pain and comfort will in fact be important considerations in Mrs. Randall's case. Although she cannot move at all, her sensation is probably intact. Without extremely skilled and, above all, experienced nursing care she will frequently be very uncomfortable. Such experience will not be available in a small city where there is probably no more than a single case of motor neuron disease each year. Thus it will be important for her to have very regular small doses of morphine to take away the *feeling* of pain and discomfort; morphine will also take away the *feeling* of thirst or hunger.

Concern for the quality of Mrs. Randall's dying and the provision of appropriate care mean that she is most unlikely to have any sensation of hunger or thirst. Starvation therefore holds no fears for her and, with her intellect intact, she can decide to refuse the nasogastric tube. In U.K. hospices, where such appropriate care is available, it is neither the physician in charge nor the patient who raises the possibility of a nasogastric feeding tube: it is usually the intern or resident. Once the possibility has been raised it will be discussed widely among the doctors and nurses, within the family, between the doctors and the patient, and between the doctors and the family. The conclusion is nearly always that a feeding tube should not be used. This accords with the principle that a doctor is under no moral obligation to do to a patient that which is of no benefit to the patient. Many people in the U.K. would regard as a refined form of cruelty any technical intervention to prolong the life of a patient whose mind and sensation are working, but who is incapable of any voluntary action and whose ability to communicate is minimal.

In the rare event that it is not possible to reach accord among the patient, doctors, and family, the outcome may be different. In Mrs. Randall's case, she and her husband agree, and no doctor would go against their combined wishes. If only Mrs. Randall refused the feeding tube, while her husband and family wanted it inserted, the likely outcome would be whatever the doctor thought best: and that would most likely be to withhold the tube. If Mrs. Randall and her husband and family all still wanted a feeding tube inserted, then it would be inserted, regardless of the doctor's opinion.

Such a case has never been to court in the U.K. If a court were ever called on to decide, it would do so under English common law according to whatever practice a responsible body of medical opinion felt to be appropriate. In other words, if Mrs. Randall refused the tube, the court would uphold that decision, since the majority of experienced doctors in this field would not wish to feed her.

In summary, this case could never have taken the course it did if it had occurred in the U.K. Ventilator support would not have been offered, and a senior physician would not have proposed inserting a nasogastric tube. Both, in the circumstances, would have been regarded as extraordinary, rather than ordinary, means of care, therefore carrying no obligation that they be used. All efforts would be concentrated instead on ensuring that routine care kept Mrs. Randall as comfortable as possible, so that the burden of her inevitable dying was kept to a minimum for her and her family. Such care would include very careful positioning, drug treatments such as hyoscine to reduce salivation when swallowing became difficult, mouth care to prevent thrush, and attention to her bowels to avoid fecal impaction.

Why such cases can and do occur in the United States is sometimes difficult for America's transatlantic cousins to understand. Can it really be explained just in terms of a desire to avoid malpractice litigation? Or does it reflect the essential Puritanism of American society, with its tendency both to demand masochism, and to reject doctrines, such as that of ordinary and extraordinary means, which sound too catholic in origin?

COMMENTARY

Hans-Georg Koch and Tatjana Ulshoefer

In the Federal Republic of Germany (FRG), the case of Pauline Randall would raise numerous legal and ethical problems, in part because the discussion about euthanasia is burdened by historical experience. The so-called "extermination of unworthy life" during the Third Reich still affects the current debate.

In the FRG one distinguishes among three kinds of euthanasia. What is called "passive euthanasia" means the withdrawal or nonapplication of life-supporting measures. The term "indirect euthanasia" describes measures with the primary purpose of minimizing the suffering of a patient, even if this implies hastening the time of death. "Active euthanasia" means all measures that actively and deliberately induce death, such as the administration of drugs with the intention of terminating life, regardless of motive.

There is a consensus that this last kind of "euthanasia" should be punishable by law. This applies even if it is carried out in accordance with the sincere and expressed wishes of the patient. (The applicable law, section 216 of the criminal code, states that killing on demand constitutes a punishable offense.)

Another preliminary remark seems in order. The discussion about euthanasia in the FRG is largely overshadowed by the debate about suicide. Most of the euthanasia cases that have reached the courts involve patients who had previously attempted to commit suicide. The Supreme Court, in several widely criticized decisions, has stated that suicide is an ethically reprehensible action. These decisions influence the evaluation of the obligations of a physician who attends a would-be suicide. In accordance with these decisions handed down by the court, the physician is liable to be prosecuted for homicide by negligence if he encounters an unconscious would-be suicide victim in a life-threatening situation and fails to administer all required and reasonable aid.

On the other hand, assisting a person determined to commit suicide is not punishable per se, nor is it regarded as suicide if a patient, being aware of his or her situation, refuses life-preserving treatment and accepts his or her inevitable death. This can, in a particular case, lead to conflicting evaluations.

A case comparable to that of Pauline Randall's has as yet, so far as we can determine, not come before an FRG court. Nevertheless, it is generally accepted that a patient has the right to refuse even part of an envisioned course of treatment—such as a specific surgical procedure. Furthermore, in medical practice the use of respirators as well as the insertion of nasogastric feeding tubes are both considered ordinary treatment. Such a wish expressed by a patient has to be respected by the physician, even if it might threaten the life of the patient and is therefore seen by the physician as irrational.

This obligation to respect the wishes of the patient results from the constitutionally guaranteed right of self-determination as well as the right to protect oneself against physical violation. This applies even in cases where a (temporary) physical violation might be medically indicated in order to save the patient from a life-threatening illness. A surgical procedure undertaken without the consent of the patient constitutes an illegal and punishable act.

This obligation to respect the wishes of the patient, however, does not obviate the duty of the physician to counsel the patient and to recommend measures which may be medically indicated. Likewise, it does not release the physician from the duty to render medical and nursing care to the patient, as well as measures that alleviate suffering, as long as the patient so desires.

Although the problem of euthanasia has been discussed in the FRG for a considerable time, there are still no clear legal provisions governing a physician's actions when a patient's life approaches its end. In view of this legal void, various medical organizations have drawn up guidelines for physicians facing a patient's approaching death.

In 1986, an interdisciplinary working group (composed of professors of criminal law and medicine as well as their assistants) produced an "Alternative Draft Bill Concerning Euthanasia" (published by G. Thieme Verlag, Stuttgart and New York). Furthermore, the subject was discussed last year by the criminal law committee of the fifty-sixth convention of the German Lawyers Association.

Given this situation, procedures in the FRG in a case similar to that of Pauline Randall's would presently be as follows:

The case of Pauline Randall would be regarded as falling into the category of "passive euthanasia," meaning the withdrawal of life-prolonging measures. The patient is fully able to express her informed wishes. In such cases, the patient's wishes are decisive, because a physician's duty is to protect life, not to force patients to continue to live against their wishes.

The positions taken by the patient's next of kin, and even more so those of the nursing staff, are irrelevant, as long as it can be assumed that the patient has made an informed decision. Differing opinions of, for instance, the patient's spouse or children do not have to be taken into consideration.

The attending physician would have to respect Mrs. Randall's wishes even if he has arrived at a different conclusion, which he regards as "medically reasonable." He is obliged, however, to counsel the patient and to recommend the procedures he considers reasonable.

Although the physician has to respect Mrs. Randall's right to reject feeding by nasal tube, nevertheless he might continue the other elements of medical care, including all nursing care.

In a somewhat different case Peter Noll, a Swiss professor of criminal law widely known in Germany, acted similarly to Mrs. Randall. When confronted with a diagnosis of cancer of the bladder, he decided against the mutilating surgical procedure recommended by his physicians, although he had a good chance to be cured. In a diary, Professor Noll recorded his thoughts and feelings for posterity. He wrote: "The will to live should not be so strong that one passively endures all pains of life-extending measures" (Peter Noll, *Diktate über Sterben und Tod*, Zurich: Peudo Verlag, 1984).

COMMENTARY

by Ren-Zong Qiu

A case like Pauline Randall's is not rare in China, even though it is a country socially and culturally quite different from the United States. In December 1986, a session of the Beijing Colloquia on Medical Ethics (a group comprised of interested professionals in ethics, medicine, and health care adminstration that meets bimonthly to address topics in biomedical ethics) discussed three cases of pain-ridden dying cancer patients who refused to accept treatment, in addition to three other cases of patients who were irreversibly comatose.

One of these dying cancer patients committed suicide as a result of the physician's refusal to withdraw treatment. The second attempted suicide after a similar denial but failed, whereupon a physician approved his request and he died peacefully. The third is still alive; he thought about suicide after his physician refused to withdraw treatment, but he has not attempted it.

Cases of this sort occur mainly in the middle-sized or big cities and other developed areas where a number of modern hospitals are located. The situation does not occur in the 10 percent of villages where people still live in abject poverty without access to health care and even without enough food and clothing, or in other underdeveloped areas.

Public officers and medical professionals are divided on the question of whether the treatment refusal of a patient like Mrs. Randall should be accepted. A survey conducted by investigators from the Central China University of Science and Technology, the Beijing Union Medical College, the Capital Medical College, and the College of Traditional Medicine in the spring of 1986 found that among 170 respondents including laymen and professionals, 39.4 percent approved of active euthanasia for a pain-ridden dying cancer patient; 31.8 percent approved of treating her with all-out efforts; 16.5 percent advocated ordinary care and food; 10 percent wanted to withdraw all treatments and food and let her die; and 2.3 percent were undecided. So far technology for electronic communication, such as was available to Mrs. Randall, is not available in China, and generally respirators and feeding tubes are classified as extraordinary care.

Although the percentage advocating passive or active euthanasia was rather high (49.4 percent), I doubt that the advocates would definitely follow through in practice. One of my friends was terminally ill with intractable pain and refused further treatment. Both the attending physician and her two children agreed that the treatment would only prolong her suffering and death. But nobody took the move. Why? The cultural climate bound them hand and foot.

The Confucian tradition is deep-rooted in China. There are twenty-four popular models of behavior of the dutiful son from various periods in Chinese history. Some of them made every effort to save their parents' lives, and they still serve as examples of filial piety. According to the Confucian tradition, if the child agreed to the parent's refusal of treatment, he or she would be charged with violating the principle of filial piety. Even if the child did not agree, he or she has to take into account the opinions of relatives, neighbors, and colleagues who may consider such an action a violation of this principle. Gossip is a fearful thing.

Most Chinese doctors and nurses were trained in modern Western medicine (in contrast to those who practice traditional medicine); they have incorporated some Hippocratic principles into their Confucian background. The former's principle of "Do no harm" and the latter's principle of "Ren" (humaneness, loving-people, or beneficence) are fused.

Moreover, their personal experience during the Cultural Revolution made them extremely cautious about this kind of case; some physicians were condemned as murderers solely because they failed to save the lives of patients suffering form fatal diseases. No legal considerations have influenced decision making so far, because courts and lawyers have been prohibited by the government from becoming involved in such cases since the 1950s on the grounds that legal professionals do not have adequate medical knowledge to give judgment. This situation is beginning to change, however, and courts are starting to consider such issues once more.

The salary of medical professionals is fixed and independent of how many patients they treat. And they do not concern themselves with the shortage of medical resources as much as the hospital managers or health policy decision makers. However, economic factors greatly influence the family's decision. If the patient were employed by the government or the military, or worked for a university or state-owned enterprise and thus enjoyed public health services (free medical care) and had a fixed salary, the family would tend to reject the patient's refusal of treatment. The families of patients employed in private or nonstate collective enterprises who are not eligible for public health care are likely to accept the patient's suggestion.

An irreversibly comatose patient who worked in a factory where I did manual labor during the Cultural Revolution has been given all-out life-saving measures in the hospital at the insistence of his children. The hospital proposed withdrawing treatment after several months, but the children rejected the idea.

In my opinion the way out of the dilemma raised in a case like Mrs. Randall's requires a conceptual shift. Medicine should be further humanized, and man's life made more humane. If a terminally ill patient refuses treatment in order to die humanely and with dignity, nobody, including his or her children or physicians, has the right to reject the patient's wishes. Instead they ought to respect the decision. An ethics committee should review the decision to ascertain if the patient is in a terminal condition and if it is his or her real wish.

Mrs. Randall is a competent patient. She understands the procedure being proposed and the consequences of refusal. She prefers a humane death to an inhumane life. Neither her children nor physicians have the right to deprive her of that final decision.

31

Active Euthanasia with Parental Consent

Hunter C. Leake III

Andrea was a nine-year-old girl who had been diagnosed as having cystic fibrosis at the age of thirteen months. Since then she had been hospitalized twelve times, eight times during the last year.

When admitted for the last time she was already receiving an experimental antibiotic, which was being administered in an attempt to control a resistant pneumonia superimposed on severely damaged lungs, a result of her underlying disease. She was at that time a severely ill, emaciated child with moderately labored breathing. She seemed to have no interest in her environment and refused to communicate with anyone but her mother.

Because of the severity of the child's illness and because the parents had accurately perceived that the experimental antibiotic was a "last ditch" attempt to control her pulmonary infection, the physician discussed with the parents their perception of "extreme medical measure" and the significance of a "no code" order. The parents indicated that in the event of a cardiac or respiratory arrest, they did not want their child to be resuscitated and the appropriate "no code" order was written. The child was not involved in these conversations or subsequent decision making, nor had the mother previously been able to answer her daughter's questions about death and dying.

As the child's condition continued to decline, the parents asked how much longer she would live and how she would die. At one point the father said: "Watching your own child die is worse than dying yourself." This comment led to a discussion of active euthanasia utilizing intravenous potassium chloride or a similar drug. The physicians pointed out that no matter how hopeless a situation or the amount of suffering that the patient and family were enduring, the law prohibits the active taking of a patient's life. They refused to consider this option.

The following day Andrea's heart began to fail. Her condition became progressively worse, and she died approximately forty-eight hours later. During these last two days her parents were appalled by her grotesque appearance, with "eyes bulged out like a frog," and were in great despair because of her steadily deteriorating condition. They felt helpless and impotent to alleviate their daughter's distress. Medical treatment was continued to the end, and no measures were taken to hasten Andrea's death.

Approximately two months after her death, the mother was asked if she would still have given permission for active euthanasia if she had been offered that option. She replied, "Yes."

Should active euthanasia be permitted to spare the patient and family from suffering when death is inevitable?

COMMENTARY

James Rachels

Active euthanasia is illegal; is it immoral as well? The American Medical Association says that it is. In its 1977 policy statement on the physician and the dying patient, the AMA condemns mercy killing as "contrary to the most fundamental measures of human value and worth."

The case presented here might cause us to doubt that judgment. Exactly what are the "fundamental measures of human value and worth" which require that Andrea suffer a forty-eight-hour period of dying, with her eyes bulging like a frog's? Her parents saw little value or worth in that sort of death. They favored active euthanasia because they thought it better for the child. If their judgment was reasonable—if in fact those forty-eight hours did Andrea no good—then insofar as medical policy should benefit patients, it should not absolutely exclude active euthanasia.

Traditional medical ethics insists upon a sharp distinction between killing and letting die. After condemning mercy killing, the AMA statement goes on to say that allowing patients to die by ceasing treatment is in some circumstances all right. Accordingly, Andrea was allowed to die but not killed. Yet upon analysis this distinction seems to have little real importance. From the point of view of the patient, the outcome is the same no matter whether she is killed or allowed to die: either way, she ends up dead. When in particular cases there is a practical difference between the two, the difference most often is that killing involves less suffering. In this respect Andrea's case is typical.

The refusal to consider active euthanasia, while at the same time allowing death by stopping treatment, also seems to involve a kind of practical inconsistency. The inconsistency emerges when we consider *why* the physicians were willing to allow death, when they could have fought it off for a while longer. Presumably it was because they felt that prolonging Andrea's life was pointless—that she would be better off not going through the longer process of dying that would take place if they stretched things out to the bitter end. But, having made *that* judgment, why should the no-code designation be preferred over the injection? If it was pointless for her to endure, say, a four-day period of dying, why should we choose a course that requires her to endure a two-day period of dying? Active euthanasia seems more consistent with the reasoning that motivates us not to prolong life in the first place.

We are taught from childhood that the rule against killing is among the most serious moral prohibitions, just as we are taught that the special task of medicine is to protect life. It is little wonder, then, that many people find mercy killing hard to accept. However, a sound moral education also includes the instruction that letting people die is wrong: thus physicians normally do *not* let their patients die when they are sick. In this case the physicians allow Andrea to die because the usual reasons for keeping people alive do not apply. But neither do the usual reasons against killing apply. The reason why killing is wrong is that, normally, to kill someone is to destroy a life, not merely in the biological sense, but in the sense of a life as an ongoing human activity. Tragically, Andrea's life in this latter sense was already over, no matter what course of action her physicians had chosen. Moreover, the reason we applaud the physician's commitment to protect life is that protecting one's life is, normally, doing one a great service. Yet in this case it is hard to see how Andrea is served by the refusal to end her life forty-eight hours earlier. On the contrary, it seems to be the parents and not the physicians who represented *her* interests at the end.

The one feature of this case that makes active euthanasia problematic is that the patient herself does not request it. If Andrea were three years old the requirement of consent would not be appropriate; if she were twenty-three, the lack of consent would be enough to stop all discussion. The fact that she is nine makes things more complicated. Children of that age are capable of understanding what it means to die, and it is unfortunate that Andrea's mother had been unable to cope with her daughter's questions. Children old enough to understand should have such situations explained to them, if only because they will figure out what is going on anyway and will need the comfort that calm and sympathetic discussion might bring. But leaving aside the earlier failure of communication, it is a different issue whether now, when death is imminent, Andrea should be asked whether she prefers an injection. My own judgment is that it would not be wise. Nothing would be gained by putting such a question to her, and it might very well make her dying all the more miserable. The consent of her parents, who obviously love her and want what is best for her, is enough. If this is doubted, it might help to ask why we are willing to issue a no-code order without first securing her consent. If one is permissible, why not the other?

COMMENTARY

Philippa Foot

In the description of this case it is assumed, quite reasonably, that it was right to allow the patient to die rather than to start resuscitation procedures when her heart began to fail. But given the hopelessness of her condition, Andrea's parents would, it appears, have chosen that measures be taken to kill the child at an earlier time. Legally it was impossible for the doctors to give a lethal injection: would it also have been morally wrong?

The decision depends on the answer to two questions. In the first place, is it morally relevant to distinguish "active" from "passive" euthanasia? Some moral philosophers argue that if it was morally unobjectionable to allow her to die then it must have been similarly unobjectionable to do what the parents desired, since the difference between active and passive—between allowing an independently established sequence to run its course and initiating a new sequence—never affects the morality of what is done. Thus, if Andrea could be allowed to die of the diseases that were slowly killing her, her death could also have been induced earlier by an injection of potassium chloride or some similar drug.

My own view is that this is a serious error. If one may, in particular circumstances, allow a man to die it does not *follow* that one may also kill him, even for his own good. Sometimes, no doubt, where passive euthanasia is justifiable so is the active form, and I do not know what would be meant by saying here that nevertheless one was "better" or "worse" than the other. It is not, however, always true that the difference between active and passive (so understood) is morally irrelevant. Sometimes it is morally permissible to allow someone to die when it would not be permissible to give him a lethal injection.

When is this distinction morally relevant? Most obviously it is in cases in which rights are in question, and this is because a man's right to noninterference usually extends farther than his right to be cared for. His rights may block our interference in his life; but if we may not intervene to bring a certain result, it does not follow that we may not allow it to come about. We could not, for example, deprive a man of his property, even for his own good, in many cases in which we would have no obligation to prevent it from blowing away. This conclusion is confirmed by the fact that permission may make all the difference in such a case. The distinction between active and passive is no longer relevant when someone is able to grant us the right to intervene in his life, or at least not directly relevant as it was before. Thinking only of the morality of the individual action, and so leaving aside such questions as that of the abuse of a practice, one might reasonably say that if someone gives us the right to kill him, for his own good, by seriously consenting to the action, it then makes no moral difference whether we do kill him or rather allow him to die.

That there is a morally relevant difference between active and passive euthanasia seems clear enough when one thinks about the crucial question of rights; and those who deny it seem simply to have misunderstood the position of their opponents. It is, however, hard to know what to say about the treatment of the patient whom we have been asked to discuss, because a second controversial question arises at this point. The case of Andrea and others like her is problematic because she was too young to be able to give valid consent to the measure that would have killed her, and so to give us the right to do what in general we have no right to do without consent. What should we think about active euthanasia in relation to children and mentally incompetent adults?

Should we say, for instance, that machinery might be set up by which guardians (though hardly parents alone) could be held to speak for the patient and to grant on his behalf the permission that a "competent" adult cold give us himself? One might believe that although no competent adult could justifiably be the subject of active euthanasia unless he himself had consented to it, others could consent for children and for mentally incompetent adults, or at least for those adults who had never been able to give valid consent. I believe that there would be no decisive objection on grounds of moral principle if it were not for the problem of the possibility of abuse. But in practice there seems to be grave danger that children and noncompetent adults would be "spoken for" by people who were really speaking for relatives, for the medical staff, or for "society," rather than for those whose rights they were supposed to guard.

The reality of the danger is, I think, vividly illustrated by the presentation of Andrea's case. First, very little is said about the one absolutely crucial factor in the situation, namely her state of consciousness and suffering. Second, the possibility is mentioned of giving the injection "to spare the patient and family from suffering" as if the suffering of others was as relevant as that of the patient. And third, much is made of the pain caused to the parents by the alteration to the point of grotesqueness in their daughter's appearance.

Now I do not for a moment want to deny that there may be cases of terrible suffering that can be ended only by death; though the subject of uncontrollable pain is, of course, one on which doctors disagree. Were we sure that active euthanasia would be practiced only where death was clearly much to be desired *for the sake of the patient,* then it could be right to allow it, even for those who had not themselves been able to give consent. But it would be quite another matter to kill such patients for the good of others, labeling it (improperly) euthanasia, and opening the way to programs such as the one instituted by Hilter before he undertook the extermination of the Jews. (See my article, "Euthanasia," *Philosophy and Public Affairs,* Winter 1977.) I am not, of course, suggesting that if Andrea had been treated as the parents wanted it would have been a case of this kind; only that the presentation of the case blurs just the distinction that should be emphasized. Moreover, there is something superficial about the thought that weighs the parents' distress at their daughter's appearance in this particular balance. For all the misery of this part of their experience it is not something to be grieved over like the loss of the child or her pain. Nor should we be impressed when we are told, as we sometimes are, that a man is treated in a "dehumanizing" way if he is allowed to become grotesque in appearance before he dies. Death is not normally pretty, and it will be no gain if ugliness in death comes to seem to us intolerable. Would Andrea's parents really have been better able to live with the grief of losing her if they thought that they had ordered the lethal injection partly to spare themselves the pain of seeing her as she would become?

It may be thought that in mentioning such matters, and not thinking only of the case or active euthanasia to put an end to a patient's suffering, I am evading the main issue. This is not true. For when we are considering a practical measure such as the permitting of active euthanasia it is a very important fact that we are apt to think about it in a confused and superficial way. This is one reason why there is so much danger in supporting any kind of active euthanasia, never mind its extension to children and noncompetent adults.

32

When the Doctor Gives a Deadly Dose

At age seventy, Mrs. R. had become severely disabled by cardiac failure due to a damaged mitral valve. With her full and appropriate consent, she underwent a risky valve replacement, which initially went fairly well. However,

within twelve hours after surgery, her cardiac output was clearly inadequate. Despite intensive care in the ICU, an adequate blood flow could not be sustained and an experimental cardiac assist device was implanted in her chest. Again, initially she seemed to improve as she was finally "waking up," though she remained moderately unresponsive. A few hours later, however, even with the assist device, her cardiac output again began to fail. No treatment arrested this downward spiral; everyone involved agreed that she would not survive. In addition to the cardiac assist device, Mrs. R. was on a respirator and had seven different tubes going into her body for fluids, medications, and monitoring.

Her surgeon, Dr. L., had remained in the hospital throughout the twenty-four hours since surgery. He talked with the family frequently and encouraged them to discuss their concerns, to visit the patient, and to call in other family members and their pastor.

Since Mrs. R. was vaguely aware and seemed quite uncomfortable, with her family's knowledge she was given morphine. Dr. L. turned off the cardiac assist device and stopped the medications regulating her blood pressure. Since she still seemed uncomfortable, jerking at intervals and furrowing her brow, Dr. L., gave her another dose of morphine. When that had no discernable effect, he asked a nurse to draw up 10 cc of potassium chloride. Then, within sight of most of the ICU staff, he injected it into Mrs. R.'s intravenous line.

Within minutes, she lay still and the cardiac monitor showed no heartbeat. Dr. L. turned off the respirator and went to tell the family that Mrs. R. was dead. The ICU nurses and house staff were very concerned. Had Dr. L. behaved appropriately? What should happen now?

COMMENTARY

Howard Caplan

Dr. L.'s actions in this case are tantamount to euthanasia and therefore illegal. Nevertheless, my opinion is that Dr. L. did nothing morally wrong. He had attempted all reasonable interventions to save Mrs. R.'s life, but not with the purpose that she should experience misery in an intensive care unit for the remaining days of her life. It is most probable that he performed surgery on Mrs. R. with the hope and goal that it provide a resumption of the life she enjoyed prior to cardiac failure. Upon determining that the outcome of the operation was poor, and that further interventions were turning futile and useless, Dr. L. did the humane thing. He provided a quick, painless death, a good death, which is what "euthanasia" really means.

This conflict between law and morality indicates that there ought to be a law permitting mercy killing in appropriate cases, and this case would certainly fall under that category. It is true that the Oath of Hippocrates demands that no doctor ever administer a lethal drug. However, the advances of modern technology require a modification of this principle; reliance on medical technology has brought much pointless suffering to people whose lives can be sustained only with much concomitant suffering. The general principle to guide decisionmakers ought to be that if there is no hope that medical intervention will restore the patient to comfort, then euthanasia should be available as a choice.

Who should make this choice? We should strongly encourage people to spend some time considering what they would want done should they ever be confronted by circumstances prognostically similar to Mrs. R.'s. Certainly, middle age is not too early to develop a personal philosophy about life and death, and to assess how much life-extending technological intervention is desirable in situations of terminal illness.

The psychological defense mechanism of denial prevents many people from thinking about such matters. Yet human beings are the only creatures on Earth who know they are destined to die. If we refuse to contemplate our eventual death, when illness or old age herald the impending end, we may find ourselves in an intensive care unit, sustained by a variety of life-support systems that do nothing to enhance the quality of our lives.

Dr. L. should be left alone. If any witness to the "crime" is inclined to notify the district attorney, the public will be inundated yet again by journalists, waxing pontifical regarding the ethics of mercy killing, the time-honored sanctity of life principle, and the arrogance of doctors who "play God." If there are people who work in intensive care units who have not yet accepted the inevitability of death, and especially the desirability of death as a means to end pointless suffering, they should find new work in some other area of medicine. My conjecture is that a national referendum on euthanasia would result in the passage of a humane law, offering hopelessly ill patients and their families the right to choose a good death, rather than having no alternative but to experience a bad death.

COMMENTARY

Nancy Dickey

Attending to a dying patient and interacting with the family are always emotionally difficult. Compassion and mental vigilance exhaust physicians both mentally and physically. However, succumbing to the pressures of the moment by "helping" a patient over the final hurdle is neither ethically justifiable nor legally acceptable. The current opinions of the Council on Ethical and Judicial Affairs of the American Medical Association clearly state that a physician may alleviate pain and cease or omit treatment but *should not intentionally cause death.*

Dr. L.'s behavior may be viewed as homicide. Whatever his justification, his behavior is unacceptable by legal, social, and ethical standards. Ethics may at times require one to attain a higher standard than that required by law, but ethical standards should not be lower than legal ones.

Despite recent changes in social perception, the law continues to view Dr. L.'s behavior as homicide. Though the penalties exacted for such behavior have been minimal, the action of taking someone's life, even in the name of mercy, has not been legally sanctioned. Physicians do not have the legal right to actively end someone's life.

Moreover, citizens who know that a crime has been committed have an obligation to report that information. Thus, the health care professionals in attendance with Dr. L. have an obligation to report his action—both to hospital personnel for evaluation and action by the medical community, and to the police for civil action. Dr. L. would then be subject to the legal process of evaluation and to peer review of his behavior.

Some people would argue that there is no difference between allowing an illness to take its course and not instituting all means of treatment versus actively intervening to speed the time of death. I believe that we must maintain our vigilance and carefully safeguard the very fine line that does separate those two notions. We must not allow ourselves to become deities who decide that a particular quality of life is not worth maintaining, that the disease process is too slow or tedious, and that therefore we shall omnisciently choose the moment of death. When treatment no longer benefits the patient, there is no ethical obligation to continue it. When there is little possibility for extending life under humane and comfortable conditions, a physician may permit a terminally ill patient to die. He may allow a relentless course of an illness to proceed to death, but taking a giant step beyond that and *choosing* the moment of death by active intervention is unacceptable.

The physician is regarded by society and individual patients as a fiduciary, a trusted advisor whose duty it is to safeguard the well-being of the patient. Withdrawing technological support and allowing a disease process to proceed to death must be done with great care. To allow a physician to become an executioner, justified by whatever eloquent references to quality of life and patients' rights, would place at risk the role of the healer and the trust of the society in the guardians of health. At no point has medicine, the profession, or its organizations, spoken in favor of euthanasia or intentionally causing death in the form of mercy killing by any name, nor should we now.

Many mechanisms have come into use in the last decade to aid physicians in making these very difficult decisions. Ethics committees and rigorous Do-Not-Resuscitate protocols have been developed in an effort to safeguard the decisionmaking process from capricious or premature decisions. However, the process is that only—a process. If a physician chooses not to follow it, it cannot benefit either the patient or the physician. More widespread knowledge about such processes and increasing opportunities to utilize these mechanisms should enhance their effectiveness for the profession and the public.

One response to Dr. L.'s behavior would be to report it as a crime. However, I believe that our response should be to educate doctors regarding the ethical nuances of limited treatment versus active euthanasia. This could be done through the peer review mechanism, the hospital executive committee, or the ethics committee.

Desite all of the movment toward death with dignity and rights of patients to terminate treatment, life should be cherished—despite disabilities and handicaps. The uncertainties of medicine should be considered and unless it is clearly established that the patient is terminally ill or permanently comatose, a physician should not be deterred from appropriately treating the patient.

In "making . . . decisions for the treatment of . . . persons who are severely deteriorated victims of injury [or] illness, the primary consideration should be what is best for the individual patient. . . . Quality of life is a factor to be considered."

Statements, currently expressed or previously formulated by the patient, regarding his or her treatment preferences should prevail in treatment decisions. Finally, the compassionate physician, while carrying out the treatment (or nontreatment) plan, should respect the comfort and dignity of the patient. Physicians should be advocates and advisors to their patients, not executioners.

COMMENTARY

Joanne Lynn

This is a very troubling case. Dr. L. has clearly erred. Mrs. R. could have been comforted in ways that are conventional and widely accepted, such as giving more morphine. To use a dose of potassium that will paralyze the heart seems more like giving a poison than giving a pain reliever. It thus seems reasonable to construe his action as being within the statutory definition of homicide. Yet prosecuting Dr. L. for homicide would probably lead to no good for anyone and might make it more difficult to provide justifiable and conventionally acceptable symptom relief in other cases. The wrong in itself does not warrant the penalty that would attach, yet it needs to be condemned so that it will not be repeated.

What should happen? First, Dr. L. should be offered the opportunity for careful consideration, reflection, and counseling. He has been working for too long and was probably too involved in the case, perhaps even too sympathetic to Mrs R.'s plight. He may well be quite resistant to recognizing that others may view his behavior in a negative light and should be granted some time, perhaps a few days, in which to examine his own action and to decide how to make amends.

Second, the family should be supported, as they always should be, through this time of crisis. There should be no deception in the first few days after death, but the exact circumstances should probably be spelled out in a conference with the family a few weeks later. The nurses and others who were witnesses should be asked to write down their observations immediately and the medical record should be carefully guarded against loss or alteration.

The institution's responsible parties should also be involved. These include the chief administrator, attorney, and ethics committee or consultants. All parties should have recurrent discussions over several days.

If all involved, including the family, are satisfied that nothing warrants referral to a criminal prosecutor and if the experience has led to apologies and revised policies that make it clear that this action has not been condoned, then I believe the issue need never be referred to the prosecutor, or even to those who regulate medical licensure in the state. The potassium injection is, to my mind, "over the line" that demarcates acceptable professional behavior; but it is so close to that line that I am loathe to encourage testing its locus and support.

But if anyone involved feels otherwise, or if those responsible for ensuring quality care in the institution feel that there are substantial possibilities of recurrence, the case should be referred to the criminal prosecutor and to the licensure authorities. Most likely, this referral would lead to a dismissal of charges or to acquittal at trial, as the cause of death will be so difficult to prove. However, the experience of a criminal charge and investigation will certainly serve to chasten those who might think of injecting potassium in their patients. Even a conviction might be good for the profession, though devastating for Dr. L.

Granted, there is little analytic difference between giving potassium or morphine in this setting. But there is a strong perceived difference, based largely upon history and the convenience of mixed motives in using morphine. That perceived difference is very important in defending a reasonable range of options for practitioners who are attempting to relieve the symptoms of dying patients. The backlash from prosecuting Dr. L. could well increase physicians' reluctance to provide adequate symptom relief, for fear that deaths accelerated in this way, which already fit within the bare language of homicide statutes, may be construed as homicide.

If this case goes to public investigation, there is probably strong reason for responsible practitioners to step forward to defend other justified and ordinarily accepted trade-offs that can be achieved between the length of a life and the attributes of that life. They would need to proffer examples of good behavior, to help to differentiate it from Dr. L.'s behavior. They would also need to instruct the public that, although wrong, Dr. L.'s behavior should not be penalized severely under criminal law. This sort of case is certain to arise from time to time and is essential in allowing society and the medical and nursing professions to define the bounds of good practice. While Dr. L. will have to bear the weight of the censure, his burden should be lightened by those of us whose range of acceptable behaviors is made more certain and more protected by his being censured.

Selected Bibliography

Part III: Death and Dying

Battin, M. Pabst, and Mayo, David J., eds. *Suicide: The Philosophical Issues.* New York: St. Martin's Press, 1980.

Beauchamp, Tom L., and Perlin, Seymour, eds. *Ethical Issues in Death and Dying.* Englewood Cliffs, NJ: Prentice-Hall, 1977.

The Hastings Center, *Guidelines on the Termination of Life-Sustaining Treatment and the Care of the Dying.* Bloomington: Indiana University Press, 1988.

Horan, Dennis J., and Mall, David, eds. *Death, Dying and Euthanasia.* Washington, DC: University Publications of America, 1980.

Kuhse, Helga, and Singer, Peter. *Should the Baby Live? The Problems of Handicapped Infants.* New York: Oxford University Press, 1985.

Lynn, Joanne, ed. *By No Extraordinary Means: The Choice to Forgo Life-Sustaining Food and Water.* Bloomington: Indiana University Press, 1986.

Murray, Thomas H., and Caplan, Arthur L., eds. *Which Babies Shall Live? Humanistic Dimensions of the Care of Imperiled Newborns.* Clifton, NJ: Humana Press, 1985.

Perlin, Seymour. *A Handbook for the Study of Suicide.* New York: Oxford University Press, 1975.

President's Commission for the Study of Ethical Problems in Medicine and Biomedical and Behavioral Research. *Deciding to Forego Life-Sustaining Treatment.* Washington, DC: U.S. Government Printing Office, 1983.

Rachels, James. *The End of Life: Euthanasia and Morality.* New York: Oxford University Press, 1986.

Ramsey, Paul. *Ethics at the Edge of Life.* New Haven: Yale University Press, 1978.

Shelp, Earl. *Born to Die: Deciding the Fate of Critically Ill Newborns.* New York: Free Press, 1986.

PART FOUR

Research with Living Subjects

INTRODUCTION

The cases in the three previous parts have focused on medical therapy, and the ethical dilemmas that arise in the context of a doctor-patient relationship, choices about reproduction, and decisions about death. In Part Four a new element enters the picture: Research involving human or animal subjects is an activity that is not carried out primarily for the benefit of the subject (although that may indeed be a result) but for the benefit of society. Research is the pursuit of knowledge that will be generalizable to other members of society, such as patients suffering from the same disease as the subject, or other scientists involved in the same general field, or the public in general.

For this reason the basic ethical principles governing research have stressed that the subject must volunteer for the study and not be coerced, that he or she must give informed consent to participation, and that the subjects must be selected equitably so that no individual or group unfairly bears the burdens (or reaps the benefits) of research.

The cases in the first section—"Consent to Research"—examine the complex questions that occur when trying to determine what constitutes *informed consent.* They cover such issues as parents' right to consent to a study of their teenage children's sexual activities, the possibility of a mentally ill patient giving consent while competent for research that he would refuse while incompetent, and the cultural and value differences between the concept of consent in the West and in the developing world.

The second section—"Selection of Subjects and Protection of Their Welfare"—illustrates the conflicts that arise between a subject's interest in obtaining optimal therapy and a researcher's interest in completing a statistically valid trial, in determining voluntariness, and in assuring confidentiality of the subject's identity. Can, for instance, a person who volunteered for an experimental bone marrow transplant program be contacted by a desperately ill person who wants her to serve as a donor for him? Can a healthy subject volunteer to be injured in research that will not benefit him but may provide knowledge about his wife's condition?

While most concern about the use of subjects in research has centered around human participation, the use of animals as research subjects has become a highly controversial area. Can animals—who can neither volunteer nor consent—be used ethically in research to benefit human beings? The case study in this section about the use of chimpanzees, an endangered species, as heart donors in transplant experimentation raises this issue in a pointed way.

Research is a highly regulated activity, with many levels of ethical and scientific review. The abuses that were prevalent as recently as thirty years ago have clearly diminished. Yet the absence of flagrant violation of human rights only highlights the much more nuanced problems that remain.

33

Studying Grief Without Consent

Linda M. Rhodes

John Clark, a graduate student at a major university, wanted to research the emotional needs of families who had a dying relative. He decided that the best way to conduct this research was to work as a participant-observer in a hospital. He already had training and experience as a counselor, and he added to his qualifications by taking a course to become a nursing assistant.

A small community hospital interested in family care allowed him to volunteer for ten hours a week as a nursing assistant and counselor. The hospital had never conducted medical research before, and had no committee for the protection of human subjects. In fact, none was required by state or federal law at that time. Clark informed the administration and staff of his research intentions and received their approval for his work.

Working in the intensive care unit and the emergency room, Clark gave basic care, took vital signs, and assisted the nurses. When a critical care patient was admitted to the unit, he was assigned to work with the family. He provided counseling, helped them deal with the hospital administration, acted as an information liaison between staff and family during nonvisiting hours, and stayed with the family when they were told of the death.

Following each death, he wrote a case history and maintained a check list of common grief reactions. He showed these reports to no one. After a period of three months, he wrote a paper reporting his findings. From this study, the staff developed a course to teach nurses how to deal with the critical care patient's family.

The families Clark counseled were told only that he was a nursing assistant and counselor working with the hospital to give special attention to their needs. They responded very positively to the services that he provided. They were not told that a research project was being conducted or that a study would be written.

Clark later decided to use his study as a central part of his doctoral dissertation, and to extend his research where necessary. The university at which he was enrolled had an active research review committee for the protection of human subjects, which was required to examine all research conducted under its auspices.

Should Clark and the hospital have obtained the consent of the families to participate in the research even though it was not legally required? Should the chairman of Clark's department now send the research study to the university's review committee? If so, what should the committee recommend?

COMMENTARY

Michael Jellinek

I find it difficult to apply the current sophisticated and sensitive guidelines on human experimentation to studies done years ago, in small hospitals, reviewed by administration and staff, and integrated into a program of therapeutic and humane care; therefore I do not believe it was necessary for Clark to obtain the consent of the families he studied. However, present standards clearly define Clark's work as research. He is planning, prospectively, to collect data using systematic methodology as part of a doctoral thesis. If further research is planned that includes patients or their family as subjects, then the departmental chairman has an obligation to send the proposal to the university research ethics committee.

Within a traditional view of medical ethics, Clark by definition is not exclusively oriented to the clinical needs of his subjects. The nature of the clinical interview and Clark's empathetic response may be significantly influenced by the demands of his research design. Further, the patient must give the physician permission to discuss the nature of the illness with the family. Only in unusual circumstances dictated by clinical necessity or urgency should the physician disclose information to the family without the patient's consent. Beyond consent requirements, the university committee will have to review the study's methodology to determine if the risk to the family members' psychological well-being (for example, a structured interview meant to test the subject's defenses) is worth the potential gain in knowledge about the grieving process. Mr. Clark will be discussing very sensitive material with his subjects and therefore the committee will have to be sure that their confidentiality will be protected.

Within a contractual perspective, Clark has an obligation to respect the autonomous functioning of the patient and the family. The committee must assure that both have the opportunity to exercise free will. Without consent patients and subjects may well wonder why they are receiving special attention or additional services. If they discovered a covert research project was the basis for these additional services rather than Clark's or the hospital's therapeutic concerns, they may well feel angry, hurt, and devalued. I would also ask the committee to consider whether the therapeutic counseling service should not be offered even if a research subject declines to participate.

If Clark's goal was to report retrospectively some of his experiences, assuring confidentiality, and in an experiential rather than systematic manner, then conceptually his work could not be distinguished from those physicians whose recognition of patterns of disease has served as the basis for modern clinical care and research. It is virtually impossible to burden physicians who retrospectively organize clinical impressions with consent requirements. If Clark reviewed computerized hospital records and maintained confidentiality, then again consent would not be necessary. Further I do not want to stifle physicians' curiosity and creativity within the context of optimum patient care, and therefore have them ponder every new question or marginal laboratory test to see if it conforms rigidly to common practice and, if not, requires research level consent.

The only certain assurance that research will not result in a loss of trust between physician and patient is the integrity of the investigator. I would ask the committee to review Clark's past work and the departmental chairman's recommendation. Given the area of research, the committee's risk/benefit review of the proposal, and the likelihood that Clark is sincere, I believe that a brief oral consent from both patients and subjects would be appropriate to the clinical setting of the seriously ill individual and anxious family. Clark should submit a written form of a proposed oral consent, and should use the approved consent early in the interview.

COMMENTARY

Ruth Macklin

Few moral rules are without exceptions. The widely accepted principle requiring those engaged in research or therapy to gain informed consent from subjects or patients rests on fundamental ethical precepts: respect for the privacy of individuals; protection of confidentiality in settings where privileged information may be divulged; and preventing harm from befalling innocent persons.

Does this case violate the moral imperative that people should be treated as ends in themselves, never solely as means? I shall argue that it does not. Should Clark and the hospital have obtained consent from the families even though it was not legally required? No, provided that all appropriate steps were taken to protect the identity of those whose case histories were written up and whose grief reactions were recorded.

As unpopular as this conclusion may seem to those who zealously defend the need to gain informed consent for every activity that might properly be termed "research," I think both common-sense morality and leading principles of ethics can support such a conclusion.

First, consider what the families whom Clark studied were told. It is true that he was a qualified nursing assistant. It is also true that he was a trained counselor working with the hospital to give special attention to the families' needs. What they were *not* told is that in the course of providing his services, Clark was writing up their case histories as part of a research study.

Does this act of withholding information amount to a form of deception? Arguments could be offered in support of either a "yes" or a "no" answer. It is surely true that an important piece of information about the nature of Clark's overall activity was intentionally omitted. On this count, it could be argued that the activity was deceptive. On the other hand, nothing in the description of Clark's behavior suggests that he intended to mislead these families in some way crucial for getting significant results. Unlike the myriad examples of social science research in which subjects are deliberately lied to or manipulated in ways the researcher deems necessary for obtaining his results, this case embodies the blandest form of deception—if it can properly be described as deception at all.

But let us grant, for the sake of argument, that an element of deception *is* present when a portion of the facts is withheld. Does this automatically make an activity morally wrong? Only the most rigid adherents of the rule "Don't deceive" would say "yes" to this general question. Clearly, these families were not being treated *solely* as means to another's end. Clark counseled them, helped them deal with the hospital administration, stayed with the family when they were told of the death—all actions that signify treating persons with dignity and respect.

Suppose Clark *had* sought to gain consent for his study from these grief-stricken family members. Is it likely that consent would be both fully voluntary and rationally informed? Probably not, given our knowledge of human behavior in time of grief. Some families might have granted consent but it is questionable whether any consent gained under such trying circumstances could meet the test of being freely and rationally given. Some families might have refused consent, possibly lessening their chances of receiving the services Clark was so ably providing.

Clark's failure to obtain consent from these families would amount to a violation of moral principle only if the identity of the individuals were not kept confidential. Recording common grief reactions and reporting anonymous case histories is no more a violation of moral precepts, when confidentiality is preserved, than writing a piece of fiction based on real-life incidents where the names and places are changed to protect the innocent. The families were helped—not harmed—by Clark's services. It appears incidental, from a moral perspective, that he was conducting a study in the course of his counseling and other helping activities. Had he manipulated these families, or treated some differently from others in order to observe varying reponses to his own actions, it would have been a different story—an experiment in social psychology requiring consent of the subjects. But none of these families was used as an "experimental control." Current concerns over the protection of human subjects of research may have swung the pendulum too far in inducing the belief that every activity labeled "research" morally requires the consent of those studied.

These conclusions notwithstanding, the chairman of Clark's department should send the research study to the university's review committee. This would not only be expedient, but also an honest way to proceed. The committee in turn should recommend that the previous studies be accepted. Finally, the extension of Clark's research should be approved so long as it succeeds in meeting the morally necessary conditions: that the identity of the subjects be kept strictly confidential; that no manipulation or deliberate lying take place; and that these suffering families continue to be treated as ends in themselves, never solely as means to a researcher's ends.

34

Parental Consent and a Teenage Sex Survey

E. James Lieberman

A research team has designed a project; one essential element is a prospective study of adolescent sexuality. The study will gather information about the transition from sexual innocence to experience among teenagers by surveying sixteen- and seventeen-year-olds. According to other research, a large number of young people of this age are sexually inexperienced or somewhat experienced. The data collected will be recorded by an identification system that will maintain the subject's privacy. The information from the survey is expected to give doctors, teachers, parents, and counselors a better understanding of adolescent sexuality and to provide a sound basis for designing sex education programs and clinical services for teenagers.

The research team is faced with a serious dilemma in seeking consent. While they plan to seek consent from the young people being surveyed, they cannot decide whether to seek parental consent as well. Previous attempts to conduct such surveys have foundered on this issue. One study in which a great many parents of a randomly chosen pool of teenagers failed to give consent was criticized for being unrepresentative. Furthermore, since adolescents do not need parental permission for sex-related medical care, why should it be sought for a survey? On the other hand, this is a sensitive issue between parents and their adolescent children as well as in the communities where the surveys will be done. What should the research team decide?

COMMENTARY

Donald Richard Nilson

The research team has decided to seek the consent of participants in this well-designed prospective study because they will record and maintain information by personal identifiers until the data-collection phase of this project ends. Consent is necessary to protect the subjects from harm that might arise through the unauthorized distribution and use of these self-reports.

The teenagers who have personally consented to be subjects in this survey (and others) should be allowed to participate without interference, in particular, *without* the consent of their parents or legal guardians. Support for this judgment arises from at least two sources: one *social* in character–the free acquisition of information pertaining to social issues; the other essentially *individual-centered*—the research subjects' right to self-determination, privacy, and free expression.

Intelligent social action presupposes positive knowledge about society and the role of the individual. Seriously facing and realistically attempting to solve societal problems requires that carefully acquired, reliable information concerning the causes and conditions surrounding these problems be available to policy- and law-makers, educators, counselors, and so on. Wherever possible, the social scientist (acting on behalf of society) must be free to conduct research without interference, except where supervening or overriding interests are at stake. Any measures which interfere with the process of acquiring data, or for that matter other phases of such experiments, are *prima facie* unacceptable and should be resisted by the scientist, if necessary, through social-legal action, unless the measures can be shown to be necessary for the protection of the subject.

Studies of adolescent sexual experiences have shown excellent response rates and no evident adverse effects when minors were allowed to participate without parental consent. When parental consent is sought, response rates fall to an unacceptable level.

Minimal changes in behavior (about 2 percent of participants report direct effects) can be attributed to participation in surveys on human sexuality, and the benefits resulting from greater reflection and increased knowledge clearly outweigh any potential damages. The collective significance of these empirical studies is that potential negative effects on subjects arising from their participation in the type of study described in the case are minimal and clearly are insufficient to justify requiring parental or guardian consent.

The argument for this same conclusion based upon individual rights is even more straightforward. Individuals much younger than the potential subjects of the adolescent sexuality survey are entitled to the free expression of their opinions and a full measure of privacy, morally and constitutionally. While the topic of the rights of children involves many troubling, unresolved, and fundamental issues, clearly minimal rights of children include their own personal control of information about their lives, beliefs, and actions. Of course, the rights and privacy of parents and guardians must also be protected through confidential handling of survey results and legal sanctions.

The research team is responsible for assuring the subjects that the data they provide will be handled with discretion, but at present there are limits to which this assurance can be made. If data are released by the research team and can be traced to individual respondents, current legislation and regulations suggest that the research team is liable to lawsuits by the respondents and will suffer damages. If data are demanded by the state through writs of subpeona and not released by the research team, again they can be penalized. If physicians can enjoy testimonial privileges with their patients, and lawyers with their clients, then we believe that researchers should enjoy testimonial privileges with their subjects. This dilemma of limited assurance needs to be resolved, but sufficient reasons now exist for the research team to handle these data very cautiously.

Centering the discussion in this case study upon surveys of sexual behavior is nescessary, but it is fundamentally misguided to tie the issue of informed consent exclusively to research pertaining to sexual behavior, and genital sexuality in particular. We regard sexual behavior as continuous with general and total self-expression. Thus, interpersonal behavior and a wide range of forms of expression are as much in need of social scientific study and adequate protection of the subject-participant as is the narrower, but presently more socially sensitive, range of behavior treated in this case study.

COMMENTARY

Margaret O'Brien Steinfels

Federal regulations designed to protect research subjects have been vigorously criticized by social science and behavioral researchers. They argue that the kind of research they do entails minimal or no risk and, therefore, does not require the degree of subject protection which biomedical research may require and for which the federal regulations were intended.

In the light of these regulations, the researchers conducting this survey of adolescent sexuality might argue that since they are not exposing a minor to risk, that is, "to the possibility of injury, including physical, psychological, or social injury," they are not required to seek parental consent. They might further argue that young people, certainly sixteen- and seventeen-year-olds, are developmentally capable of giving consent, a point supported by their reference to the adolescent's right to obtain sex-related medical care without parental consent. (Note, though, that the Supreme Court struck down parental consent requirements in this area on privacy grounds without ruling on the adolescent's capacity to consent.)

Seeking therapy is a significantly different act from participation in non-therapeutic research; equating the two because they are both sex-related ought not obscure the relatively different balance between risk and benefit in each case. And precisely in examining the possible risks in the research survey does it become clear that most adolescents do not have the experience or critical faculty to adequately judge risk to themselves. Therefore their parents' consent as well as their own should be sought.

Two arguments can be made in favor of requiring parental consent for all research on minors. First, most parents are better able to calculate the actual risk to an individual child and protect him or her from it than a researcher who can only predict probable risk to a group. Indeed, a statistically minor risk for a group, like 1 or 2 percent, could mask a significant risk for an individual in that minority. Second, the regulation requiring parental consent for research on children recognizes, as a matter of public policy, that parents ought to be the final judge in matters concerning their minor children.

Although parents may not know the exact state of their child's knowledge or experience, particularly in sexual matters, they are likely to know their child's vulnerabilities; they can find out how intelligently and carefully the researcher or interviewer will respond to any question or concern their child may raise during the survey. They can also ascertain whether the child understands the nature of the survey and the kinds of questions that will be asked before the child gives his or her own consent.

Depending on the setting, parents may be concerned about the degree of privacy and confidentiality their child will enjoy. If the survey is conducted in a school setting, will school personnel have access to the responses? Will the fact that any particular child has participated in the research be a matter of public knowledge even though individual responses will be kept in confidence? After the data are analyzed, will the researcher sufficiently disguise the settings and individuals so that publication will not breach the confidentiality or anonymity of the subject?

Other more general risks may concern a parent but may be ignored, minimized, or denied as being relevant issues by the researcher.

Most researchers regard data-gathering as a value-free activity; they are seeking information or opinion in as neutral a manner or formulation as possible. But the mere act of asking a question suggests interest, not neutrality. "How many times have you had sexual intercourse in the last week? month? year? How many times have you had sexual intercourse with a person of the opposite sex? same sex?" Such questions to an adolescent are about as neutral as the classic "When did you stop beating your wife?" They imply an attitude and an opinion, which may leave even the most sophisticated adolescents in a quandary about what his or her values and practices ought to be. Information flows both ways in survey research and precisely because the message that comes from the researcher is ambiguous and subtle, parental concern is justified.

Matters of sex (as of other serious matters like violence, politics, drug use, work habits, racial attitudes, and religion) are likely to be subjects about which most parents do not feel neutral, and they do not want their children to be neutral either. Will the family's own values be subtly undermined by the "value-free" formulations of the questions and the authority under which the questions are asked, including, by virtue of their consent, parental authority?

Under whose auspices and for what purpose is the research survey being conducted? There are differences between Planned Parenthood, Right-to-Life, *Hustler* magazine, Parke-Davis, Columbia records, and the manufacturer of Trojans—all organizations potentially interested in adolescent sexuality. Parents might reasonably see greater risk in sponsorship by some rather than others. Or, in a survey of racial attitudes, parents might want to distinguish between research sponsored by HEW [Health, Education and Welfare, the former name of the federal Department of Health and Human Services], *Time* magazine, the NAACP, and the United Arab League.

And what of the purpose of the research? We are told that this survey of adolescent sexuality will lead to improved sex education programs and clinical services for teenagers. Should parents refuse to consent, if they see these purposes, or those of any research project, placing their family values at risk? Although, "a fair explanation of the procedures . . . and their purposes" is the first requirement of informed consent in the HEW regulations, researchers may argue that the *purpose* of the research should not be subject to scrutiny under consent procedures and that to refuse consent on these grounds unreasonably hinders their efforts.

But let us shift the issue to areas other than adolescent sexuality. Black parents might reasonably refuse consent for a survey conducted by Arthur Jensen, or those who hold his views, on the grounds that the outcome of the research undermines their efforts to secure equal education opportunities for their children.

Parents of developmentally impaired children may be reluctant to consent to a survey whose purpose is to develop a tracked system in local schools.

If parents see risk where researchers see none, these examples suggest why. What the researcher regards as disinterested information gathering may be seen by parents as jeopardizing their ability to protect their child from harm and as undermining the family's moral, political, or social values. What is a factual issue to the researcher may be a moral one for the family.

Given the value-free and scientific premises proclaimed by most research, it is impossible for researchers to acknowledge the fact-value paradox in the way they work. The best protection then for children and family autonomy in child-rearing is to maintain the parental consent requirement for research with minors.

35

Can a Subject Consent to a "Ulysses Contract"?

J.S., a twenty-four-year-old male schizophrenic, has been taking antipsychotic medication regularly since the age of fourteen. Four years ago he was admitted to a private mental hospital, where he was treated with moderately high doses of Prolixin, a powerful neuroleptic. He progressed to the point of being treated in the day treatment program while he lived with his parents. Recently, J.S. started to complain of difficulty in swallowing and increased involuntary movement of his legs, arms, and tongue. When symptoms became acute, he was diagnosed to have tardive dyskinesia—an iatrogenic, usually irreversible, and progressive syndrome caused by neuroleptic medication. There is no known successful treatment.

The doctor recommended that J.S. should be placed on a less powerful antipsychotic medication, Mellaril, which he hoped would prevent the tardive dyskinesia from getting worse. After a month on this new medication, however, J.S.'s psychosis deteriorated so severely that he had to be hospitalized again. Five days later, the patient was squatting in the corner of his room smearing feces, spitting on himself, refusing to eat, and burning himself with matches. He refused all medical interventions. When his health and safety became dangerously affected, the hospital invoked the emergency exception to the informed consent law, which permitted physicians to temporarily administer antipsychotic medication against the patient's will. Within a week, J.S. emerged from his profound psychosis and again became affable. In a few weeks, he was able to comprehend his situation: the medicine that prevented him from "going under" was causing him to suffer from tardive dyskinesia, and this condition was likely to worsen so long as he remained on this medication.

At about this time, J.S.'s therapist heard of an experimental program for the treatment of tardive dyskinesia at a nearby research facility. J.S. was accepted into the program, and signed consent forms for treatment with experimental drugs. In the experimental unit, J.S. was first taken off all medication. Within a week he again regressed into an acutely psychotic condition and he refused the experimental medication. Some researchers suggested that J.S.'s parents be asked to invoke a state law that provided for limited guardianship of a patient in need of special services, but the research unit's lawyer counseled against this approach. The researchers then suggested going ahead with the treatment anyway. Since the patient had consented during his competent hours, they argued that it didn't matter if he changed his mind later; the "Ulysses contract"was binding. (Ulysses had asked his men to bind him to the mast of his ship before sailing past the Sirens, and to refuse his requests to sail nearer while he was under the irresistible influence of the Sirens' lovely song.) Again legal counsel did not agree and the research team finally decided to exclude J.S. from the project. He went back to the hospital where Prolixin was administered. When he returned to "normal" and learned what had happened, he begged for another chance to try the experimental medication.

Who ought to be able to consent to experimental treatment for J.S. ? Should the subject's wishes during his competent period be recognized as valid?

COMMENTARY

Morton E. Winston and Sally M. Winston

Two distinct but related ethical issues are raised by this case. The first concerns the decision to contine using a medication that has known harmful iatrogenic effects. Since there is no effective treatment for tardive dyskinesia (TD), decisions to prescribe neuroleptic medications must be made on a case-by-case basis.

Among the possible benefits are the potential for deinstitutionalization and self-sufficiency; the alleviation of suffering; cessation of suicidal, self-destructive, or antisocial behavior; and amenability to other forms of therapy. The risks and costs are the potential iatrogenic symptoms: disfigurement, discomfort, social ostracism, and eventual threat to life. In each patient, physicians must weigh the probable level of functioning with and without medication, speed of progression of symptoms, degree of dose-relatedness, reversibility of the syndrome, and the degree to which the symptoms of TD are masked by the medication that causes it.

Generally, patients and/or their legal guardians are informed of these risks before they consent to treatment. However, because of significant individual differences in responding to these medications, and the progressive nature of the iatrogenic syndrome, clinical judgments need to be continuously reevaluated. In the case of J.S., the physician apparently decided that the danger produced by J.S.'s own psychotic behavior was a graver and more immediate risk than that produced by the iatrogenic syndrome. Since the more powerful neuroleptic will tend to mask the symptoms of TD while causing the underlying syndrome to worsen, the decision does not solve the problem.

The most interesting issue raised by this case, however, concerns the patient-subject's consent to and subsequent refusal of the experimental treatment. We think it is reasonable to interpret J.S.'s initial consent as constituting a Ulysses contract in which he, in effect, instructs others to disregard his deranged protests and to carry out what he had indicated in his competent hours to be his authentic desires.

The function of informed consent is to insure that the individual's own choices and preferences, where known, be given priority in decisions concerning treatment. In cases like this, where a patient is intermittently competent, the most responsible policy is to regard statements made during the most lucid and competent periods as best expressing the patient's true intentions. Given that J.S. predictably regresses into florid psychosis when unmedicated, his refusal of the experimental treatment is probably itself a symptom of his illness, a part of the general negativism of schizophrenia, and should not be interpreted as a withdrawal of consent.

Like Ulysses, J.S. appears to realize that he will need someone instructed in advance to ignore his deranged opposition and steer him under protest into treatment. Unlike Ulysses, however, J.S. did not explicitly indicate in advance that his protests were to be disregarded. However, foregoing the experimental treatment is not in the best interests of J.S. or the research team. Therefore, a "reasonable person" standard would suggest that, if able to do so, J.S. would have acted prudently had he followed Ulysses' course.

Once J.S. refused the experimental treatment, the research team had several options. If the research team had sought to have him declared legally incompetent and placed under the limited guardianship of his parents, they would have had to show that he was unable to make a competent and responsible decision concerning his participation in the experiment, and that the experimental treatment would be likely to benefit him directly in a way unobtainable by any other means. It seems unlikely that a court would have granted guardianship, since the patient was clearly competent when he entered the experimental program, and there was no evidence that the experimental treatment would in fact benefit him, or benefit him more than his normal medication. This is probably why legal counsel advised against this course. On the other hand, to ignore the patient's refusal would appear to abrogate his right to withdraw consent; hence counsel advised against forcing participation.

Since the treatment was experimental, the hospital emergency rule could not be invoked, except to administer an approved medication. To give J.S. the experimental treatment along with his normal medication would violate elementary principles of research design which typically aim to control for possible drug interaction effects. Thus, no doubt regretfully, the members of the research team felt that they had no alternative but to exclude J.S.

Cases of this kind could best be handled if there were a regular procedure for drawing up Ulysses contracts, allowing patients to specify in advance the precise conditions under which their requests or protests are to be disregarded, and to designate someone to act as their proxy under those conditions. Ideally, such agreements should not involve complicated legal procedures, but they should provide safeguards to allow competent persons to change their minds. One possibility would be to have the IRB appoint a person to monitor both the subject's initial consent and subsequent behavior in order to determine whether the terms of the Ulysses contract are being fulfilled. Without such agreements, it will be difficult to successfully treat patients such as J.S. who are caught between the Scylla of psychosis and the Charybdis of tardive dyskinesia.

COMMENTARY

Paul S. Appelbaum

The history of regulation of medical research involving human subjects demonstrates a primary concern with two issues: the right of subjects to act autonomously in deciding on participation, and the imperative to protect subjects from harm. Can both these concerns be justified in a manner that would permit J.S. to participate in a research project that holds the potential for substantial benefit to him?

Considering first the autonomy issue, our task is to determine which of J.S.'s decisions—the nonpsychotic decision to participate in the study or the psychotic decision to refuse—represents the most authentic manifestation of his will. I use authentic here to mean the decision that is most congruent with his life history and his sense of himself as a person (see Bruce Miller, "Autonomy and Refusing Lifesaving Treatment," *Hastings Center Report*, August 1981).

Given the distorting effects of psychotic illness on persons' usual modes of thought, behavior, and communication, J.S.'s decision to participate in the experimental program, which was made while he was nonpsychotic and in a state that the law would define as "competent," is much more likely to represent his authentic desires than his subsequent refusal in a state of psychosis and legal incompetence. This conclusion is bolstered by the fact that although J.S. experienced severe consequences as a result of his initial decision to participate, namely regression to a psychotic state, he chooses to take part in the study when he is competent again. Such first-hand experience with the risks of participation approximates the level of knowledge we would like to see in all subjects who consent to research. Although there may be technical legal problems in honoring J.S.'s previous competent consent at a time of subsequent, even incompetent refusal, allowing him to participate would seem to be the proper ethical course.

Note that no one else needs to decide what constitutes J.S.'s best interests or, at the time of refusal, how he would have decided if he were competent. Like any other competent individual, J.S. has told us his wishes and we must honor them.

Proceeding along these lines, however, raises an additional concern. Ordinarily, one of the most important mechanisms for preventing harm to subjects is to permit them to withdraw from a research project at any point during the study. In the name of protecting J.S.'s autonomy, however, we have deprived him in part of this right. Clearly, some additional means of protection are called for. In such circumstances, an individual independent of the research team—perhaps associated with the IRB that reviewed the project—should be empowered to monitor the situation and withdraw J.S. from the study should significant, unforeseen risks arise.

I conceive the powers of this monitor to be strictly limited. The role does not call for substitute decision making, or for a reassessment of J.S.'s participation unless there is imminent danger from risks of which the subject was unaware at the time of the original consent. As a competent decision maker, J.S. has as much right as any other person to consent to known risks, particularly when the possibility of personal benefit exists. (Many cases of TD do improve or remit with the cessation of neuroleptics, and it is unclear if the syndrome is inevitably progressive even when neuroleptics are continued.)

The implications of this discussion are not limited to situations such as J.S.'s in which the possibility of a competent consent exists. Given the importance of further research on conditions found only in people who can never be expected to give a competent consent—such as patients with advanced senile dementia or severe chronic psychoses—it is crucial to explore means of allowing these individuals to participate in research, while simutaneously ensuring their protection. I am not addressing the question of obtaining initial consent. But once participation has been approved, the presence of an independent individual, charged with monitoring unexpected risks, may provide an important measure of protection to the subjects involved.

COMMENTARY

Nancy K. Rhoden

The distinguishing features of the proposed Ulysses contract are that a person, while competent, embarks on a course of action but suspects that strange, mind-altering forces may come into play and thus explicitly instructs those nearby to ignore future decisions that reflect such unnatural influences. J.S., we must assume, did not initially give a consent even remotely resembling a Ulysses-type contract: regulations governing federally supported research require that subjects be told they can withdraw at any time; in any case, people entering an experimental treatment program rarely agree not to withdraw. Thus legal counsel were correct in refusing the researchers' request to render J.S.'s consent retroactively binding. It would be dishonest, and indefensibly paternalistic, to justify overriding a refusal (even an incompetent one) by reference to a prior consent when the consent lacked the features of a true Ulysses contract.

But even though J.S.'s prior consent could not appropriately be transformed into a Ulysses contract, such a contract could be a prime candidate for getting J.S. back into the experimental program and for ensuring that further incompetent attempts to withdraw will be ignored. A binding consent, particularly for experimental treatment, is highly unusual. But the pecularities of J.S.'s situation, and those of others like him, present the strongest possible justification for such an approach. The case suggests that J.S. is one of those schizophrenic patients who responds quite well to neuroleptic drugs such that, when taking them, he is in fact reasonably competent, in contrast to his condition when unmedicated. Because of this we can feel fairly confident that his consent while medicated represents his true wishes, like Ulysses' request prior to succumbing to the Sirens' strange spell. Thus the principle of respect for persons would support ignoring J.S.'s refusal and honoring the decision that most accurately reflects his "real" wishes. The principle of beneficence would probably yield the same result, since the experimental treatment is most likely in J.S.'s best interests (unless its risks are unusually high).

But we should not rush headlong to embrace Ulysses contracts for the treatment, experimental or otherwise, of the mentally ill. Our society has a long and shameful history of ignoring mentally ill patients' refusals of treatment and complaints of side effects. Particularly in our understaffed and underfunded state mental hospitals, doctors have treated patients with unnecessarily high doses of neuroleptics without monitoring the patients' responses or attempting to reduce the dosage, and have then ignored patients' complaints of neurological abnormalities until irreversible damage was done. Should we now so readily sanction a binding consent that allows doctors who are experimenting upon victims of this iatrogenic disorder to unhesitatingly ignore patients' attempts to withdraw from the project? We must remember that some attempts to withdraw may be due to unpleasant side effects of the experimental drugs. (Suppose Ulysses had asked that his bonds be loosened because they were choking him.) In addition, many mental patients may be rendered unusually docile, dependent, and easy to control by neuroleptic drugs. Thus an initial consent to treatment may not always represent their true wishes.

Clearly we cannot have a Ulysses contract that makes the consent absolutely binding without regard to the reasons behind a subsequent refusal. It is easy enough to say that a subsequent refusal that is competent—e.g., the patient lucidly states that the new drug is causing severe dizziness and he would rather live with the tardive dyskinseia (or schizophrenia)—will override a prior Ulysses-type consent, while a subsequent incompetent refusal will not. But competency is notoriously difficult to define and determine. Some mentally ill persons, plagued by side effects, may subsequently refuse in such an unusual, oblique, or paranoid manner that their refusal appears thoroughly irrational. Moreover, physicians faced with a patient's attempt to withdraw from an experimental treatment program may be tempted to underestimate the competency of the person who questions their medical judgment (as they may have overestimated the patient's competency when he or she originally consented).

A completely psychotic refusal should not override a valid consent, but we must provide safeguards that will recognize legitimate revocations of consent. Perhaps physicians could give mentally ill patients the option of appointing, during their lucid intervals, a relative, friend, attorney, or other individual (not a member of the treatment or research team) who could act as a substitute decision maker in the event the patient again lapses into incompetency. The various persons involved might still disagree about the patient's competency, but such a modification would allow an independent person, who presumably has the patient's best interests at heart, to consider a subsequent refusal of treatment in light of the patient's mental state at the time of consent, his or her present mental state, any side effects from the experimental treatment, other options, and so forth. Alternatively, patients could choose to make a modified Ulysses contract in which consent would be binding for a specified time period and then reviewed, or in which a subsequent incompetent attempt to withdraw could be overridden, but only after review by an independent psychiatrist or hospital ethics committee. Such modifications could allow valuable treatment programs, experimental or otherwise, to proceed despite psychotic attempts at withdrawal, while building in safeguards to ensure that a patient's legitimate desires are not ignored.

36

Informed Consent in the Developing World

The government of a North African Islamic republic has called upon an American physician, Dr. Arthur Bosley, to determine whether hydatid disease is a serious health problem. This infectious disease is caused by the larval form of the tapeworm *Echinococcus*, whose eggs may develop into numerous large, fluid-filled cysts in the lungs, liver, and other organs. These cysts, which can attain a diameter of 6 inches or more, may distort or displace vital organs or may rupture, causing an immediate and sometimes fatal toxic reaction. Under natural circumstances the tapeworm lives part of its life cycle in sheep and part in dogs. Because sheep play a prominent role in Islamic religious life, a large proportion of the population comes into contact with the parasite.

While there is no effective treatment for most forms of the disease (other than surgery in advanced cases), other sheep-rearing countries have prevented infection by eliminating the parasite. These control measures require expensive regional or national programs for the discovery and proper disposal of infected sheep and for the killing of stray or feral dogs, which might spread the infection. To determine whether it should deploy the resources necessary for such a program, the government wants Dr. Bosley to conduct an accurate survey of the distribution of the disease in humans.

Dr. Bosley believes that the best way to undertake this survey is to test a few drops of blood taken by finger prick and to perform a skin test of the type used worldwide to diagnose allergy. Together with his North African colleagues, all of whom were trained in Europe or America, Dr. Bosley decides to conduct the survey among adult patients attending public clinics, where as many as 100 or 200 patients can be seen each day. A preliminary survey convinces Dr. Bosley that these subjects have an understanding of disease and its causation that is very different from his own. Many of them believe that a disease is caused by the activities of malevolent spirits or persons, and that therapy depends upon removing or placating these beings. However, they also recognize the power of Western physicians to influence symptoms of disease. Dr. Bosley finds that his subjects are particularly pleased with his use of needles as this practice conforms to their own notions of the efficacy of puncturing as a therapy. And it is therapy—not participation in research—that they are seeking at the clinic.

Recognizing that informed consent is a basic tenet of research ethics, Dr. Bosley faces a dilemma. In this particular society and with these particular subjects, can he fully inform them and obtain their consent? Are different standards of informed consent appropriate in different settings?

COMMENTARY

Ebun O. Ekunwe

There are two vital questions raised in this case: Is the proposed study the most effective way of assessing the size of the problem? And, are the tests similar to tests that a doctor may ordinarily perform in diagnosing and managing a patient who comes to the clinic?

Currently, the two tests that Dr. Bosley proposes appear to be the safest and surest means of diagnosing the individual cases of hydatid disease. These data will enable him to determine the distribution of the disease in the study population. Therefore, Dr. Bosley needs to carry out his study as proposed. In answer to the second question, it is quite likely that many patients have had patch tests for various allergies and even more have had blood drawn for "tests."

Accordingly, Dr. Bosley should obtain what is best described as "uninformed consent." In most developing countries, the germ theory of disease causation is yet to be accepted, particularly among the not-so-educated members of the population. Dr. Bosley and his team could spend a considerable amount of time and energy explaining the cause of hydatid disease and still not succeed in getting the people to understand. Since he cannot convince them of the true etiology and pathology of the disease, he should not waste his time.

In most developing countries, a blood test is considered a good thing—if your blood is good, then you are all right. If Dr. Bosley tells the patients attending the clinic that he wishes to do a blood test on them, they would readily consent. In this case, the patient consents without having all the available information at his or her disposal. The researcher is informed on the patient's behalf as he (the researcher) knows that: (1) the procedure is essential to the health care policy decision and (2) the risks involved are tiny and no more than the risk of having regular clinic tests.

Suppose Dr. Bosley and his team were to write out all information on a piece of paper and request that each patient should sign (as in developed countries). He would encounter two major problems. First of all, his population may not be able to read. Even those who can read may not understand all the medical terms that such information is bound to contain. Fear and rejection usually attend a lack of understanding. The second problem is the signature. People are afraid to sign or thumbprint any document. They feel, rightly, that the writer of the document has a hold, usually sinister, on them once they have signed.

If, on the other hand, he spends time verbally informing them, they are going to be suspicious of his intentions. They would consider him the obstacle between them and the services offered by the clinic. In addition, they would feel that he has something to hide—"Many words hide a multitude of sin." Those who have not actually heard him will know him by reputation, through the grapevine. They will in turn stay away from the clinic. In this sense, trying to obtain informed consent may be reverse ethics, as it will keep patients away. Then Dr. Bosley's sample will not be truly representative of the population and the distribution that he arrives at may be vastly different from the true distribution. Besides, he will lose a lot of skin test results, because the patients whose skin has been tested will not all come back to have the result read.

However, Dr. Bosley owes it to his patients and himself to explain that the finger prick will not make them better. If he fails to confess that he does not possess magical powers to use his needle to make them feel better, his program will soon be in disrepute. Before long, patients are going to notice that there is no difference between the health of those who have had the finger prick and those who have not. Finally, even in developing countries, if the proposed tests are different from routine tests, and carry risks of complications and/or pain, then informed consent must be obtained either verbally or in writing.

COMMENTARY

Ross Kessel

This case raises important questions concerning the special problems of obtaining informed consent in a transcultural setting and in particular of the possibility of forcing Western values upon non-Western societies. Many of the same questions may be faced in transcultural settings within the United States.

In considering whether to conduct this research study, Dr. Bosley must weigh the costs and benefits. In considering the best interests of those he is attempting to benefit he must ask how and by whom the seriousness of health problems is ranked; how medical resources are allocated; and whether marked inequalities in access to health care influence the moral choices to be made. Moreover, in arriving at estimates of the risks and benefits of his research he must determine who shall make such estimates. This in turn will lead him to examine whose standards and values need to be considered, and whether local or Western standards of institutional review should prevail, particularly in obtaining informed consent.

Whose standards should operate here? Should Dr. Bosley enforce essentially Western notions of consent upon local physicians with different, and perhaps even hostile, values? Or should he accept some local standard of consent, even if it fails to meet all the guidelines of his American Institutional Review Board (IRB)? He will not receive specific help from the International Guidelines proposed by the World Health Organization.* These accept the principle from the Declaration of Helsinki, revised in 1975, that "each potential subject must be adequately informed of the aims, methods, anticipated benefits and potential hazards of the study and any discomfort it may entail . . . and . . . the doctor should then obtain the subject's freely-given informed consent, preferably in writing" (Recommendation 9, page 38). However, the Guidelines recognize that ". . . those who are *totally* unfamiliar with modern medical concepts" (page 24, emphasis added) and "vulnerable social groups" (page 26) present special problems; and, indeed, state that the involvement of human subjects is only contingent upon freely-elicited informed consent "*when feasible*" (page 7, emphasis added).

Turning to the current federal regulations, issued in January 1981, concerning the protection of human research subjects (45 CFR 46) Dr. Bosley will find them similarly flexible. The regulations leave room for American investigators to explore with their overseas counterparts appropriate forms of obtaining consent, without negating the responsibility of IRBs and the Department of Health and Human Services to oversee such research protocols.

For example, a signed consent form need not be obtained if the research presents no more than minimal risk of harm to subjects and does not involve a procedure for which written consent is normally required outside the research context. Moreover, an IRB may approve a consent procedure that omits or alters some elements of informed consent—*or waive the requirement altogether*—if the IRB finds and documents that the subjects are at no more than minimal risk or that the research could not practicably be carried out without the waiver or alteration.

Regardless of these formal requirements, Dr. Bosley will find that the elements of free and informed consent are the same in this study as they would be within the United States. Dr. Bosley's subjects must be both competent and free to give consent, and they must both be given and comprehend enough information to make consent meaningful. However, special moral and sociological problems arise within a transcultural setting in deciding what information to impart, how to impart it, and whether it has been understood.

Dr. Bosley must decide who shall give consent, and under what conditions. He will surely decide that his subjects are fully competent and ought to consent for themselves, and will reject the notion of group or proxy consent whereby a local leader gives consent for all.

Even if the issue of competency is put aside, obtaining individual consent that is free and uncoerced may be no small task in a public clinic. When hundreds of patients must be seen each day there may not be much time or

*Anonymous, "Proposed International Guidelines for Biomedical Research Involving Human Subjects," WHO/CIOMS, Geneva, 1982.

inclination for careful explanations and questions. Moreover, patients in the public clinic will likely believe that they are not in a position to refuse consent.

Perhaps the most perplexing questions facing Dr. Bosley are how to adequately inform his subjects of the nature and reason for his study and how to determine whether they have adequately comprehended this information and can therefore provide informed consent. Moral problems arise in deciding what information to impart; sociological problems arise in the method of communication and in determining whether it has been comprehended.

To inform his patients of the purposes and benefits of his study Dr. Bosley will have to enter the belief system of his subjects. In the case of hydatid disease he will find that while they may accept the notion that dogs (animals generally held to be "unclean") may be accepted as a cause, they will have great difficulty accepting his view that so holy an animal as a sheep could be responsible for human disease. Moreover, many of his subjects are likely to be convinced that the final cause of disease is the result of the evil eye rather than the accidental passage of a parasite from animal to man. Dr. Bosley may also have difficulty informing his subjects of the risks of his procedure. He may find, as Teitelbaum* has done, that whatever he may say, diagnostic skin testing and finger puncturing will be "known" by his subjects to be therapeutic. Within their view of illness and its management, the "risks" of skin testing may well be perceived as "benefits," which provide treatment for the unrelated illnesses that brought them to the clinic in the first place. Thus, in trying to inform his subjects about the purpose of his study and the methods to be employed, Dr. Bosley may find himself "lying" in order to stay within, and avoid damaging, their belief systems.

How will Dr. Bosley determine that his subjects have understood the information he presents? Even if he finds competent translators, the cultural gap is likely to prove wide. His best alternative is probably to provide an opportunity for his subjects to ask questions, even though his subjects may have difficulty framing them. Only by this means will Dr. Bosley assure himself that his subjects are adequately (though surely not fully) informed.

In conclusion, Dr. Bosley must proceed upon the belief that his research subjects are fully competent to give free and informed consent. He must develop procedures in the setting of his study that will minimize, if not eliminate, coercion and undue influence both from his own words and actions and from the clinic setting itself. He will need to develop a setting in which his subjects are encouraged to explore with him their understanding of the nature of his enterprise and especially its risks and benefits. He may well decide that his description of the nature and causation of hydatid disease be within the framework of these subjects' views of disease and of their understanding of the benefits to be derived from the study.

*J.M. Teitelbaum, "The Social Perception of Illness in Some Tunisian Communities," *Psychological Anthropology*, ed. T. Williams (The Hague: ICAES, Mouton, 1975); and J.M. Teitelbaum, "Humoral Therapy in Tunisia," *Anthropology and Mental Health*, ed. J. Westermeyer (The Hague: ICAES, Mouton, 1976).

37

When Research Is Best Therapy

Mr. S, a forty-eight-year-old male, was referred to the oncology clinic with a histologically proven diagnosis of renal cell carcinoma, that is, cancer of the kidney. Lung metastases present at the time of original diagnosis have grown. Although there is a small percentage of spontaneous remission with this disease, no curative radiation therapy or chemotherapy is available. The response rate to standard progestational (hormonal) agents or chemotherapy is about 5 percent and those responses usually involve only modest shrinkage. Mr. S informed his physician that unless some form of treatment would improve his quality of life or extend his period of survival he would prefer to postpone treatment, particularly if a proposed therapy would risk reducing the quality of his existence.

The physician knew that a drug company was financing a randomized trial that would compare gamma-interferon to Depo-provera, a standard progestational agent. As with almost all studies of anticancer drugs, both physicians and patients would be aware of the treatment. Two-thirds of the patients were to receive interferon; those who received Depo-provera and did not respond to it would not be "crossed over" to interferon.

Although no interferon of any kind was then available for nonresearch uses, studies of alpha-interferon in renal cell carcinoma had indicated a 5 to 30 percent response rate. A Phase I trial of gamma-interferon designed to determine toxicity and recommended dosage level had resulted in six responses from among thity-six patients with renal cell carcinoma at various dosage levels. No regular Phase II study had been done. On the basis of this evidence, the physician believes that gamma-interferon would be the most promising treatment she could offer Mr. S.

Should the physician ask Mr. S to participate in this study? If she does, should she make certain he understands that: (1) In her best clinical judgment, only gamma-interferon offers any real hope for his disease; (2) He has the right to withdraw from the study at any time and therefore a right to withdraw if he is randomized to Depo-provera? Does Mr. S's agreement to participate in the study entail an obligation to accept either therapy? Finally, should the drug company have conducted a regular Phase II study of gamma-interferon before financing this randomized study?

COMMENTARY

Don Marquis and Ron Stephens

Mr. S's physician faces a serious dilemma. She believes that gamma-interferon is the best drug available for his renal cell carcinoma. The only way for him to receive it is by participating in the clinical trial. Since physicians have an obligation to give their patient what in their judgment is the best treatment that can be obtained, it might be argued that the physician has an obligation to enroll Mr. S in the study.

Yet Mr. S is disinclined to accept ineffective treatment and the physician evidently believes that Depo-provera is very likely to be ineffective. What, then, should she tell Mr. S? Should she enroll him in the study? One possibility is to suggest that participation is tantamount to a contract between Mr. S and the drug company; Mr. S would participate in the study even if he receives Depo-provera in exchange for a chance to receive gamma-interferon. However, this characterization obscures the patient's right to withdraw from the study at any time.

Another possibility is to obtain Mr. S's written informed consent to participate in the study, but remain silent concerning both the supposed contract and his right to withdraw in the event of randomization to Depo-provera. Yet since patients frequently do not read consent forms carefully and often do not understand them when they do, it is questionable whether such "consent" would be informed. If the physician is properly concerned with Mr. S's autonomy, she should explain that he can withdraw from the study at any time for any reason without his care being compromised, and make certain he understands that this provision holds even if he is randomized to receive Depo-provera.

There are, however, substantial arguments against withdrawing the patient if he does not receive the desired therapy. If every physician adopted this alternative, the study presumably could not be completed. Further, this seems tantamount to *using* a drug company protocol to obtain experimental therapy for a patient while at the same time frustrating the purposes of the protocol.

While it might damage a physician's career in academic medicine, this last course of action is morally preferable. It is the only course of action that does not violate the physician's duty to her patient. The moral bind experienced by physicians who consider enrolling patients in the study suggests that the study itself is ethically flawed. Is this so?

This is a Phase III study of anticancer drugs designed to show that a proposed treatment regimen is better than or at least as good as, but less toxic than, standard therapy. A physician should ask her patient to participate in such a randomized study only if good evidence that one treatment is inferior to the other is not available. Only randomized clinical trials that satisfy a condition of therapeutic equivalence should be conducted.

The physician in this case *believed* that the gamma-interferon versus Depo-provera trial did not meet this standard, not because she was convinced that gamma-inferteron was a proven therapeutic agent for metastatic renal cell carcinoma, but because she had no confidence in the "standard" therapy for the disease, Depo-provera.

There is considerable justification for her conclusion. For some oncologists, Depo-provera has been the drug of choice for metastatic renal cell carcinoma only because there is no other potentially effective treatment. Many would offer it to a patient only if he or she really wanted chemotherapy and then only because Depo-provera does not have serious side effects. In addition, poorly designed studies of the efficacy of Depo-provera have yielded mixed results. Hence the physician's belief that gamma-interferon offered Mr. S the only real hope of benefit for his disease was probably quite sound.

The trial was badly designed. A Phase III study on gamma-interferon should not have been conducted because there was no established efficacious treatment. The drug company instead should have run a regular Phase II study of gamma-interferon involving fifteen to twenty patients with renal cell carcinoma who would receive gamma-interferon at a dosage schedule suggested by the Phase I trial.

COMMENTARY

Ethel S. Siris and M. Margaret Kemeny

One of the realities of medical practice is that there are some diseases for which no good treatments exist. The difficult question of whether to enroll a patient such as Mr. S in a clinical trial, with all of its attendant risks and uncertainties, must be faced by both the patient and the physician. Defining the roles and ethical and legal obligations of the three participants involved in the decision to enter a cancer patient into a clinical trial—the personal physician, the patient, and the clinical investigator—provides insight into the issues that arise in this setting.

The personal physician's role includes an obligation to inform the patient of the existence of the clinical trial and to give an objective opinion as to whether enrolling in the study would be in the patient's best interest. There are many considerations in deciding whether to recommend participation in a randomized trial in oncology, including possible inconvenience and considerable expense to a seriously ill patient, the loss of the primary doctor's control of treatment, and the possible risks and discomforts of untested therapies.

Unfortunately, Mr. S's doctor is not being objective about the study. Though there are only minimal data on the safety and effectiveness of gamma-interferon in treating metastatic renal cell carcinoma, she has a strong conviction that it is the treatment of choice. She may take this position in part because the results with standard treatment—Depo-provera—are so dismal. However, she also appears to feel that gamma-interferon is intrinsically a better choice, a treatment that she believes should work and be safe. Given the preliminary nature of the studies, some of which examined a different agent (alpha-interferon), her certainty seems premature. The clinical trial is being conducted to provide a more objective basis for evaluating the data.

The physician's beliefs pose a serious problem for her and her patient: She wants Mr. S to enter the study, but in light of his stated wishes concerning treatment and her strong conviction about the best therapy, she wants him to participate only if he is randomized to receive gamma-interferon. In our view this position is flawed. The physician may certainly convey her impression that gamma-interferon is promising, but she should be careful to avoid creating a situation in which her patient will suffer emotional anguish if he is randomized to the "wrong" treatment arm. Her role is not to make a judgment about which arm of a particular study she hopes her patient will receive, but to decide whether to recommend this or any appropriate study.

The patient's role in deciding whether to participate in the clinical trial also entails certain obligations. The process of obtaining informed consent should make it clear to Mr. S that he has the right to withdraw from the study at any time. This right includes the option to leave the trial solely because he is disappointed about the treatment to which he has been randomized. We would hope, however, that a patient would not enter a study with the unstated intention of leaving if he doesn't receive the treatment he wants.

It is the investigator's responsibility to be certain that the trial is designed so that it is scientifically and ethically valid, one in which all treatment arms offer equivalent risk/benefits ratios. If the patient understands this and has not been unfairly influenced by unsubstantiated opinions regarding different treatment modalities in the study, he or she should be able to accept his or her assignment in good faith. Though we strongly agree that the patient has inviolate rights, we would also argue that he or she has some obligation to remain in the study out of fairness.

The patient entering a clinical trial in oncology is typically anxious and frightened. The informed consent process, though imperfect, should convey enough information about the study and alternative management strategies to allow the patient to make a rational choice in what is invariably an emotionally turbulent setting. The researcher has the obligation to inform these individuals not only objectively, but also compassionately. All of this takes time, both the patient's and the researcher's. In fairness, Mr. S should agree to enter the study only if he reasonably believes that it is in his best interest to participate and is committed to fulfilling the protocol requirements in good faith.

Finally, should the drug company have performed a Phase II rather than a Phase III study? Both typically involve controlled trials, with Phase II studies looking for a promise of efficacy of the study therapy in a small number of subjects and Phase III trials seeking definitive evidence of efficacy when the experimental agent is compared with current therapies in a larger number of subjects. When a treatment arm proves significantly more effective than the control arm, the study can be stopped and the new treatment used on a wider range of patients. All new drugs eventually go through the Phase II-III process, since all drugs must be compared to existing treatment regimens. There is no way to assess the efficacy of one arm over another before the clinical trial has been implemented.

The medical community's scientific obligation is to continue searching for better treatments for solid tumors and to test these treatments with an established empirical scientific method. Individual patients and their personal physicians must also recognize their responsibility to society as a whole. Without individuals who freely participate in such studies, many advances in cancer treatment modalities in such varied areas as lymphomas, testicular tumors, ovarian cancers, and some lung cancers could not have been made. Mr. S and his physician should carefully consider these issues in the context of his personal needs and wishes as they work together to do what will be best for him.

SELECTION OF SUBJECTS AND PROTECTION OF THEIR WELFARE

38

The Last Patient in a Drug Trial

A thirty-year-old man was admitted to the hospital for chemotherapy. Eighteen months earlier he had had an above-the-knee amputation for a malignant tumor of the right foot and was considered free of disease. A month before admission a chest X ray showed multiple areas of metastatic tumor throughout both lungs. For several weeks he was treated with a combination of conventional chemotherapeutic drugs that are sometimes effective against this type of tumor. This patient had no response, however.

Normally, he would now be a candidate for treatment with an experimental drug. In this instance, the drug currently being tested has shown no antitumor effect in any of the eighteen patients with this form of cancer who have received it. Toxicity has been typical for an experimental anticancer agent. All the eighteen patients experienced significant nausea and vomiting for about forty-eight hours after taking the drug. Several patients developed sores and ulcerations in the mouth for several days, and almost all had temporary severe decreases in their blood counts. Two patients developed pneumonia as a result, and were treated with antibiotics.

If no responses were seen, the trial of this drug was originally designed to end for this type of cancer after nineteen patients. The physicians in charge of the trial could then say with 95 percent confidence that the drug would be effective in less than 15 percent of patients with this kind of tumor, and thus that this drug had little usefulness against this form of cancer. This patient is the "last" patient in the trial—unless he responds, the trial will be closed. The patient wants to be treated. The physicians in charge of the trial are anxious to finish the study so a definitive judgment can be made on the usefulness of the drug.

Is the physician obligated to treat the patient with another drug that "might" work rather than to complete the trial? Does the fact that the research team "knows" the drug is ineffective affect the patient's informed consent? Do the physician's obligations to perform scientifically good research conflict with his obligations to this patient?

COMMENTARY

Peter P. Sordillo

The physician who enters a patient in a Phase II trial of an anticancer agent has two goals: to evaluate the usefulness of the Phase II drug* against a certain

*A Phase I trial attempts to establish the safety of an agent rather than to assess its effectiveness.

form of cancer and to offer the patient another chance after he has failed to respond to conventional chemotherapy. Occasionally, a patient in whom standard chemotherapy has not worked will respond to a new drug, and sometimes these responses are marked. Likewise, there is no way to assess the value of a new agent other than to test it on patients with cancer, since the effectiveness of a drug against animal tumors frequently does not correlate with its effectiveness against tumors in humans.

The case dramatizes the potential conflict between these two goals. Certainly, the physician does not want to expose his patient to a drug that is likely to make him sick but is unlikely to help him. On the other hand, the physician feels obligated to see that the scientific trials that he conducts are rigorous and valid so that it can be determined which of the hundreds of new drugs being tested every year are useful.

This conflict does not arise only when the "last" patient in a trial is to be treated, however, and cannot be resolved merely by ending the trial at an earlier point. Even after nineteen patients have failed to respond, by the criteria outlined in the case history, there is still a 5 percent chance the drug may be an active agent. Others have argued that it is a much greater error to conclude that a potentially active agent has no value than it would be to conclude that an inactive drug is active. The latter will be quickly discovered, but if a trial finds an active drug to be inactive, that drug may be lost forever. So even after nineteen patients have failed to respond to a drug, the physician may feel he has not "proven" the drug inactive, and may be reluctant to end the trial. Further, even a hint of antitumor activity in such a trial may mean the drug has usefulness for a group that has not been tested (for example, patients not previously treated with standard chemotherapy) or in combination with other drugs. Conversely, even midway through a trial of a drug that has not produced responses (and most new anticancer drugs produce few or no responses), the physician may believe that this drug is *less* likely to benefit his patient than another drug that has not been tested.

Thus, the obligations of the physician to the patient and to do good research, may be in conflict not only when the "last" patient in a trial is being treated, but throughout the trial. Can this conflict be lessened? I would argue that whether a physician advises his patient to participate in the trial of a new drug must depend both upon the status of the trial and the condition of the patient at that particular moment. For example, a physician may feel that a patient who is not healthy enough to live through more than one trial of a drug that proves inactive should not waste his "last chance" on a drug less likely to help him; thus he may recommend that the patient receive something else. On the other hand, there may be less objection to a patient who is expected to have a long life span being one of the last subjects in such a trial. Currently, these distinctions are not made. The toxicity encountered during the trial and the potential harm to the patient must also be weighed. The severe discomfort and the risk of serious infection that often accompany these drugs seem easier to accept early in a trial when there is still a significant hope of benefit than when the hope of benefit is small.

One might claim that imposing such conditions detracts from the scientific validity of the drug trial since we are "selecting" those patients who participate. While this argument may be valid for controlled trials, it does not apply to the noncontrolled Phase II trials of experimental agents as currently conducted. The major purpose of these trials is to detect any sign of activity by a new drug, and the exclusion of sicker patients (who are less likely to respond to agents that are useful) could actually make it less likely that the drug will falsely be called inactive.

Providing information on the status of the drug trial is clearly an essential part of giving informed consent. In current practice, what the last patient in a trial is told about the potential value of a drug is usually the same as what the first patient learns. But the information necessary to provide true informed consent must include not only a description of the drug's toxicity, but also some idea of the success or failure the investigators have encountered during the trial. This need not be a precise statistical statement, but something on the order of: "This drug has been very useful against animal tumors, although so far it hasn't worked on any of the patients on whom we have tried it. We'd like to try it on one or two more people with this form of cancer before giving up on it. If this drug doesn't work, we have other, newer drugs with which we can try to help you." A statement of this sort would provide the patient with some of the information he needs for deciding whether to take the new drug, without foreclosing the possibility that informed patients would agree to participate in these studies.

COMMENTARY

Kenneth F. Schaffner

Medical research represents a quest for useful *warranted* assertions about human beings and their illnesses. Over the centuries many therapeutic regimens of questionable benefit and often considerable harm have been inflicted on patients, from ancient enemeta and bloodletting to more recent gastric "freezing" for duodenal ulcers. Various statistical methods have been developed to test scientifically whether the observed effects of a new drug (or other treatment) are attributable to the drug and not due to chance, biological (including genetic and environmental) variability, clinicians' bias, a placebo effect, or spontaneous remission.

It will not be possible in this short commentary to discuss all the different designs for clinical trials, such as randomized, fixed sample, sequential, double-blind, matched pairs, and the like.* (The trial discussed here is what is termed a nonrandomized Phase II trial.) Suffice it to say that all such trials

*The reader is referred to E.A. Gehan and E.J. Freireich, "Non-Randomized Controls in Cancer Clinical Trials," *New England Journal of Medicine* 290 (1974), 198–203; and more generally to H. Wulff, *Rational Diagnosis and Treatment* (Oxford: Blackwell, 1976), esp. Chapters 9, 10 and Appendix; and to A. Feinstein, *Clinical Biostatistics* (St. Louis: Mosby, 1977). See also D.L. Sackett, "The Competing Objectives of Randomized Trials," *New England Journal of Medicine* 303 (1980), 1059–60.

have as their objectives *validity* or statistical soundness, *generalizability* or wide applicability, and *efficiency* or cost-effectiveness. In my comments I shall focus primarily on the issue of validity and its relationship to the ethics of patient care.

In part, because of biological variability, there are few completely deterministic processes or therapies that are 100 percent efficacious in medicine. In order to detect, in as rational a way as possible, those clinical procedures that might be useful, statistical reasoning must be invoked. A clinician who reasons statistically asks whether an observed pattern of patient responses can provide a valid inference for a clinically important effect at some level of probability. (Similar reasoning comes into play in the *design* of a trial.) Sound statistical methodology in a clinical trial is a sine qua non for grounded knowledge of the utility or disutility of a drug. A clinical trial of a drug that is methodologically unsound and/or statistically unconvincing will not persuade other physicians to use (or to discontinue) a particular drug.

Clinical trials, especially the large randomized ones, are essentially a post–World War II innovation. From their inception, investigators have had to wrestle with difficult ethical issues of patient assignment, risks and benefits and more recently with the complexities of informed consent. Clinical trials also illustrate the ethical conflict of the physician as researcher and the physician as therapist.

Statistical validity and the ethical dilemmas inherent in medical research coalesce in this case study. The research physicians wish to be able to conclude with "95 percent confidence that the drug would be effective in less than 15 percent of patients with this kind of tumor, and thus that this drug has little usefulness against this form of cancer." They need one more negative response to achieve these percentages, presumably the patient in question.

Little information is provided about additional features of the research design or why the 15 percent figure was chosen. Apparently this is the control percentage for currently available therapy for this type of tumor in patients at similar stages of disease. The size of the trial needed to achieve the 95 percent confidence level (or analogously a significance level or P value $\leq .05$) can be obtained from what is known as a binomial distribution. To use a loaded coin-toss analogy, the investigators have asked themselves: how many times do I have to toss a coin, which I believe in the long run will turn up heads (therapeutic successes) less than 15 percent of the time, to be sure that I will get this result ($<$ 15 percent) nineteen times out of twenty ($19/20 = 95$ percent)? More specifically, if we assume a constant run of tails (therapeutic failures), how long must the trial be? The simple binomial formula shows that for eighteen failures the desired probability is .054, whereas for nineteen failures, it becomes .045, thus crossing the "magic" threshold of "significance" or "confidence."

Significance levels of 5 percent or less and confidence regions of 95 percent or more have been adopted, often without question, by investigators and by journal editors who may not publish a trial unless the threshold is crossed. The 5 percent level is conventional but not completely arbitrary since in a normal distribution approximately 95 percent of the probability falls between +2 standard deviations from the mean. Still, some researchers, such as A. Feinstein, are critical of its dogmatic character.

These considerations underlie the case in question but do not provide any clear answer. Only additional information and ethical principles will provide the necessary guidance. The main ethical principle operative in this case—one accepted by essentially all investigators—is that no patient should be assigned to a trial if he or she and the responsible attending physician justifiably believe that harm will result. If there is another experimental drug available with more likely beneficial results, the patient should be advised of the option or options. If such a drug is not available, there is still a *higher* than 5 percent chance (actually 15 percent) that the drug currently under investigation will work in 10 percent of the cases. This chance is calculated on the basis of probability but should be adjusted to take account of other biochemical, physiological, pharmacological, and clinical information relevant to *this* patient. The attending physician should provide the patient with a summary of this complex and updated knowledge in terms the patient can understand. This summary should include a clear statement of the anticipated side effects of the drug and a report on the efficacy of the drug to date. Should the patient elect the current drug and should it not work, the investigators will have achieved their 95 percent level; but clearly a patient cannot be expected to enter such a trial to achieve "statistical significance."

39

Mrs. X and the Bone Marrow Transplant

Arthur L. Caplan

William Head, a twenty-seven-year-old leukemia patient from Louisiana, requested that a district court in Iowa intervene in his behalf with the University of Iowa Institutional Review Board (IRB). He wanted to have the board make a third effort to contact a potential bone marrow donor. The University of Iowa hospital has an experimental bone marrow transplant program in which six individuals have participated. None of the recipients of tissue from nonrelated donors has lived for more than a few months. The transplant procedure involves some inconvenience and a good deal of discomfort for the donor.

Mr. Head himself contacted the various medical centers around the United States doing research on bone marrow transplantation among nonrelated donors in order to determine whether a suitable donor existed. In a telephone call a technician informed him, without authorization, that a possible matching donor did exist in the computer files at the University of Iowa. Mr. Head then requested that the institution contact the individual about the possibility of aiding him by a transplant.

His request was referred to the IRB at Iowa. After long deliberation about the rights of subjects to consent voluntarily and without coercion, the IRB decided to send a letter to the prospective donor—"Mrs. X." She is a California woman whose records had been included in the computer data because she had been tissue-typed as a possible donor for her three-year-old son, who later died of leukemia.

The letter described the program in general terms and was accompanied by three newspaper articles describing successful bone marrow transplants among related donors. When Mrs. X did not respond to this letter, the IRB chair followed up with a telephone call restating the general request. Mrs. X said that she had understood but was not willing to participate as a donor unless "it was for a relative."

Mr. Head was informed of her decision, at which point he retained a lawyer and went to court. He wanted the court to compel the IRB to try once more to recruit Mrs. X by telling her that a specific patient might be helped by her donation. What should the court's decision be? How should Mr. Head's need for this experimental procedure be balanced against the need to protect the interests of the potential donor?

COMMENTARY

Charles W. Lidz, Alan Meisel, and Loren H. Roth

This is a complex case with many issues to weigh, but the court clearly should decide against Mr. Head's request. The moral ambiguity of this case rests primarily on the fact that we do not like the outcome. While it would be much nicer if Mrs. X would simply agree to be a donor, the concept of autonomous and free choice that is embodied in the doctrine of informed consent is designed to protect her decision. We are faced with two issues. First, we must decide whether the IRB proceeded in the correct way to produce the decision; and second, whether or not the result is so wrong that we are willing to attempt to override the potential donor's decision by putting pressure on her. For there is no question that that is what Mr. Head proposes to do.

Although the primary issue in this case may seem to be the question of invading the potential donor's privacy, we believe it is actually the protection of her initial decision from harassment and pressure. Although the right to privacy is an essential principle, we frequently countenance minor violations of it in the interest of important substantive goals. Indeed, the IRB has already invaded Mrs. X's privacy (quite correctly providing her with an opportunity to behave altruistically), and another letter per se does not constitute a substantially greater invasion. Rather, the ethical difficulty with another letter from the IRB concerns its proposed contents and its consequent effect on Mrs. X's free choice.

The right to make an informed decision about what is to be done with one's body can be overridden only if the decision maker is incompetent or the decision coerced. Since neither of these exceptions apply in this case, Mrs. X presumably has the right to decide about whether to participate in the transplant. For her decision to be rational, Mrs. X must at least have access to the relevant information. Since her child had leukemia and she received information from the IRB about the research, she presumably had enough general information to make a rational choice. But is this enough? Does Mrs. X also need the further information that there is a specific individual who needs her bone marrow?

Whether such information is relevant to her decision and thus promotes rationality is debatable; but the pressure that such a letter would place on her certainly compromises her autonomy. Her statement that she would be a donor only for a relative seems perfectly clear and implies that if someone else needed her bone marrow, she would refuse. All the additional "information" would do is to engender guilty feelings about possibly being responsible for someone else's death. This type of information no longer promotes informed consent. Rather, it is a form of psychological coercion.

This raises an interesting theoretical point. We usually think of the doctrine of informed consent as requiring the disclosure of information to patients. However, if information is coercive or serves primarily to undercut the individual's ability to make a rational decision, it conflicts with the requirment that such decisions should be voluntary. In this case, the new information only turns a clear hypothetical decision into a decision which places her under substantial emotional stress. The IRB, by refusing to contact her again, acted in accordance with the spirit of federal regulations requiring efforts to "minimize coercion and undue influence" (*Federal Register* 46 [January 26, 1981], pp. 8366, 8389–90, to be codified at 45 CFR Section 46.116).

Of course, one might still argue: "Even though, in principle, Mrs. X's decision should not be tampered with, this decision would create such an unfortunate outcome that she should be contacted anyway. After all, this is a life and death matter. Against such matters, principles such as informed consent and the right to privacy seem trivial." Whatever the general merits of such ethical pragmatism, it is not an adequate argument in this case. While it is hard to deny Mr. Head any potential treatment, there is no evidence that this procedure would save his life and little evidence that it would substantially prolong it. Moreover, the procedure would be painful and a substantial inconvenience to Mrs. X.

There is one final reason for allowing the decision to stand. IRBs have been accorded responsibility for managing problems of this sort, and their institutional integrity will be maintained by respecting the decisions they render. Decisions should be overturned only if it can be clearly shown that IRBs abused their discretionary powers, failed to conduct themselves in accordance with their own procedures and those imposed upon them by law, or clearly failed to apply established substantive standards of law or medical ethics. Except under such conditions, courts should not substitute their own decisions for the IRB's. To do so would be to undermine the authority of the IRB and thereby discourage other IRBs from making hard choices.

COMMENTARY

David Zimmerman

Most of us will agree, I suspect, that it is crucial for tissue and organ banks jealously to protect the privacy of potential donors. But that is not the issue facing the court, since Mrs. X's existence (though not her identity) has already been revealed to Mr. Head. The question is whether the Iowa IRB should persist in its attempt to secure Mrs. X's cooperation, this time by informing her that there is a specific dying person whose marrow type matches hers.

I believe it would be wrong for the IRB to approach Mrs. X a second time, but only because in this case the probable benefits do not outweigh the probable harms, not because it is a case of coercion or because rights would be violated. Of course, if the facts were substantially different—if the probability that the marrow transplant would succeed were at least as great as it is with related donor and donee, thus shifting the cost-benefit calculus—I might well encourage the IRB to try again.

If the approach were made and Mrs. X were to agree to serve as a donor, then she would suffer considerable inconvenience and discomfort; and if she were to refuse to serve, then she might well suffer some psychological discomfort at refusing aid to another human being, for example, pangs of conscience. But even though life itself is far weightier than mere inconvenience and discomfort (physical or psychological), the probability that Mr. Head will be helped by the operation seems to be so vanishingly low, and the probability of harm to Mrs. X so palpably high, whatever she decides to do, that the expected benefits of making the second approach are far lower than the expected harms.

Many would argue this case in another way, including, even stressing, the moral relevance of considerations other than probable harms and benefits—rights, for example, or justice and fairness. I am not among them.

It is not that I believe in the adequacy of an exclusively utilitarian approach to moral questions: such an approach often leaves out crucial moral considerations. But I do not believe that there are any weighty rights in this case or considerations of fairness to be balanced against considerations of probable consequence. Why do others feel differently? Perhaps they believe that a second approach by the IRB would be coercive. After all, Mrs. X has already been approached once (twice, if we count the original letter and follow-up telephone call separately), and has made clear her unwillingness to serve as a marrow donor to someone unrelated. Any further approaches, they feel, would involve coercion, or at least unfair pressure.

But I find it hard to see this as a case of coercion; and if it is a case of pressure, then it is hard to see it as unfair pressure. In the paradigm case of coercion the gunman says, "Your money or your life," thereby forcing his victim to choose between two disagreeable alternatives. The second approach to Mrs. X is superficially similar in that she too would face two disagreeable alternatives: to offer herself as a donor with all the attendant inconvenience and discomfort, or to refuse and perhaps suffer some degree of psychological discomfort and pangs of conscience.

But there is a significant difference: in making the second approach the Iowa IRB would neither be altering the structure of Mrs. X's choices nor attaching a negative sanction to one of them (refusing to cooperate) that was not there before, as they would be, for example, if they threatened to make public her refusal. The sanction is indeed real (we do, after all, speak about the "sanctions of conscience"), but it is not something that the Iowa IRB attaches to the choice; it is, rather, a feature of Mrs. X herself.

Some might ask: What real difference is there between attaching a sanction to a choice and informing a person that she has a choice, where this knowledge brings with it a sanction because she is the sort of person she is? At the very least, they might insist, the IRB would be pressuring Mrs. X by exploiting a certain fact about her moral psychology—a clear moral wrong.

But does the second approach involve moral pressure? It would, I suppose, if the IRB simply went back to Mrs. X with the same request; certainly if they went back many times. But they would be going back with some new information: that there is a specific recipient whose tissue matches hers. Granted, Mrs. X could have inferred this information from the general content of the first approach. But it is well known that we are typically more responsive to the plight of particular persons than to the plain knowledge that they exist.

The charge of exploitation, certainly of wrongful exploitation, seems to me similarly misplaced. The IRB would, after all, be "exploiting" Mrs. X's own vulnerability to the sanctions of moral conscience. Do we really want to hold that people ought generally to be spared the pangs of conscience? Surely not where we believe that they ought to go along with the proddings of their conscience, or at least where we believe that there is a real question whether they ought to.

But this means that we cannot determine whether the IRB would be wrongly exploiting Mrs. X's vulnerable conscience without first determining what she morally ought to do. And this in turn throws all the moral weight back on the other features of the case, most notably the probable good and bad consequences of her cooperating with the IRB or refusing to cooperate. Since my roughly utilitarian treatment of this kind of case yields the same conclusion as one that stresses rights, why bother trying to sort out the strongest *reasons* for the conclusion?

Because this is not the last time an IRB—and perhaps even the courts—will face this kind of choice, we need to identify the morally relevant considerations. What if the next time the question comes up, marrow transplants with unrelated donor and donee are more likely to succeed? For one who sees this approach to a potential donor as coercive, this might not alter the moral conclusion (if the likelihood of success is not *too* much greater). But for one who sees no significant rights at issue at all in this kind of case it will matter a great deal.

[Editor's note: The Iowa District Court for Johnson County that heard Mr. Head's case ruled that "a hospital's record of the tissue typing of a potential donor is not exempt from disclosure under section 68A.7 (2) of the Iowa Code (1983), and public records statute," and ordered the defendants to send another letter to Mrs. X. The Attorney General's office, representing the University of Iowa Hosptials and Clinics (a state-supported facility), appealed the decision to the Iowa Supreme Court. On March 28, 1983, that court reversed the decision, holding that "the statute requires the record to be kept confidential."]

40

Can a Research Subject Be Too Eager to Consent?

Lila Goldberg, age twenty-one, was admitted as a voluntary patient to the adult psychiatric service of a large university teaching hospital because she had lost thirty pounds in six months and extensive out-patient medical evaluation had failed to reveal an organic basis for the weight loss. After the diagnosis of anorexia nervosa was confirmed, the patient was placed on a high-calorie diet and a behavior modification program supplemented by individual psychotherapy.

One week after admission, Steven O'Connor, a psychiatrist affiliated with another ward, solicited Ms. Goldberg's participation in a research project that would measure the concentration of biogenic amines in the blood and spinal fluid of patients suffering from anorexia nervosa. This investigation was not intended to be of direct clinical benefit to the patient. However, the study could conceivably provide information about the presence of any underlying neurophysiological abnormalities in this disorder. Ms. Goldberg readily agreed to be a subject and signed a thorough informed consent form for the protocol, which already had institutional review board (IRB) approval. As a participant she would have blood drawn by vein several times and would undergo three lumbar (spinal) punctures—procedures that carry a high risk of discomfort and a low risk of infection.

Lila's psychiatric nurse, Sharon Miller, questioned her patient's inclusion in this study. Having observed that all anorectic patients eagerly agree to participate in studies despite discomfort and potential harm, Nurse Miller reasoned that psychiatric illness made an anorectic patient overly cooperative and thereby masochistic. The patient's willing participation in the protocol could be construed as another anorectic symptom. Dr. O'Connor countered that Ms. Goldberg was fully competent to volunteer. Should she be allowed into the study?

COMMENTARY

Spencer Eth and Cheryl Eth

Lila Goldberg, described as an adult who is not retarded, psychotic, or mentally incompetent, has voluntarily entered a hospital for treatment of her mental illness. There is apparently no hesitation accepting her consent for hospitalization, diagnostic procedures, and treatment. Unexpectedly, however, objections are raised to her participation in a research protocol. The argument is based on the peculiar nature of her illness—that anorexia nervosa causes a specific impairment of critical judgment, which greatly increases the likelihood of a variety of self-destructive behaviors.

Anorexia nervosa is a mental illness that primarily affects adolescent girls. Typically, those affected retain their intellectual abilities and can often continue to function until the illness has progressed to the point of serious medical complications. In fact, the contrast between an emaciated appearance and persistent dieting and hyperactivity may be the only clue to this potentially fatal illness.

A prominent personality feature of anorectic women is submissiveness. Many are described as "perfect children." The manifest need to be cooperative, even obedient, propels anorectics into perpetual self-sacrifice. Often the patient's life before the onset of anorexia has been a series of attempts to live up to the expectations of family and friends, along with fears that she will fail to be the "best little girl." Starvation may be the sole area in which she expresses her independence and mastery. The patient is locked into a behavior pattern (starvation) much as the alcoholic is compelled to abuse liquor despite the dreadful consequences.

In situations where the anorectic must satisfy her unconscious need for self-punishment, her capacity to act as a moral agent is diminished. Offering the anorectic an opportunity to participate in an experiment associated with discomfort is comparable to offering a heroin addict the chance to be in a morphine metabolism study. Two dangers of research are (1) probable risks or injuries to subjects that exceed anticipated benefits; (2) the possibility of injury to the person's autonomy and moral integrity. Dr. O'Connor's study clearly carries no substantive physical risk. But without additional protection anorectic patients are vulnerable to moral injury whenever they are solicited for research.

An additional safeguard is needed to supplement rather than replace the anorectic patient's own informed consent. This mechanism might operate as follows: if the anorectic declines to enter the study, her decision alone suffices. If she wishes to participate, then a concurring opinion is required prior to her acceptance.

But who shall serve in this role of patient advocate/guardian? We would eliminate some obvious choices. Local IRBs should not become involved in the mechanics of securing consent. The psychiatrist, whose duty is to provide treatment to Lila Goldberg, faces a double-agent problem of divided loyalties if he is also acting in his colleague's behalf. The patient's parents, if they are available, are usually concerned, but the psychological conflicts at work in anorexia deeply enmesh the family in the patient's illness. One alternative would be a patient representative or subject advocate appointed by the state or by the hospital. However, a much simpler solution is to turn to the professional psychiatric nurse. She possesses the minimum of a bachelor's degree in nursing and two years of psychiatric nursing experience, which should ensure knowledge of the research process, proficiency in interviewing, and the ability to assess the patient's capacity to function in the psychological, social, behavioral, and medical spheres.

The designated nurse should have no vested interest in the research project nor should she provide primary care to the patient. She could be a consultant who would interview the patient until key data were collected. If the patient wished to enter the study and the nurse determined that participation was self-destructive, the patient would be excluded. This independent veto power is analogous to the nurse's role in disapproving a psychiatric patient's pass to leave the hospital if the pass request is deemed clinically inappropriate.

This consent process does not guarantee a wise decision, but it does minimize the risk of collusion with an anorectic's self-destructive impulse. There are drawbacks—added expense and inconvenience, diminution of independent decision making, and the creation of an impediment to research—but the important advantage is that it protects the moral integrity of the patient.

COMMENTARY

Harold Edgar

In all likelihood, Ms. Goldberg should be allowed to participate in the research. Before so voting, I want to discuss the matter briefly with my IRB.

First, Ms. Goldberg has been admitted to the hospital for treatment. Presumably Dr. O'Connor, from a different ward, has consulted her physician to assure that this physician knows no reason—physical or psychological—why Ms. G should not consent. If not, Dr. O' acts wrongly. Does the IRB have a rule covering this situation? Is one needed? Is there any doubt about the impropriety of administering unnecessary spinal taps to patients for whom one is not responsible and about whom one knows almost nothing?

Second, commentators too often ignore nurses and other hospital personnel in discussions of medical ethics. They see patients more often, and in more varied circumstances, than physicians usually do. Nurse Miller, a psychiatric nurse, may be especially capable of discerning a particular patient's inability to understand and act with conventional rationality about a research protocol. Such a patient should not be asked to risk serious pain and discomfort in research not directly benefiting her. I believe lumbar punctures pose such a risk. Am I wrong?

Nurse M's objections, however, are not based on observations of Ms. G. She has developed her own theory of anorexia: *all* anorectics are willing to suffer in others' behalf, and this trait is part of their disease. She reasons further that consent produced by "disease" is not free and meaningful.

Her evidence is scant. From what we are told, it is simply that everyone says "yes" to Dr. O'. Are not other explanations of the patients' behavior much more likely? Is Dr. O' informing patients of the possible discomforts in a fair way? Researchers want potential subjects to say "yes" when asked to join an experiment. Researcher enthusiasm may be desirable, and is inevitable anyway. The policy problem is to temper enthusiasm in order to minimize unnecessary risk taking and to assure subjects a fair choice.

This responsibility now falls partly on IRBs. Few IRBs check systematically whether the research they approve is in fact understood by the patients who sign up. Should they? Broad questions about IRBs and whether there may be better ways of accomplishing their mission are beyond the scope of this commentary. As a practical matter, however, making sure that researchers do not inappropriately encourage volunteering is complex for reasons other than the difficulties inherent in policing a hospital. Briefly, a physician's confidence may be helpful to patients in many settings. Requiring a skeptical presentation can compromise a physician-patient relationship. Moreover, what is a physician to say when the patient asks for an opinion on whether to volunteer? These are problems of research on nonvalidated therapies however. In experiments such as this one patients should be told bluntly that there is no chance, or no reasonable likelihood, that undergoing the procedure will help them. Researchers sometimes shy away from such candor. Consent forms often include boiler plate statements such as "we hope this research may be of benefit to you" in circumstances where there is no such chance. More important, researchers may wrongly convey such impressions in seeking consent.

All the patients Dr. O' has approached have volunteered. Should this trigger another look at the protocol? Most IRBs do not keep track of such percentages with a view to rechecking the consent process if the level of volunteering seems out of line with our intuitions about readiness to take risks. We should be cautious, however, in assuming that everyone is against risk taking. Persons suffering from a baffling and life-threatening problem might well risk discomfort to help others similarly afflicted. Anorectic patients may have a special desire to learn that their problems have a direct biochemical cause.

The case assures us that the consent procedure is full and fair. Thus, it remains only to discuss with the IRB Nurse M's observation. Is it true in the experience of the medical members that anorectics uniformly sign up for research regardless of what it entails? The researchers I have questioned casually say that anorectics are pretty much like everyone else. Some say "yes" and some say "no" to research participation. If that is the case, there is no reason not to proceed with the research.

We presume adults' statements are legitimate signs of their preferences over a vast domain of activity, and we respect such preferences although we realize that people may not truly know what they want. Similarly, we act on the words they say recognizing that people often do not say what they mean or mean what they say.

To be sure, no rule is absolute. We disallow some preferences, and we correct for mistake and fraud in many contexts. But, there is no fraud or mistake here. Moreover, Ms. G does not fit a narrow category of persons whose ability to process information and relate it to themselves is so sharply limited that to credit their "statements" would undercut respect for the principle of autonomous choice. No claim is plausible that Ms. G's agreement is uniquely determined by a condition foreign to her character.

The mentally distressed have as vital a stake as the rest of us, if not more so, in assuring the conservative admnistration of doctrines that deny significance to individuals' statements of what they want. Surely we are not going to monitor all Ms. G's choices, and disregard whichever ones we think occasion more suffering than likely benefit. To assume that her choices in this context require a unique capacity beyond that required for everyday affairs is to elevate medicine and research to an undeserved status. To make informed consent the tool for finding such a capacity will convert it into an elaborate fiction.

41

Can a Healthy Subject Volunteer to Be Injured in Research?

Anthony Breuer

A sixty-three-year-old woman thought to be suffering from Amyotrophic Lateral Sclerosis (ALS), or Lou Gehrig's Disease, came to a major medical center for a second opinion. Here the diagnosis was confirmed. She agreed to participate in a basic research project directed at exploring cellular mechanisms that might cause ALS, a fatal disorder of the nervous system. The project had passed rigorous peer review, was funded by the National Institutes of Health, and had been approved by the Institutional Review Board of the medical center. During the informed consent interview the patient was accompanied by her sixty-five-year-old husband, a retired carpenter who was in good health.

Part of the research protocol required excision of the motor branch of the median nerve in her left (nondominant) severely afflicted hand. The patient and her husband understood that the removal of this small ALS nerve would permanently limit her ability to move her thumb with the same facility as before the biopsy, but would not affect her ability to flex or bend the distal part (phalanx) of the thumb. The patient agreed to the biopsy specifically because she wished to contribute her nerve to this research effort. She fully understood that this was not a treatment protocol and that her participation would be of no immediate benefit to her.

At the same time the patient's husband volunteered to undergo biopsy of a motor branch of his own normal median nerve to serve as an experimental control. He knew he would lose most of the function of the thumb in his left (nondominant) hand. But, he assured the physician, he was not doing carpentry and neither needed nor intended to work during his retirement. He wished to contribute to the research effort and to the understanding of his wife's disease.

The offering of a normal nerve as a control for an investigation into a fatal disease process raises a serious question for the physician/researcher. The husband, who is not the patient, is volunteering to be a research subject. Should the clinical researcher accept the offer and operate on his thumb?

COMMENTARY

Robert J. Levine

In this case there is an easy way out. A normal median nerve can be secured from an amputated arm (for example, from a patient with an osteosarcoma) or, in accord with the provisions of the Uniform Anatomical Gift Act, from a brain-dead person. In general, when we can, we should redesign research to replace a risk of injury (in this case, a 100 percent risk) with mere inconvenience.

But let us suppose that the research objectives can be achieved only by taking the motor branch of the median nerve from the hand of a healthy person. Why not? Principle 5 of the Nuremberg Code should cause us to hesitate: "No experiment should be conducted where there is an a priori reason to believe that death or disabling injury will occur except, perhaps, in those experiments where the experimental physicians also serve as subjects." Should we consider whether a neurologist could get by without motor function in his or her nondominant thumb? If so, then perhaps we can meet Nuremberg's rigorous standard.

This, however, is not the final answer. Consider Nuremberg's use of the term "disabling." Since this man does not intend to do carpentry in his retirement, he would not be disabled in the sense used by the Workers' Compensation Board. On the other hand, try tying your shoes or opening a pistachio nut without using both thumbs. Not impossible, but quite difficult. At a minimum, the prospective subject should be informed of all anticipated consequences of his offer.

Suppose the fully informed retiree still freely offered to donate his nerve. Then we must wonder if his offer is truly "free." Does he think that his offer will be rewarded by the doctors' paying special attention to his wife's needs? Does he see this as a means of expiation of some real or imagined sin against his wife? These are the sorts of concerns that informed the Declaration of Helsinki's Principle III.2: "The subjects should be volunteers—either healthy persons or patients for whom the experimental design is not related to the patient's illness." Admittedly, this is a principle that we violate daily without remorse.

We live in a society that disapproves strongly of pointless acts of self-mutilation: consider our revulsion from the self-laceration of the more extreme punk-rockers. By contrast, we generally approve heroic acts done for altruistic reasons. While a soldier is not required to hurl his body on a hand grenade to save his comrades, those who have done so have received posthumous Congressional Medals of Honor. In this context, the sacrifice of the ability to open pistachios easily may be regarded as reasonable if, in turn, one might save thousands from the scourges of Amyotrophic Lateral Sclerosis. In the absence of the urgency created by a live hand grenade, however, one should consider very carefully the conditions under which such a sacrifice could be considered permissible.

In order to justify acceptance of an offer of the sort made by this man, in addition to the general norms that guide the conduct of all research involving human subjects, the following conditions should be met: (1) The problem to be solved must be very important; the dreadful disease ALS qualifies on this count. (2) There must be strong theoretical reasons to predict that the research will make a major contribution to the solution of the problem. (3) There should be no alternative approaches to the solution of the problem which would result in lesser disability to any individual. (4) The subject should meet very high standards of comprehension and voluntariness. (5) The investigators should make a commitment to rehabilitate the subject to the extent they can with the aid of other professionals such as physical therapists; there should be no charge to the subject for the necessary therapy.

Having allowed the proverbial camel's nose under Nuremberg's tent, can we be sure that the rest of its carcass will not follow? No! Therefore, as an IRB member I would vote to disapprove this project until it was discussed and approved by an authoritative national ethical deliberative body such as the recently abolished President's Commission for the Study of Ethical Problems in Medicine and Biomedical and Behavioral Research or the Ethics Advisory Board.

COMMENTARY

George A. Kanoti

Is it ethical to agree to a person's free choice to undergo a nonreversible injury and thus compromise the principle of "Do No Harm"? Clearly the husband had no ethical obligation to participate in this research, but does he have the right to volunteer?

No overt coercion appears to be present, but there are subtle coercive elements. The husband's feeling for his wife and his frustration at the lack of knowledge about her lethal disease could lead him to consider sacrificing his own healthy nerve to advance knowledge. Since it has been only a few weeks since ALS was confirmed, the researchers should be cautious about the adequacy of the consent. The prestige of the researcher and the institution also can contribute to the decision to volunteer.

The physician is pulled by contrary obligations. On one hand, it is important to answer a medical question in a scientifially valid manner by comparing the activity in a diseased motor nerve with that of its exact normal counterpart. The availability of a perfect control would improve understanding of ALS. But the researcher also has an obligation not to produce harm. The husband is not ill, nor does he have a disability. He would suffer loss of flexibility in his thumb if the median nerve were surgically removed. This would limit his ability to grasp and hold objects in that hand. The physician also realizes that this proposal is freely volunteered. It is an opportunity that rarely presents itself. One benefit might be to the volunteer's self-esteem; that is, his sacrifice will further knowledge of this terrible disease.

Ethically, the volunteer's proposal falls within the category of an act of supererogation or altruism (above and beyond the call of duty or obligation). In applying the principle of supererogation to a specific case, one must be sensitive to the unique factors of the case. In this instance we have a retiree, a former carpenter, who obviously has used his hands in his trade. We also know that the loss of motion in the thumb is not total, but is limiting. We are not sure exactly how limiting the loss of the nerve would be on the manipulation of tools. We also have to make certain that the request is motivated by a genuine interest in advancing knowledge and not by some psychological reaction to the illness in his wife and the frustration of a lack of knowledge about the causes and cure of ALS.

The best solution would be to acknowledge the offer, request further information about the need for full use of the thumb, and advise a period of several months for both physician and husband to reevaluate the request. And, the researcher should make every effort to obtain a nerve biopsy from a brain-dead donor, perhaps as part of a transplant donation effort, during this period. If the effort to obtain an alternative nerve biopsy fails and all parties remain convinced that the choice is free and knowledgeable, the procedure can be performed.

COMMENTARY

Douglas P. Lackey

One could easily imagine an IRB rejecting this protocol. The benefits of the research are conjectural and distant; the harm is certain and immediate. The subject's consent cannot quash the general prejudice against deliberate mutilation, especially when the voluntariness of the consent is tainted by the stress of dealing with a spouse's severe illness.

No right of the carpenter would be violated by this refusal. In my experience on an IRB, I have encountered cases in which cancer patients have demanded access to experimental protocols and cases in which families of Alzheimer's patients have demanded enrollment of senile relatives in experimental regimens. In all these instances, IRBs have properly maintained that no one has a right to be an experimental subject.

Nevertheless, assuming that the research has scientific merit and that the nerve used as a control can only be obtained from a living subject, I think that the experiment should proceed.

In cost-benefit analyses of research protocols, the IRB should weigh expected costs against expected benefits, where an "expected cost" is the probability of a loss multiplied by its severity. No special moral weight should be given to a loss the probability of which happens to be 100 percent. (Likewise no loss should be dismissed as negligible merely because its probability is low.) There is a common psychological tendency to prefer a greater expected loss of low probability to a lesser expected loss of very high probability. This tendency is irrational and should be resisted in the formation of policy.

Far from impugning the validity of the carpenter's consent, I would give it relatively high weight. Many prospective experimental subjects, reading the list of possible side effects, reason that since the side effects have low probability, they will not occur. On this assumption they volunteer for the experiment. This amounts to rating the expected disvalue of their improbable side effects as zero, a certifiable mistake in moral mathematics. (Across thousands of experiments, some subjects who say "it won't happen to me" must be mistaken.) The carpenter cannot be making this mistake, since he knows for sure what is in the bargain. His consent to mutilation is at least as informed and rational as the consent subjects commonly give to experiments that have improbable but catastrophic side effects.

There is a tendency among researchers and many IRB members to regard people with medical problems as morally ideal subjects for research on those problems, even when the prospect that the research will produce therapy for these subjects is nil. ("They have an investment in the disease," I have heard it said.) On the other hand, the participation of normal subjects, who have no investment in the disease, is viewed as altruism verging on the irrational. There is relatively little resistance to using severely ill Alzheimer's patients as subjects in Alzheimer's research, despite the logical tangles of proxy consent. But the carpenter's sacrifice will be seen as abnormal and will be referred to journals as a problem in medical ethics.

I think that philosophers should be the last to assume that all action not directly linked to self-interest must be dismissed as irrational. The carpenter's desire to find some way to share his wife's fate is rooted in feelings, but these feelings are at the center of human life. For the bureaucracy to block this attempt on moral grounds would be a most inhumane application of humanistic ethics.

42

Transplanting a Chimpanzee Heart

A heart transplantation team at a major urban teaching hospital invariably has more candidates for heart transplantation than hearts available to transplant. The program is known to benefit both low-risk and high-risk patients. Nevertheless, 30 percent of the candidates die before a heart becomes available. Members of the transplant team, who are both medical practitioners and scientific researchers, consider alternative sources of organs and decide upon the hearts of chimpanzees.

The researchers realize that they are entering upon relatively uncharted waters, despite the close evolutionary link between human beings and chimpanzees. However, they have previously performed a series of preparatory experiments transplanting hearts between cynomolgus monkeys and baboons. Though all the hearts were ultimately rejected due to the incompatibility of the two species' tissue types, there was temporary survival—an average of eleven weeks—sufficient to "buy time" for potential transplant recipients.

If the analogy between monkey/baboon and chimpanzee/human being holds, the chimpanzee heart could serve as a temporary "bridge" to a human heart, if and when one becomes available. For various reasons, medical and otherwise, the transplant team considers the chimpanzee heart preferable, as a bridge, to an artificial, mechanical heart. Moreover, it is possible that the chimpanzee heart could become a permanent replacement, if problems of immunological rejection could be overcome. Still further, this experiment might lead to scientific knowledge allowing the use of other types of animal hearts, for example, those of pigs or cows. This would solve—practically, if not ethically—the chronic problem of the insufficient supply of transplantable hearts.

Confounding this possible human benefit and heady medical technology are certain inexorable facts. Chimpanzees are an endangered species. There are about 100,000 chimpanzees left in the world and about 2,500 in captivity in the United States. International trade in chimpanzees is banned, breeding in captivity is difficult, and capture of wild chimpanzees is "inefficient" in terms of preserving individual lives. For every wild chimpanzee captured and delivered to its destination, as many as ten other chimpanzees die.

Moreover, captive chimpanzees are much in demand for other forms of scientific and medical research. Finally, the scientific merits of using chimpanzees in research and particularly in this medical therapy carry a correlative ethical albatross. Can we, for such a purpose, ethically justify the use of such a complex and elaborate form of animal life, in several behavioral activities so close to our human selves?

Should the transplantation team go ahead with its experiment? Should the project be approved by the institution's Institutional Review Board (IRB) and Institutional Animal Care and Use Committee (IACUC)?

COMMENTARY

Strachan Donnelley

If the transplant team is embarking upon uncharted waters, the ethicists are in the same boat. There seem to be no adequate or widely accepted ethical principles with which to decide this case. We should perhaps immediately ascribe to Socratic wisdom and state frankly that we know that we do not know. Yet I think we can make some headway and point to the problems that we need to resolve.

There are numerous ethical issues surrounding this xenograft—the trans-species transplant of a chimpanzee heart into a human being. The IRB must struggle with the problem of what would constitute adequate informed consent for this unprecedented "innovative therapy" or experiment. Both the IRB and the IACUC must satisfy themselves that the medical professionals/researchers are fulfilling the ethics of good science—that the preparatory experiments were sound and that there is a reasonable expectation of good results—both for the human research subjects/patients and for the advancement of significant scientific knowledge. However, the latter question is intricately tied up with perhaps the most difficult and interesting ethical issue—this particular use of chimpanzees in scientific research and medicine.

A singular virtue of this case in animal ethics is that it bypasses the usual ethical concern with animal pain and suffering and focuses directly on the issue of the ethically legitimate and illegitimate uses of animals for human purposes. This issue hinges crucially on the relative moral status of human beings and the various species of animal life. If one tends toward extreme positions, there is no ethical dilemma. If animals have no moral status and are not objects of moral concern, we can freely use them for our own purposes (e.g., as supplying hearts as "bridges" to human hearts). If we accord chimpanzees a moral status near, if not equal. to our own, we should prohibit their use in most, if not all, painful or ethically harmful research and certainly in this particular experiment.

However, if we tend to neither extreme, but consider chimpanzees as important objects of concern, though of less ethical significance than human beings, then things become decidedly less simple. We are confronted with ultimate questions about our status in the overall scheme of the world and about our proper relation to nature and the realm of animal life. Concerning all this, there is no philosophic or ethical consensus, though I would argue for a fundamental ecological perspective and a conception of man as within nature.

From such a perspective, animal individuals and communities of individuals are understood to be essentially interconnected. Individual animal lives are lived out on various species-specific levels of activity, some more complex, elaborate, and, thus, ethically significant than others. Organic, worldly "activity" is taken to be the "ultimate good," and thus the fundamental focus of ethical concern. Our final ethical duty is therefore the protection of the ongoing realm of life as a whole, with its various interlocked levels of animate being. Our penultimate ethical duty is concern for finite and mortal individual lives (the concrete instances of life), relative to their unequal status of ethical significance.

According to this philosophically speculative and tentative position, it would be unethical to use chimpanzees for merely therapeutic purposes—that is, to use individual chimpanzees for the sake of individual human beings. Given the open-ended demand for "bridge hearts," this already endangered species of richly significant life would soon be extinct. Human life would remain finite, mortal, and vulnerable to all the vicissitudes of worldly, metabolic existence, while the particular and complex goodness of chimpanzee being would have vanished from the world. The ethical costs of such human self-concern, both for human beings and for the animal kingdom as a whole, seem unjustifiable.

However, if this procedure were deemed a potentially significant scientific experiment that in no way threatened the presence of "chimpanzee being" in animate nature, then it might be ethically justifiable. If there was the real potentiality of the use of animal hearts of nonendangered species (e.g., pigs or cows), if we deemed this an ethically appropriate use of individual animal lives, and if the chimpanzee experiments were crucial to the possible realization of this novel therapy, we could ethically justify the use of a limited number of chimpanzees—if this were an adequate allocation of a very scarce animal research resource and if we satisfied the ethical demands of experimentation on human research subjects.

These are all very big "ifs." Ethical caution should here carry the first word, in the face of parochial human self-interests and medical technological hubris. However, a possible ethical justification could be based on the intrinsic goodness of organic, worldly activity and the varying ethical significance of different levels of animate being. This, of course, would be to ascribe to a substantive speculative vision of the world. Yet this seems the fate of all ethical positions—that they are ultimately based in some particular metaphysics.

COMMENTARY

Willard Gaylin

Following the wisdom of the Queen of Hearts ("Sentence first—verdict afterwards") I will start with my conclusions. Although trees may have standing, animals have no "rights." In the world of morality—as in the world of politics—the animate (and the inanimate) exist, are valued, respected, esteemed, judged, considered, dealt with or destroyed, all in service of the purposes and interests of humankind.

This position has in the past been attacked as being unfairly anthropocentric. I acknowledge my bias, although I would point out to critics that the position was most firmly established in the religious tradition of the Old Testament and confirmed in that same tradition by such modern philosophers as Kant. With the inherent self-confidence of his Lutheran morality, Kant said, "The first time he [man] ever said to the sheep, 'Nature has given you the skin you wear for my use, not for yours,' . . . he became aware of the way in which his nature privileged and raised him above all animals." We stand above the general animal host.

I oppose the attribution of rights to animals because I fear it diminishes the special status of Homo sapiens. The respect for human beings demands a dignity granted our species beyond any qualitative comparison with others. We are *sui generis*. We also pay a price. This unique nature imposes a special moral obligation on our species, which is why only we human beings are able, and willing, to agonize about other species.

There is no way to defend or argue the special dignity of humankind within the brief context of a case history. But even within the severity of my position the case of the chimpanzee hearts raises moral dilemmas. It *is* directly within the purposes of humankind to treat animals with compassion, empathy, sensitivity, and understanding; to have reverence for those common qualities we share with the higher primates; and to be aware that with the mutability of our nature the way we honor and revere other creatures and other things will define the degree to which we have been true to our humanity. If human nature is so perverted as to be indifferent to suffering and blind to beauty, what is left of that nature is no longer "human"—therefore not worthy of its special role in the moral universe.

This does not mean that living things may not command respect. But all animals are not created equal. This is recognized implicitly in the Animal Welfare Act. In this act "animal" is defined as "warm-blooded animal." As Sarah Swenson has noted, the word "animal" itself is here defined in anthropocentric terms of the animal's usefulness/relationship to human beings, rather than by criteria such as intelligence or biological complexity.

Some animals have less value than inanimate structure; some animals have negative value. I do not grieve for the destruction of T. pallidum, that beautiful and delicate spiral organism that is the cause of human syphilis. To destroy this entire species would be a blessing, whereas if someone were to blow up the Grand Tetons or willfully destroy Botticelli's "Primavera," a greater moral crime would have been committed through the destruction of these inanimate "things."

Nonetheless, this case is a difficult one. Heart transplantation is not necessarily my highest priority of research in this period of limited resources. But in this specific case it deals with the survival of children which, indeed, is high on my priorities. However, it places at risk that creature most nearly human, and therefore most worthy of respect, the chimpanzee.

To debate the principles, beyond the case history, let us now not concern ourselves with the value of heart transplants, or other specifics of the current state of scientific knowledge. Let us assume a valuable and available technology, and go straight to the heart of the moral dilemma.

Chimpanzees have enormous charm, sensitivity, great intelligence and a strong kinship with humanity. Should this be sacrificed for human ends—and with what limits? The implicit issue evolves into the following dilemmas: Given a promising or proven procedure would you sacrifice a chimpanzee for a trivial human need? I suspect most of us would not. Would you sacrifice a chimpanzee for a child's life? I suspect most of us would. Would you sacrifice the entire species of chimpanzees for the entire species of Homo sapiens? I suspect most of us would. And now finally the hard question. Would you risk sacrificing the species of chimpanzees to relieve the pain and suffering and premature death of many children? Here, I, at least, emphatically would. Others would not.

Our current understanding of anthropology is replete with the suggestion of humanoid species—higher than the chimpanzees—which have died out for unknown causes of climate or competition. Such is the "cruelty" or actually the moral indifference of nature. It is only with the introduction of human sensibility, human empathy, and human contacts for identification that we—alone among creatures—consider the "rights" of other species. It is the nobility of the human being that some of our misguided members might sacrifice their own children for the preservation of a kindred, living creature. I am pleased for the presence of such advocates (they honor our species) even while I reject their sentimentalities. I am, however—even with my coarser sensibilities as expressed by my willingness to sacrifice the chimpanzee—still, I hope, within the limits of decency that define that glorious discontinuity—Homosapiens.

Selected Bibliography

Part IV: Living Subjects Research

Annas, George J., Glantz, Leonard H., and Katz, Barbara F. *Informed Consent to Human Experimentation: The Subject's Dilemma.* Cambridge, MA: Ballinger Publishing Co., 1977.

Barber, Bernard. *Informed Consent in Medical Therapy and Research.* New Brunswick, NJ: Rutgers University Press, 1980.

Beecher, H.K. "Ethics and Clinical Research." *New England Journal of Medicine* 274 (1966): 1354–60.

Fried, Charles. *Medical Experimentation: Personal Integrity and Social Policy.* New York: American Elsevier, 1974.

Jones, James H. *Bad Blood: The Tuskegee Syphilis Experiment.* New York: Free Press, 1981.

Katz, Jay, Capron, Alexander M., and Glass, Eleanor S., eds. *Experimentation with Human Beings: The Authority of the Investigator, Subject, Professions, and State in the Human Experimentation Process.* New York: Russell Sage Foundation, 1972.

Levine, Robert J. *Ethics and Regulation of Clinical Research,* 2nd ed. Baltimore: Urban and Schwarzenberg, 1986.

National Commission for the Protection of Human Subjects of Biomedical and Behavioral Research. *The Belmont Report: Ethical Principles and Guidelines for Protection of Human Subjects of Research.* DHEW (OS) 78–0012. Bethesda, MD: US Government Printing Office, 1978.

President's Commission for the Study of Ethical Problems in Medicine and Biomedical and Behavioral Research. *Protecting Human Subjects: The Adequacy and Uniformity of Federal Rules and Their Implementation.* Washington, DC: US Government Printing Office, 1981.

Regan, Tom. *The Case For Animal Rights.* Berkeley: University of California Press, 1983.

Rowan, Andrew N. *Of Mice, Models, and Men: A Critical Evaluation of Animal Research.* Albany: State University of New York Press, 1984.

PART FIVE

Mental Incompetence

INTRODUCTION

While decision making is difficult enough for the competent person, as the cases in the previous parts have shown, decision making for an incompetent person—one who lacks the mental capacity to understand the situation and to make informed choices—presents clinicians and ethicists with a range of troubling questions. The ethical principle of beneficence—to protect the welfare of others—supports interventions that might offer improvement in the quality of the incompetent person's life. However, another important ethical principle—that of respect for persons—supports an acceptance of a person's wishes to control basic aspects of life, whether or not that may be perceived by others as the best choice.

The cases in the first section—"Involuntary Treatment"—pose these dilemmas in their sharpest form. Depriving a person of the freedom to live in society or forcing him or her to undergo medical treatment are among the most extreme forms of control that society can impose. But, when faced with a person who is demonstrably unable to make rational decisions, what should clinicians and judges do? These cases discuss that dilemma in the context of neurological and psychiatric treatment and involuntary commitment of the homeless.

Just as troubling are the cases in the second section—"Decisions on Behalf of the Incompetent." Is sterilization of a severely retarded child in her interest or largely in the interests of her caretakers? Should the interests of others weigh heavily in that decision? And, on a policy level, if a sheltered workshop for mentally retarded clients can serve only a certain number, should its programs be designed for long-term benefit of a few or the short-term benefit of many?

These cases demonstrate the difficulties of making decisions for vulnerable persons who deserve respect for their individual worth but who also deserve the benefits of life, insofar as is possible, available to their fellow human beings.

INVOLUNTARY TREATMENT

43

"Ain't Nobody Gonna Cut on My Head!"

A fifty-six-year-old farmer, accompanied by his wife, consulted the Neurology Service of Veterans' Hospital because of memory difficulty. For two years the patient had been having increasing trouble with technical aspects of farming. More recently he had been talking about his brother George as if he were alive although he had died two years earlier. He gave his own age as 48 and the year as "1960, pause . . . er, no, l970." Examination revealed that the patient walked with a wide-based gait (a standard sign of brain pathology) and decreased cerebral function but was otherwise normal. The patient had no difficulty with simple coin problems and could repeat six digits.

Pleading pressing business, the patient declined hospitalization to determine the cause of his decreasing cerebral function. His wife tried to persuade him to enter the hospital, but when the resident suggested that she might assume guardianship for her husband through court action she declined.

Six months later the patient's condition had worsened. Through the urging of the county agent the patient had leased most of his farmland to his neighbors and now did no work. His gait had become so wide-based that acquaintances mistakenly thought him inebriated. He urinated in his pants about once a week, and recently seemed not to care. He sat watching television all day, but never paid any attention to the program content.

Examination at this time showed an apparently alert man without speech difficulty but with considerable mental deterioration. The patient gave his age as thirty-eight, the year as 1949, the president as Eisenhower, and the location as a drug store in his home town. He failed to recognize the name Lyndon Johnson, but upon hearing the name John F. Kennedy he spontaneously volunteered knowledge of his assassination. The patient could not subtract 20 cents from a dollar but could name the number of nickels in a quarter. He could recite the months of the year and could upon request from his wife give fairly long quotations from the Bible.

The resident and the attending physician urged hospitalization. They told the patient they would evaluate him for treatable causes of mental deterioration and memory deficit. In view of his wide-based gait and urinary incontinence in association with dementia, it was likely he had occult hydrocephalus. It was explained that this disorder caused decreased mental abilities by interference with absorption of cerebrospinal fluid. The mental deterioration in these patients is partially (as in his case now) or completely (as in his case six months ago when first seen) reversible. The treatment is to place a plastic tube through the skull to drain the cerebrospinal fluid from the brain to the vascular system; this was explained to the patient with diagrams. The patient immediately rejected the surgery, summarizing his thoughts with these exact words: "Ain't nobody gonna cut on my head." The patient's wife again attempted to persuade the patient to accept hospitalization and, if tests confirmed the clinical impression, surgery. The attending physician argued to the wife that the patient did not have the mental competence to decide his own fate and the wife should become the patient's legal guardian through court action and force hospitalization. The wife politely but vigorously rejected this course of action, pointing out that in her family the husband made all important decisions.

The resident and the attending physician differed in opinions at this point. The resident thought the patient should be followed in the outpatient clinic until he perhaps changed his mind. The resident pointed out that though the patient had decreased mental abilities he still retained enough intelligence to decide his own fate. The attending physician wished for court action to make the patient the ward of one of his relatives or, if necessary, the temporary ward of the hospital, and to force hospitalization and therapy.

COMMENTARY

James M. Gustafson

The principal substantive moral issue in this case is the status of the right of the patient to determine his own bodily destiny. He refuses to consent to a procedure which is likely to relieve his disability, though apparently he understands in lay terms what is involved in the surgery. At his level of competence he is "informed," but he refuses to give "consent."

The principle of informed consent is based upon one moral assumption and upon one philosophical judgment. The moral assumption is that individuals have a right to refuse treatment even when in the judgment of others that treatment is in the patient's own best interests. A person has a right to determine his or her own destiny. The ground of this assumption is historically located in the libertarian tradition of Western culture; it stems from the same tradition that values civil liberties, that believes that the state exists properly only on the basis of the consent of the governed, and so forth. The philosophical justification for the individual's right to self-determination has been made in various ways: the right is "natural"; capacity for self-determination is what makes humans distinctive as a species and from this is derived both its value and the right; individual rights are conferred by God; excessive incursion on self-determination leads to repression and in turn to social unrest, and for this reason the right is to be protected.

The serious philosophical judgment on which the principle of informed consent is based is that persons actually have a capacity to determine their own destinies. Every case of this sort opens the historic debate about "free will" if the case is carried beyond the immediate clinical circumstances.

This case can be analyzed on the basis of two questions which follow from the two previous paragraphs. 1) Are there *moral* grounds for exerting persuasive, or legal and coercive, measures to override this man's presumed right of self-determination? Do his obligations to his family and to the community (or, to make the point in a weaker way, do the interests of his family and the community) provide a sufficient basis for intervention without his consent? How one would answer this question would depend upon the status of the right of self-determination in relation to the claims of communities (his family, the neighbors, etc.) to limit and even override that right. 2) Are this man's capacities to judge rationally and to act in accordance with a rational judgment impaired by his illness to the extent that he cannot properly exercise his moral right to self-determination? Is he, to use the common term, really "competent?" Does his impairment provide "excusing conditions" so that just as he is not held accountable for his wide gait, so he is not accountable for his rejection of the proposed therapy? Given the assumption of "free will" in the consent procedure, can his will be judged to be "less free" than is necessary and sufficient to make a sound judgment? The attending physician could justify his "wish" for court action on the basis of either or both of the matters raised by these questions.

In this case I would argue in favor of the attending physician's "wish." My principal argument would be on the basis of the patient's limited capacities to exercise his right of self-determination. Note that an empirical judgment about those limits is involved. A hypothesis (and that is all it is) would be required to support the argument, namely, if this man's capacities were not so impaired he would consent to the surgery. Procedurally, I would support the steps taken in the report of the case; that is, first seeking voluntary consent of the patient, then of his family, and only as a last resort seeking a court order. I am prepared also, however, to argue that this man has obligations to his family and to the community that he ought to take into account in making his own judgment. His failure to consent is, it appears, costly to others; others are dependent upon him and, thus, also have a claim on him to consent to a procedure that would permit him to fulfill his duties to them. Procedurally, if such a line of argument failed to persuade him, and then his family, there would be a moral justification for court action. At the base of my conviction here is a significant qualification of the individual libertarian tradition in the direction of a more "social" view of persons and of duties and obligations of persons to other individuals and to communities.

COMMENTARY

Francis C. Pizzulli

At first blush, the attending physician presents a fairly convincing case for initiating state intrusion into the patient's brain. As the title of the case implies, the proffered therapy is fairly characterized as "brain surgery" and thus avoids categorization as "psychosurgery," replete with its politically value-laden premise of experimental treatment for the purpose of controlling socially deviant behavior. If, indeed, the preliminary diagnosis of occult hydrocephalus is sound, the operation would be tailored to rectify an accepted organic brain pathology. Though this entails the concomitant effect of controlling aberrant behavior (e.g., urinary maintenance and dementia), the presence of excess cerebrospinal fluid calls into play a well-defined medical/disease model which makes less persuasive the need to inquire into the motives of the physician as a check against the potential transmogrification of psychiatrists into thought-controllers.

If one were to accept the physician's evaluation of the mental incompetency of the patient, coerced institutionalization and treatment could be defended on a number of grounds. The procedure is relatively non-intrusive; to wit, it is a safe, non-experimental operation which involves no destruction of brain tissue and is intended to control behavior that ranks rather low on the continuum of volitional and autonomous functions. Not only is this intrusion minimal, but an array of humanitarian and utilitarian impulses militate for intervention. Does not the state have a moral obligation to the patient's former self to restore it? Or an obligation to construct a new self for the person, at which point he would be released to exercise his autonomy to its fullest potential? And would not this restoration to optimal functionality redound to the benefit of his family and community?

Even if we were to assume the patient's competency, the cost of overriding his competent judgment would be measured in terms of a single interference with personal autonomy at a particular time, presumably to be outweighed by the personal and social interest in a long-term increase in autonomy achieved by effective treatment.

Is there a decisive rebuttal to the physician's benevolent despotism? From a traditional legal perspective the case for involuntary commitment (i.e., enforced hospitalization) in this instance is rather weak. There is no mention of antisocial activities by the patient, which would warrant a finding of "dangerousness to others." To say that occasional urinary incontinence and mindless fixation upon the boob tube—behavioral traits found in many "normal" persons—constitute dangerousness to oneself reflects a most extreme paternalistic bias.

Even if the criteria for involuntary commitment are met, the case against intervention by no means falls. We cannot conclude that because an individual may no longer be competent to care for himself generally (e.g., due to memory deterioration), he is thereby incompetent to pass informed judgment upon such an intrusion as the proposed organic therapy. The notion of limited competency, besides having legal recognition, is rooted in the empirical observation that certain mental illnesses do not completely obliterate a person's ability to make decisions. While the patient may no longer recall dates and ages, it is hard to envision how memory deficit can totally discredit the capacity to understand the consequences of an operation, and to immediately summarize the resident's explanation and conclude with a refusal, as the patient has done. Even if we were to adopt the simplistic view that there is no competency where the refusal only occurred because of the mental deterioration, there is no evidence to indicate that the patient is other than strongly individualistic, and would not have decided likewise prior to the onset of deterioration. Moreover, the competent spouse's concurrence in his decision might be construed as evidence of agreement with his lifelong views on brain surgery.

To respond to the invocation of a classic Benthamite calculus that would override limited, albeit informed, judgment to refuse therapy, we might profitably view the case from a rule-utilitarian perspective. While it may be true in this particular case that only a minimally intrusive operation is needed to arrest mental deterioration and partially restore memory function, we should ask what the consequences would be of a practice of substituting the state's judgment for individual informed consent in order to achieve the incremental gain in utility involved in curing those who suffer from marginal mental impairment. Is it too far-fetched to conclude that the result would be a society in which democratic values of personal autonomy, freedom, and privacy would be subjugated to the ideal of state control over various kinds of behavior?

There is one final barrier to coerced surgery, assuming for the sake of argument that there are grounds for civil commitment and that the patient does not have the limited competency to give informed refusal to treatment. Shall the next-of-kin be designated as the proxy, with the power to give or withhold consent? To argue in the negative, because it is suspected the spouse will only rubber-stamp the incompetent's decision, conflicts with the legal presumption of identity of interests among kin. Likewise, to propose a third-party guardian who will rubber-stamp the physician's decision, on the ground that it will enhance the well-being of the patient and his family, arrogates to the physician the right to define that well-being, instead of allowing it to be defined within the privacy of the family.

In sum, only a highly paternalistic society could tolerate the intrusions upon autonomy and privacy that would flow from a practice of coercion in cases such as that at hand.

44

The Woman Who Died in a Box

One frigid January day Rebecca Smith, age sixty-one, was found dead of hypothermia in her makeshift home—a cardboard box covered by a rug—on a New York City street. The Red Cross had reported her unusual living arrangements to the police two weeks earlier. Social workers had visited her, offering food and help in moving to a city shelter. A mobile unit designed to help geriatric patients had approached her. A psychiatrist had visited her and declared her an "endangered adult," part of the procedure that would have allowed the authorities to hospitalize her under seventy-two-hour protective custody. But before the order could be carried out—the first time the city had attempted its implementation—Rebecca Smith died.

Before she joined the ranks of New York's homeless street people, Rebecca Smith had lived a rather different life. One of a family of thirteen children in

Virginia, she had graduated from Hampton Institute as valedictorian. But she was hospitalized as a schizophrenic for ten years and underwent electroshock therapy. When she was released from the hospital, her daughter said, she was a changed woman.

In 1959 Mrs. Smith came to New York to live with her sister and then entered a mental hospital in Long Island. She was later released from the institution and decided to strike out on her own. That meant living on public assistance, taking Thorazine, and going to a medical clinic. In 1981 she failed to appear for recertification interviews with social workers and from then on—until her death—she lived on the streets.

Could Rebecca Smith's death have been prevented? How far do society's obligations extend toward those who are in need but who refuse to conform? Does society have different obligations to intervene in protecting those it considers mentally ill?

COMMENTARY

Kim Hopper

On March 19 this year [1982], I joined a hundred others across from the White House in a memorial service for the homeless poor who had died on the streets of six American cities this winter. Forty crosses were driven into the ground of Lafayette Park, joining over 500 already in place, the reported toll of the last five years or so in eleven cities. As it happened, the name on the cross I carried, the name I shouted out in the bright sunshine that day, was Rebecca Smith.

Rebecca Smith's death has drawn much more attention than her life ever did; it has been the subject of two editorials in the *New York Times,* another in the *Washington Post,* and of several commentaries on local TV news. But listen for a moment to the words of Betty Higden in Dickens's *Our Mutual Friend*: "You pray that your Granny may have the strength enough left her at the last . . . to get up from the bed and run and hide herself, and sworn to death in a hole, sooner than fall into the hands of those Cruel Jacks we read of, that dodge and drive, and worry and weary, and scorn and shame, the decent poor" (cited by Steven Marcus, "Their Brothers' Keepers," 1978).

What little we know of Rebecca Smith's life suggests that she may well have read about, and directly encountered, "Cruel Jacks" in the course of her institutionalized life. Mental hospitals were forbidding places in the 1950s and 1960s, and patients often fared as badly there as the "decent poor" had a century earlier in England.

There is a danger in discussing Rebecca Smith's death—that it will be taken for more than it should be, as emblematic of a general refusal of assistance on the part of the homeless. From there, it is a small step to reviving the stale myth that the legions of the homeless poor on our streets are there because they choose to be. The recent history of New York's sheltering efforts suggests otherwise.

Since the *Callahan v. Carey* suit* was filed in October 1979, more than 1700 new emergency shelter beds have been provided by New York City. All were filled this winter. An additional 175 homeless men and women avail themselves each night of the twenty-four-hour drop-in facilities at the Moravian Church and Olivieri Center. Dozens more found respite this past winter, courtesy of the churches and synagogues that opened their doors to the wandering poor. Did these people materialize out of thin air? Or, as appears to be the case, were most of them making their way wretchedly until a more decent option presented itself?

It is difficult to attribute the recent surge in the sheltered population to more rational behavior by the homeless. If anything, observers agree that recent recipients of shelter have more tenuous mental health than traditional clients of the public shelters. The decisive difference appears to be the range of options offered the homeless poor: as that range has increased, so has their demonstrated willingness to come in out of the cold. It takes some flexibility, a modicum of decency, and respect for the heightened sense of self-protection that life on the streets can breed. It takes patience—but that is all.

But exceptions do occur. We don't know exactly what Rebecca Smith was offered, or what she understood the offer to be. A lot of people tried, but there was neither world enough nor time. City attorneys waited until a Friday afternoon to file papers in court, assuring inattention for another two days. Does that imply misgivings about their own resolve? This was, after all, the maiden application of the Protective Services Law. The process has since been streamlined to minimize gratuitous delays. Thus, several people may subsequently have been spared death by exposure. Clearly, once the protection of due process is secured, it is a civil obligation to take emergency action to save from imminent death one who is unaware of the peril.

But in the unforgiving light of hindsight, more than "what should have been done" is illuminated. Private shelters are filled with wary, once-desperate men and women who formerly saw no alternative to the degradation and danger of the public shelters than to live apart from them and to die decently when that failed. Betty Higden would have been one:

> Comprehending that her strength was quitting her, and that the struggle of her life was almost ended, she could neither reason out the means of getting back to her protectors, nor even form the idea. The overmastering dread, and the proud stubborn resolution it engendered in her to die undegraded, were the two distinct impressions left in her failing mind.

Betty Higden's prayer—"to die undegraded"—was heard. She died, alone and unseen, by the roadside one night, the money to pay for her burial sewn

*This class action suit successfully argued that conditions in the public shelters for men were so dangerous, dirty, and degrading as to constitute a genuine deterrent to their use by homeless men. It was settled in August 1981 by means of a negotiated consent decree that not only recognized a legal right to shelter but also established certain qualitative standards that public shelters must henceforth meet.

into her gown. There is a defiant dignity in such a death, one that refuses to exonerate a society inured to her suffering. It was as if she had demanded, not justice at last, but injustice consistently applied. There were to be no eleventh-hour "heroics," no final capitulation to the indignity of a pauper's death. This recognition, that even the desperately poor may prize self-respect above a forced and servile dependency, should arrest easy ruminations about "what should have been done."

Rebecca Smith's is not a "right to die" case, anymore than Betty Higden's was. It is rather an object lesson in how comfortably we tolerate routine misery and how quickly we will pounce to sequester evidence of that fact.

Of course, there is an out. One could argue that others have found their way to refuge before death, that it needn't be shameful, and that were more decent shelter available, Rebecca Smith might not have had to die to force the issue. But to raise the question of intervention only at the hour of her death is seriously to cheapen the worth of her life.

COMMENTARY

Nicholas N. Kittrie

Despite my continuing concern for the excesses of the "therapeutic state"—which has permitted involuntary sterilization, lobotomies, electroshock, and indeterminate incarceration for those suffering from mental illness, while forbidding these procedures to be applied to convicted criminals—I believe that New York has failed in its duty toward Rebecca Smith. This conclusion follows from general principles of enlightened jurisprudence, which are applicable community-wide, regardless of the psychiatric status of Rebecca Smith or the mental illness laws of New York.

The balance between personal autonomy and communal responsibility is difficult to strike. Excessive stress on autonomy is likely to reinforce individualism, but also to introduce alienation and community disintegration. Emphasis on communal responsibility, on the other hand, while strengthening collective bonds, could result in paternalism and possibly even in authoritarian suppression. Different societies strike the balance differently. While American jurisprudence, in its commitment to liberty, has not usually articulated "Good Samaritan" laws for the community or individual citizens, both the Italian and French Penal Codes specify penalties for "any person who neglects to afford the necessary assistance" to a "person wounded or otherwise in danger."

One may doubt the desirability or effectiveness of decreeing that an individual citizen become a Good Samaritan under the penalty of criminal law or of interfering with an individual's voluntary exposure to danger—including motorcycle riding, smoking, or sky diving. Yet one can readily concede the importance of communal efforts on behalf of those who appear to be *involuntarily* stranded or in danger.

Rebecca Smith was exposed to evident, continuing, and increasing danger on the public streets of New York. Suppose she had stepped into the middle of oncoming traffic. Would the state agencies have felt the need for a complex and time-consuming procedure to remove her to safety? Would it have mattered whether or not she suffered from one mental illness or another, or from none? In a reasonably humanitarian, welfare-oriented society, at the moment of risk the state must step in, at least temporarily, to rescue those disabled from their own pursuit of "life, liberty and property." This rescue the state owes to its citizens regardless of color, creed, sex, fortune, or mental ability.

What if the citizen for a second time marches into the middle of the traffic, climbs onto the rooftop, or threatens to jump from the bridge? Even for a person who is sane, the state is expected to make a second rescue effort. Moreover, under common law such willful citizens could be charged with disturbing the peace, attempting suicide, or some other obscure legal violation, thus affording the state the justification for temporary restraint.

If minor sanctions are to be attached to deliberate, repeated risk takers, they should apply whether the risk takers are competent or incompetent. But I am strongly opposed to attaching a psychiatric label to people in order to permit greater intervention and control over their lives than over the community at large.

Rebecca Smith died before New York City authorities could implement her hospitalization under its new protective custody law. Yet for at least three decades, under special laws, the mentally ill, alcoholics, and drug addicts have been confined on the basis of psychiatric labels, without complying to the standards of "due process" and "probable cause" required under the criminal law. At the height of the therapeutic state, in the 1950s and 1960s, efforts were made to greatly and unduly broaden the insanity defense, as well as to altogether prohibit criminal sanctions against public drunkenness. But the late 1970s brought an antitherapeutic movement of similar extremity. While therapists of two decades ago called for voluntary and involuntary "treatment" of all deviants, today's therapeutic nihilists wish to totally abolish the insanity defense and to condemn to benign neglect those who require assistance.

Neither extreme supplies even and civilized justice for America. Rebecca Smith's life should have been saved, even at the cost of a temporary loss of freedom. But the same conclusion should apply to all citizens similarly situated, regardless of their psychiatric diagnosis. The New York seventy-two-hour temporary custody law, designed exclusively for those allegedly mentally disabled, proved not only unjust, but also ineffective.

DECISIONS ON BEHALF OF THE INCOMPETENT

45

Sterilizing the Retarded Child

A retarded eleven-year-old girl from the city of Sheffield, England, had been booked to enter a hospital on May 4, 1975, for a sterilization operation. The girl, known as "D," suffers from Sotos Syndrome—also called cerebral giganticism—an unusual group of congenital abnormalities including epilepsy. Characteristics of the disease include large hands, feet, and skull; poor coordination; and endocrine problems of unknown etiology. Intelligence ranges from normal to severe retardation, with most mildly retarded. ("D" had a normal intelligence range, a fair academic standard, and the understanding of a nine- to nine-and-a-half-year-old.)

While authorities in the genetics of Sotos Syndrome are uncertain about its inheritability, they believe that it is not one disease but a heterogeneous group of disorders, and that it may be either a recessive trait or a new dominant mutation. Most cases of Sotos Syndrome have been sporadic, occurring equally in both sexes. Those afflicted do not seem to have a higher incidence of relatives affected than does the normal population, and the risk of genetic transmission is not known. There have been reports, however, of its occurrence among first cousins, identical twins, and between father and son.

"D's" father died in 1971, leaving the mother to raise the girl and two other daughters in very difficult circumstances. The mother, a part-time cleaner, is very hard-working, sincere, and devoted. The girl sleeps with her mother in one bed; their two-bedroom house has no toilet; and they live under conditions described as appalling.

In 1973 "D" was transferred to a school specializing in children's behavioral problems, a move reported to be a success. Her progress in education and behavior was evident. But by the time "D" reached puberty at the age of ten the mother had grown concerned, fearing her daughter might be seduced and have an abnormal baby, for which she would then have to care. She stated: "I don't think my daughter will ever be responsible enough to bring up a family. I don't think she will improve enough to look after children." However, "D" had not yet shown any interest in the opposite sex, and her opportunities for promiscuity were virtually nonexistent since her mother was always at her side.

Dr. Ronald Gordon, a consultant pediatrician at Sheffield Northern General Hospital who had taken an interest in the family, said that there was a risk that any child borne by "D" would be abnormal and that the girl's epilepsy might cause her to harm a child. He thought that she would always remain so substantially handicapped that she would be unable to care for herself or any children she might have. He maintained that his recommendation to operate was based on his clinical judgment; furthermore, he claimed that he and the gynecologist, Dr. Sheila Duncan, should be the sole judges of whether surgery should be performed, provided that there was parental consent. Dr. Gordon also asked the mother, who consented to the sterilization, to discuss the operation with her daughter.

Mrs. Margaret Dubberley, an educational psychologist at the school the girl attended, strongly opposed the operation and brought legal proceedings aimed at having the girl made a ward of the court. The headmaster at the girl's school believed it was unrealistic to be dogmatic about "D's" future, a view supported by some medical evidence. Mrs. Dubberley was further supported by the National Council for Civil Liberties and by a movement in the House of Commons opposing the operation.

COMMENTARY

LeRoy Walters

Before we examine the normative issues in "D's" case, it will be useful to analyze precisely what kind of sterilization is being proposed on her behalf. Since there is no evidence to indicate that the sterilization of "D" is medically required for the diagnosis or treatment of an existing illness or injury, the proposed sterilization can be categorized as *nontherapeutic.* A more complex question is the voluntariness of the proposed procedure. The surgery envisioned is clearly not compulsory, or involuntary, in the sense of being performed against the expressed wishes of the daughter. However, "D" is legally a minor and is probably not mentally competent to provide voluntary consent to the surgery on her own behalf. Perhaps a third category is required—nonvoluntary sterilization, or sterilization in the absence of the prospective sterilizee's consent or refusal. The proposed sterilization in "D's" case would seem to correspond most closely to this third category; that is, if performed, the sterilization would be nonvoluntary and would be authorized by the substituted judgment of the mother and the two physicians.

Under what conditions can nontherapeutic, nonvoluntary sterilization be morally justified? I would like to suggest three formal requirements which should be applied to this and similar cases. First, there should be *just cause,* or a sufficiently weighty reason, for the proposed sterilization. A just cause is required because sterilization in the absence of consent constitutes a significant invasion of the body and a rather massive intrusion into the sphere of reproductive privacy that has recently been recognized by Anglo-American law. The second requirement is that sterilization should be a *last resort,* since it is generally irreversible and since equally effective, reversible contraceptive techniques are available—for example, the pill. The third formal requirement is *due process,* or an adequate procedure for representing the interests and protecting the rights of all parties concerned.

The proposed sterilization of "D" satisfies none of these formal requirements. First, there is no just cause for the sterilization of "D." It is not clear whether sterilization was recommended by the mother and the pediatrician primarily for the benefit of "D" herself, for the benefit of her mother and sisters, or for the benefit of a child which might potentially be conceived and born to "D." (Another logical possibility, not mentioned in this case, would be sterilization for the benefit of society as a whole.) However, no convincing arguments are presented to support any of these possible justifications. The evidence concerning the probability of "D's" producing handicapped children is inconclusive at best. In addition, the prognosis for "D's" own intellectual development is uncertain. It is at least possible that with the aid of continued special education she will one day be able to make informed decisions concerning her reproductive capacities.

Second, the proposed sterilization of "D" is clearly not a last resort. In the case report there is no evidence to indicate that reversible contraceptive techniques were either considered or tried. Until such alternatives have been demonstrated to be infeasible, consideration of an irreversible surgical procedure is premature.

Third, the proposal to sterilize "D" also fails to satisfy the due process requirement. Quite possibly the physicians and the mother based their decision primarily on the best interest of the child, as they perceived that interest. However, the "clinical judgment" of the physicians extended far beyond the bounds of the medically indicated. Even the mother, whose response in very difficult circumstances is understandable, did not sufficiently consider the rights of her child. In cases where the performance of an irreversible, nontherapeutic procedure on a child is contemplated, due process seems to require either the appointment of a guardian for the child or formal approval by an independent review committee. This at least seems to be the view of the U. S. Department of Health, Education and Welfare (as expressed in the sterilization restrictions published in the *Federal Register*, February 6, 1974) and the British Department of Health and Social Security, as outlined in a discussion paper, "Sterilization of Children under 16 Years of Age" (cited in the *British Medical Journal*, November 8, 1975, p. 356).

It is easy to forget that the momentary act of nonvoluntary sterilization has lifetime consequences for the person undergoing the procedure. A sociological study by G. Sabagh and R. B. Edgerton in *Eugenics Quarterly* (December 1962) reported that, of forty retarded persons who had been sterilized prior to their release from the institution, many understood "the meaning and implications of sterilization" and 68 percent "disapproved of the sterilization procedure which they had undergone."

In sum, the proposed sterilization of "D" in this case fails to fulfill the requirements of just cause, last resort, and due process. The preferable alternative would be to employ nonpermanent contraceptive techniques as necessary, in the hope that one day "D" will attain sufficient intellectual maturity to make her own reproductive decisions.

COMMENTARY

Willard Gaylin

When analyzed in terms of the specific data presented in this case, a court decision to prevent irreversible surgery seems reasonable enough; and that is, in fact, what took place. The child is, after all, still young; the nature of the mental impairment is still unclear; the degree of retardation (and possible maturation that can be expected) has yet to be defined. There will be a time for a reevaluation when the facts of her destiny become clearer.

The actual response the court's decision elicited, however, was not what one would expect for a prudential compromise, but more like that which is accorded a victory of the forces of good over those of evil. The applause in Britain and elsewhere was as unanimous and hearty as though Tinkerbell's life depended on it. One suspects that it was not the eleven-year-old girl and her future that were being judged, but a cliché. For years sterilization of the mentally retarded has been an issue fraught with emotion. The ominous implications of genetic engineering, cast in the shadow of the recent Nazi past, make the problem too easy by evoking an instinctive and intuitive response to the connotation of the words employed rather than their explicit meaning. Here was an issue that managed to unite educational psychologists, the medical establishment, the civil libertarians, and the House of Commons on one side—with only the unfortunate girl's mother in opposition. Any moral issue in biomedicine these days that commands such unanimity warrants a reexamination.

What is needed is some understanding of the value of sterilization in the mentally retarded. An automatic negative response is not warranted; and the reason is precisely the one sometimes relied upon by opponents of sterilization—that we now recognize the mentally retarded as a broad spectrum of individuals who, while limited in their capacity for certain functions of the healthy mature adult, are not limited in all.

One of the great disadvantages of IQ as the measurement of retardation is that it forces us to see the retarded of all ages as children. We describe them as "having the mentality of a six-year-old." No mentally retarded individual has the mentality of a six-, eight-, twelve- or fourteen-year-old. A six-year-old is a learner par excellence, with unbounded intellectual curiosity, and a potential for mastery of new material that a thirty-six-year-old would envy. He is, however, immature, childish, and incapable of making the decisions which his profound intelligence might imply. A thirty-six-year-old with severe retardation to a point where he can neither read, write, count, tell time, nor follow street directions, can still be a mature adult in a host of ways beyond the capacity of the six-year-old. The price we make the retarded pay for their incapacity in one area is the sacrifice of capacity in certain other areas which could be compensatory if allowed to develop.

Because we cast mentally retarded adults as children we are appalled, for example, at the thought of their having a sexual or even a social life. Deprived of the joy and privilege of parenthood, for which they may have no capacity, they are punished further by being denied the privilege and pleasure of affection, tenderness, romance, and sexual contact for which they may indeed have a capacity.

A mentally retarded individual ought not be given the responsibility of raising a child, and indeed a mentally retarded woman could be terrified of the changes in her body which pregnancy would produce. Sterilization could allow for the kind of innovation in social living lacking at most facilities for the mentally retarded. There is no reason why community living, even a family-type living, that involved affection, tenderness, and sexuality could not be a fundamental part of their lives and partly compensate for their lack of ordinary intellectual pleasures. Instead we punitively add one deprivation onto the other.

Sterilization is, after all, simply a word. There is nothing in the procedure itself that is innately evil. We allow sterilization when its benefits for the individual outweigh its costs. It is a legitimate procedure, offensive to some for religious reasons but not to others. In this matter society ought to respect the individual conscience and the individual value.

When, as with the retarded, the concepts necessary for intelligent decision making are beyond a person's intellectual grasp, we would be wise to leave the power of the delegated autonomy in the hands of the family. If that is abused all sorts of legal mechanisms exist for rectification. What state right warrants intrusion into the decision making? If it is established (first by the family, then if there is suspicion of abuse, by courts), that the mental retardation is of a degree that precludes the role of parent, the young woman will be deprived only of the "privilege" of conception and, presumably, abortion. She will gain, however, new freedoms, and her parents will gain peace of mind.

The incursion into the powers of the family by the state, here as in other places, is often cast in the noble language of rights. What is really at issue in many arguments about "fetal rights," "infant rights," and so on is in reality the relocation of delegated autonomy and power from one institution—the family—to another—the state. Too often the kind of government intervention we have been seeing in these difficult cases, where right and wrong are too finely balanced for comfort or confidence in any decision, represents arrogance rather than compassion. It is unseemly and demeans the state, for more often than not the state is acting not *in loco parentis* but simply as Nosey Parker.

If "D's" incapacities to be a mother are still evidenced when she is fifteen years of age, she, through the agents of her care, that is, her family, ought to have the right to exercise the privilege of sterilization.

46

Which Clients Should a Sheltered Workshop Serve?

The Lynngrove Association for the Mentally Retarded (LAMR) is a nonprofit organization that receives public money to operate a sheltered workshop called Deuce Industries. Deuce provides a training program to take developmentally disabled clients through a series of increasingly complex and demanding tasks in preparation for regular employment, as, for example, cleaners, orderlies, messengers, and file clerks.

An ongoing discussion about Deuce's aims and objectives has centered on two controversial areas: first, the possible elimination of current client-workers from Deuce to make room for new workers; and second, the level of wages Deuce pays its workers and the amount of outside funding Deuce receives. In the first area, two groups of workers pose the problem. One group includes those workers who have completed the program and are now ready for regular employment. Even though some of these workers are reluctant to leave Deuce, some staff workers have suggested that they be "pushed out of the nest" to make room for new clients. Others have argued that at least in some cases these workers should be retained. It is often difficult for them to find regular employment; even when work is found, it is usually at the most menial level, far below what the worker was doing at Deuce. Moreover, many of these workers have for the first time in their lives found a home—friends, a caring community, and a sense of purpose.

The second, fairly large, group of problem workers involves those who "get stuck" in the program and apparently never will be able to graduate from Deuce to regular employment. Some of these workers have been at Deuce since the organization was founded ten years ago. Should they be removed from Deuce to make room for new clients?

On the question of wages, currently Deuce pays its workers only 32 cents per hour, whereas normal workers would earn at least the $3.85 per hour minimum wage. Some of the staff argue that this low wage devalues retarded people, since LAMR is committed to the practice and goal of *normalization*—which has been described by psychologist Wolf Wolfensberger as "making available to the mentally retarded patterns and conditions of everyday life that are as close as possible to the norms and patterns of the mainstream of society." But other staff workers point out that if the minimum wage were paid, the number of workers at Deuce would have to be reduced drastically. At best only one third of the current work force—the most productive—could be kept on.

What policy should the agency adopt on these two issues?

COMMENTARY

Michael McDonald

The most immediate moral issues presented here involve tradeoffs: in the first instance between actual and potential clients; and in the second, between fewer workers at higher wages and more workers at lower wages.

To decide whether a tradeoff is moral, one must consider what minimum standards and functions are acceptable. I am inclined to take a utilitarian view that the overall welfare of the client population in the area served by Lynngrove ought to be the most important consideration. But because welfare considerations are complex, it is useful to try some more indirect and concrete approaches to this issue.

One promising approach is to look at the nature and function of the sheltered workshop program. What does Lynngrove expect to accomplish with Deuce Industries, and beyond that what does Lynngrove's funding agency, the government, expect of such associations for the mentally retarded? Are sheltered workshops intended mainly as *training* or *maintenance* programs? If Deuce is primarily a vehicle for training retarded people, then one would be disinclined to retain either "graduates" of the program or those who are unlikely to graduate. A more maintenance-centered perspective would lead in the opposite direction.

In the second instance the results would be less clear-cut. However, taking the training view, it would be harder to argue that the workers should receive the minimum wage if trainees in ordinary apprenticeship programs normally do not receive the minimum wage (on the ground that apprentices in their work are receiving, rather than providing, a benefit).

Maintenance-centered considerations could cut either way, depending on the minimum level of maintenance in question and the degree to which wages from Deuce make a difference in the client's welfare. Some workers at Deuce would likely be recipients of other services provided by Lynngrove, such as residing in group homes. For these workers the wages received would be a much less important component of their total welfare than for those who do not receive such services.

My own, albeit limited, contacts with staff members of such agencies lead me to believe that Lynngrove would be likely to favor a more training-oriented perspective over a maintenance-oriented view. This is not surprising given the historical development and current context of such organizations. They are seen and see themselves not only as providing a noninstitutional alternative to large-scale public institutions, but also as the main element in the progressive deinstitutionalization of society's treatment of retarded people. This is very much bound up with the Scandinavian philosophy of "normalization" advocated by Wolfensberger and others. Moreover, because such institutions compete for those public resources earmarked specifically for the care of retarded people, they tend to emphasize what makes them distinct, namely, their concern with training.

Without denying the importance of either normalization or deinstitutionalization, I would caution against endorsing an exclusively training perspective. First, if pushed to an extreme, the logic of concentrating on the most trainable marginalizes and devalues the remainder. Second, it is very difficult to uncouple training and maintenance even when dealing with a "normal" population. Consider children in primary schools or special skills programs for the chronically unemployed, and imagine ignoring maintenance considerations to concentrate solely on training. A closely related third consideration is that the sheltered workshop offers its clients more than a work experience; it provides them with the intrinsically valuable experience of being a functioning part of an ongoing, productive community in which the values of contribution, cooperation, and concern are crucial.

If normalization has a moral justification, then surely a central principle is that such a process helps clients to see their lives as worthwhile. If we recognize that humans are social beings, this sense of being worthwhile is only likely to be acquired as a vital part of a significant community, which sheltered workshops are or at least can become.

This has a special bearing on the issues in this case, in which the wholesale removal of current workers at Deuce and their replacement by new workers is contemplated. Such steps may well destroy whatever sense of community exists in Deuce and so reduce the overall benefits Deuce can provide to current and replacement workers alike. So barring any large increases in budget, I would recommend staying with lower hourly wages and only a gradual turnover in client population.

COMMENTARY

Stanley S. Herr

Sheltered workshops have organizational needs that often conflict with the rights of their "client-workers" and the progressive ideologies of their staff. In the United States, this is a large, fast-growing, and poorly regulated industry with over 3,800 workshops and 200,000 clients. For persons with developmental disabilities, workshops also fulfill a variety of counseling, educational, recreational, and job placement functions. But industrial and habilitation aims often clash, and sheltered workshops must struggle with a mixture of missions and motivations. This case study typifies those conflicts and the challenges of bringing workshop roles and client rights into better fit.

The staff of the workshop and its sponsoring organization profess to adhere to a philosophy of normalization. In essence, normalization is the use of culturally valued means to achieve culturally valued ends so that handicapped individuals can lead lives as normal and integrated as possible. For most persons with mental retardation, work in the mainstream of society at a decent wage, or preparation for such work, is a critical component of that process. For the minority unable to work in a competitive employment environment, there is a need for alternatives to the traditional transitional workshop. But program staff at Deuce Industries have given consideration neither to the development of those alternatives nor to the participation of "client-workers" in overall policy decisions or their own vocational plans.

In addition, the staff should consider the workshop's responsibility to place its clients in appropriate settings and the Lynngrove Association's capacity to mobilize public support for external changes in government and business that would increase the vocational choices available to persons with developmental disabilities. If they neglect these larger issues, can they really achieve normalization and habilitation for their clients in an insular setting?

Turning to specifics, Deuce Industries should adopt a policy of assisting its fully trained workers to find and to adjust to real jobs on the outside. Although job placement is a major workshop role, it is often performed ineffectively, with the result that less than 10 percent of workshop clients enter competitive employment each year.

Part of the reason is that sheltered workshops tend to underestimate the work potential of their clients, to create dependencies, to overlook on-the-job training methods and standards, and to neglect job development, follow-up, and counseling aspects of vocational rehabilitation. At an individual level,

Deuce staff can ease the transition for the reluctant client through the use of trial visits, creation of alumni groups for its "graduates," and other forms of ongoing social support.

Staff and the Lynngrove Association should also vigorously lobby the government for such measures as adequate recreational and other daytime programs for handicapped adults who are leaving workshops, and tax credits for businesses that train and hire handicapped workers. Since the public is funding such nonprofit organizations to bring handicapped adults into the labor force, it can reasonably expect them to spearhead that objective.

As for long-stay clients who are not trained even after ten years of exposure, there is a question of whether the clients or the programs have failed. Vocational training specialists, such as Marc Gold, have convincingly demonstrated that workshops should invest more effort in the technology of instruction, the details of task analysis, and the design of structured learning environments that enable clients to acquire competence and self-esteem.

If these particular clients have gotten "stuck" in a program that is supposed to turn out service workers, how do we know they will not succeed in a production-oriented workshop? For example, studies show that with sophisticated behavior modification techniques severely retarded adolescents can be trained to assemble a twenty-four-piece bicycle brake.

In light of new knowledge on habilitation, Deuce Industries might well adopt other strategies for helping these lagging learners, such as diversifying its own programs, transferring these clients to a more innovative agency, or creating a work activity center for clients in need of prevocational skills. In any event, sudden and mass expulsion of long-term clients would raise troubling ethical, legal, and programmatic questions.

The payment of a flat 32 cents an hour for all Deuce workers—less than one-twelfth of a minimum wage—is not even a close question. Under the laws of the United States, this practice would violate the Fair Labor Standards Act, which permits sheltered workshops to pay subminimum wages only if those payments to disabled workers are based on productivity norms and commensurate wages for similar jobs in private industry.

Unfortunately, outside verification of these rates is infrequent and lawless practices are rampant. According to the *Wall Street Journal* (October 17, 1979) and a congressionally mandated study, wage earnings are dismal and slipping with inflation, with a third of workshop workers with disabilities that did not interfere with or only slightly hampered work performance receiving less than half the minimum wage. In this context, the notion that token wages should be paid in order to engage more mentally retarded persons is an invitation to open-ended exploitation of those individuals. Imagine the uproar if this were proposed as a solution for unemployment among nonhandicapped workers!

The argument that these worker-clients are really only paying for their apprenticeship is also unconvincing. First, workshops receive government grants and charitable contributions to defray unusual training expenses. Second, long-term "training" programs that go on for years and years are a far cry from valid apprenticeships. Third, such token payments demean workers and supervisors alike, and deprive the program of powerful and normal incentives for working.

Finally, if workshops must charge their clients for genuine, short-term intensive programs of vocational preparation, it would be sounder practice, in terms of normalization, candor, and client dignity, to do so on a direct rather than a disguised basis. As long as the workshop has remunerative contracts and produces goods and services, workers should receive authentic wages and enjoy fair, tangible rewards for their productivity. A greater measure of client participation in the making of these policy decisions is surely part of the solution. In the past, workshops have been characterized by paternalism and sweeping discretion over the lives of their clients. In the future, workshops must equip their worker-clients to enter the world of work and to live more independently. If we really intend for this to happen, these workers must learn to make decisions, to bargain collectively, and to gain social competence. These are lessons that workshops must demonstrate as well as teach.

Selected Bibliography

Part V: Mental Incompetence

Chodoff, Paul. "The Case for Involuntary Hospitalization of the Mentally Ill." *American Journal of Psychiatry* 133 (May 1976): 496–501.

Culver, Charles M., and Gert, Bernard. *Philosophy in Medicine: Conceptual and Ethical Issues in Medicine and Psychiatry.* New York: Oxford University Press, 1982.

Edwards, Rem B. *Psychiatry and Ethics: Insanity, Rational Autonomy, and Mental Health Care.* Buffalo, NY: Prometheus Books, 1982.

Gutheil, Thomas G., and Applebaum, Paul S. *Clinical Handbook of Psychiatry and the Law.* New York: McGraw-Hill Book Co., 1982.

Macklin, Ruth. *Men, Mind, and Morality.* Englewood Cliffs, NJ: Prentice-Hall, 1982.

Macklin, Ruth, and Gaylin, Willard; eds. *Mental Retardation and Sterilization: A Problem of Competency and Paternalism.* New York: Plenum Press, 1981.

Szasz, Thomas. *The Myth of Mental Illness: Foundations of a Theory of Personal Conduct.* New York: Harper Row, 1974.

PART SIX

Allocation and Health Care Policy

INTRODUCTION

Although modern medical technology has created many ethical dilemmas for practitioners and patients, as the case studies in the previous parts have shown, it is, by and large, a boon to society. But the kinds of sophisticated medical care available today are expensive, thus raising a new series of questions concerning the allocation of these scarce and highly desired resources. The involvement of the public, through government agencies, in decisions about allocation brings to the forefront the ethical questions of obligations to distribute these resources fairly and to create health policy that takes into account both the patient's and the public's interests.

The case studies in the first section—"Allocation of Scarce Resources"—focus on issues of equitable distribution. Who, for example, should be admitted to the last bed in an intensive-care unit? If two people on a hospital unit have cardiac arrests at the same time, and there is only one medical team to handle this emergency, which one should get the life-saving treatment? Increasingly, as these cases suggest, the cost of care plays a role in allocation decisions.

The second section—"Organ Procurement and Transplantation"—considers questions of allocation of human organs, a resource that until the past few decades was unusable in medical therapy. Hearts, kidneys, corneas, and other organs can now be transplanted, but there are still too few available to meet the ever-growing demand. Who on the waiting lists should receive these scarce resources? And how far should we go in creating new sources of organs. For example, should we allow the use of aborted fetuses conceived expressly for their organs or newborns doomed to die because they are born lacking a full brain?

The final section—"Health Care Policy"—turns to questions about the role of regulation in mediating between individual and public interests. For example, should drinking on the job be handled as a medical problem or as a moral failure? Should mentally retarded persons carrying the hepatitis

B virus be allowed to attend public schools? Should potential risks to their health deprive individuals of the opportunity for occupational advancement?

As the final section in this volume, these cases broaden the initial focus of biomedical ethics on individual patient-doctor relationships to include questions of the public's role in establishing norms and policies. But the importance of the individual moral agent—whether as professional or patient—does not diminish. A complete biomedical ethics values both perspectives.

ALLOCATION OF SCARCE RESOURCES

47

Forced Transfer to Custodial Care

Lawrence Hessman

Mrs. B, seventy-four years old, has diabetes and is partially blind. She has lived in a nursing home for the past ten years, and the state Medicaid agency pays her expenses. She feels secure in the home, and she has made many friends there.

The state is trying to save money by caring for its elderly medical patients at the lowest possible cost. Many patients are being transferred from nursing homes to less costly facilities that basically offer only custodial care. The goal is to move as many patients as possible out of facilities providing inappropriately intensive medical support to institutions offering maintenance meeting state-approved standards of quality, but without the medical services now deemed unnecessary.

An arbitrary grading system has been established to evaluate nursing home patients to determine their suitability for transfer. Patients are assigned a certain number of points according to their ability to dress, feed, clothe themselves, and the like. If the number of points the patient receives is higher than a designated total, officials feel that the patient can be transferred without any harmful effects.

When she is evaluated, Mrs. B receives more than the designated number of points, and the decision is made to transfer her. She is not consulted, nor is she given a voice in the decision. She is simply moved—forcibly and against her wishes—to a custodial care institution. The evaluation does not take into account the psychosocial impact of the move or the personal dimensions of Mrs. B's adjustment to the home she had been in for the last decade.

Is the state's conduct ethical? Since it is paying the costs of care, and since it has assigned a higher priority to other areas of medical care for funding, does it have the right to disregard individual patients' wishes concerning the location of their care?

COMMENTARY

Charles Fried

This case is sad and appealing, but raises no difficult questions of principle at all. Presumably the nursing home from which Mrs. B would be moved is deemed inappropriate to her care because it provides a more intensive level of medical supervision than she requires. And, obviously, overall costs of any program cannot be contained if a patient's friendships and preferences require that that patient continue to occupy space in a medically more intensive (and therefore more expensive) environment than is medically indicated.

The situation must arise fairly regularly with patients who would be more comfortable in the more pleasant, caring, and competent surroundings of an acute care hospital than in a nursing home. Surely, however, to be moved by such considerations and, thus, in effect to turn acute care hospitals into nursing homes would make the present disastrous situation regarding hospital costs even worse.

The state agency has to do what it is doing (assuming that it is doing what it is doing intelligently and fairly). If it did not, then some portion of its limited health care budget would be wasted, and persons with more acute needs would be inadequately treated. In other words, if Mrs. B were to win, we must assume that there would be losers in even more desperate straits than she is.

Of course nothing requires the state to act without consulting Mrs. B nor hearing her side of the case. But this is not the same thing as giving her "a voice in the decision." Competing beneficiaries of limited funds would of course all love to have a "voice in the decision," when that means giving them a veto over unfavorable decisions. Mrs. B should certainly be able to present her case and to explain why either an exception should be made or why the state agency's guidelines when applied to her case do not require that she be moved. But to allow the matter to depend on her choice is preposterous.

Of course her physician should make every *proper* effort to have her remain in those circumstances which are most favorable to her. He should make sure that the appropriate agency is aware of the extent to which a move might be detrimental. But it is no part of his duties as her physician to falsify the facts (as doctors sometimes do in efforts to procure certain governmental benefits for their patients) nor to use irregular pressures on her behalf. It would be wrong for a lawyer—and it would certainly be wrong for a doctor—to do this. In the end, if the state agency does move her, the responsibility is not her doctor's but that of the agency. It is no more his responsibility than would be the decision of the Social Security Administration to deny a disability benefit when a patient's doctor was unable in all honesty to come forward with a diagnosis justifying such benefits.

COMMENTARY

Robert Michels

Institutions make decisions that affect the lives of individuals and may affect them adversely. When this occurs (as it did with Mrs. B), we must ask whether it was "ethical," whether it should have happened, and, if not, what should have been different.

This case is simple enough. Mrs. B is old, sick, disabled, and lives in a nursing home. Yet life is not all bad; she feels secure and has many friends. The state is paying her bill, and the state wants to save money. For administrative reasons it wants to move her, judging that she is "suitable" for transfer to a cheaper setting. Against her will, and without her participation in the decision, she is moved.

The case is sad as well as simple. On the face of it, it should be otherwise. Mrs. B should be allowed, at age seventy-four, to finish her days where she feels happiest. State-supported nursing homes are hardly palaces, but this one is Mrs. B's home, and the state should forcibly remove a citizen from his or her home only under extreme circumstances. True, it is paying the bill, but one of the marks of a civilized society is that even dependent citizens have rights and privileges.

However, that is not the whole problem. Health care is expensive, and the resources allocated to it force us to make choices. Perhaps if Mrs. B stays in the nursing home, a young man with asymptomatic hypertension will not be detected by a screening program, or a slum child with cerebral palsy will not have two weeks at a summer camp, or the Methadone Maintenance Center will have one fewer social worker. These are the real effects of budget cuts and reallocations.

What are we to do? Mrs. B earns our sympathy, but the needs are greater than the resources. Somewhere choices must be made. Are cases like Mrs. B's the inevitable result? Are there ethical guidelines as to how the choices should be made?

First, the question of resource allocation cannot be ignored. The public must constantly be reminded of Mrs. Bs as it decides how much should be devoted to health care and how it should be distributed. It might be that the state should not be forced to choose between Mrs. B's life and other alternatives, but that citizens should support, or demand, that it provide all of them, sacrificing other goals in the process. But the recent trend of political decisions has not been in that direction.

Second, there are guidelines that should apply to state decisions that directly affect the lives of individuals. The state is planning a transfer of patients from one institution to another, but Mrs. B is an individual who lives in her home, and the state's procedures should recognize that to one who lives there, institutions are homes and each individual is different.

The decision-making process should be able to make individual decisions about individuals, not simply apply "arbitrary" systems of classification. The noxious character of institutions stems from their tendency to classify people arbitrarily rather than to respond to their individual needs and desires. Further, Mrs. B should be able to participate in the process—in fact, her participation should be required. This is part of recognizing that she is a person, not a line on a state budget. Finally, the state's guidelines should take into account the meaning of the move to Mrs. B, as well as her physical capacity to adjust to it. There are at least two reasons for this: the less important is the clinical fact that her ability to function in the new institution is largely determined by the meaning she attaches to going there. The more important one is that she is a person, and to consider her physical capacity without concern for her psyche is to treat her solely as an organism.

It would seem that the state fell short on several of these, and, therefore, was "unethical." However, we should recognize that the state might have followed ideal procedures and reached the same conclusions, forcibly wrenching Mrs. B from her home, if its citizens have other priorities that are higher than the care and comfort of the needy.

COMMENTARY

Steven Sieverts

One would wish that this pathetic case were purely conjectural, but, alas, it reports a scenario which has played many times in the past few years. The imperative of health care cost containment has become excessively dominant in some government agencies, seemingly overriding all other considerations. All too often, the Mrs. Bs have indeed suffered as a consequence of how some public administrators have behaved under that kind of pressure. Cost-cutting, when it becomes obsessive, can offend human decency.

From an ethical standpoint, however, I suggest that the issue in this case is misrepresented. The question is not whether the Medicaid agency has the right or obligation to assure that beneficiaries are receiving at public expense only appropriate services to which they are entitled under law. Clearly it has both.

Rather, the issue is the unacceptable manner in which the state officials and the health professionals seem to have behaved in this case and in other cases like it. The Medicaid law and the state regulations simply do not instruct bureaucrats to force our nurses and social workers to carry out sudden and inhumane transfers of elderly poor patients without any prior consultation. They also do not require the negligent public administration and professional management that kept this patient in too intensive a facility for a decade, not only wasting money but probably making her more dependent and less self-reliant than was necessary. They do not force procedures that ignore common decency.

This case presentation asks: since (the state) is paying the costs of care . . . does it have the right to disregard individual patients' wishes on the location of their care? Let us ask the question another way: do individual citizens have the right to receive, on demand, publicly financed services to which they have no entitlement? The answer, when it is phrased that way, seems clear: obviously not. Any health insurance program—public or private, categorical or universal, limited or comprehensive—must employ procedures to assure that beneficiaries receive only that to which they are entitled.

Those of us who are health care administrators and those of us whose jobs involve the financing of medical care have a constant obligation to assure that our front-line personnel do not implement necessary policies in ways that trample on patients' rights and sensitivities. This requires clearly written policies and rules as well as sensitive management. In this case, the ethical issue may be in part that the public administrators' instructions to the social workers and nurses in the field may have been so poorly phrased (or poorly intended) that insensitive or brutal behavior was subtly encouraged. The crux of the matter, however, is that health care professionals charged with a demanding task—arranging for the timely and humane transfer of a patient to a more appropriate facility (or finding a legitimate and appropriate alternative course of action)—chose to behave in a way that violated not only basic standards of civilized human behavior but also strongly established ethical principles governing how health care professionals are to act with respect to patients.

If the law or the rules tend to promote unethical behavior, it is an ethical obligation of the administrators and professionals to get them changed—and failing that, to interpret them humanely and even to ignore or disobey those aspects that violate basic principles.

The state regulations were indeed badly written, but that is not the main issue. The central point is that the administrators at the top and middle, and the professionals who actually deal with patients, have an overriding obligation to care about the welfare of those patients. When the implementation of rules, even stupid rules, is done in ways that deny basic human rights, such as the right to be consulted and heard about one's own health care, primary blame must be affixed on the people responsible for that implementation, not on an impersonal "state."

48

The Last Bed in the ICU

At the age of seventy, Mrs. A has been admitted to the hospital for the fifth time in as many years for treatment of respiratory difficulty. The last time she was in the hospital she had nearly died. She has severe emphysema, and when she developed a cold, her deterioration was so rapid that only artificial respiration in the emergency room saved her life. However, it proved very difficult to wean her from the respirator. She spent four weeks in the Intensive Care Unit and required constant care from the medical staff, principally Intern B. After she was discharged, she remained short of breath even while watching television.

Now, five months later, she has contracted another cold, but this time Intern B has managed to treat her without resorting to the ICU and the respirator. During her illnesses, Mrs. A's two sons have been in constant contact with the medical staff. They have been anxious, agitated, and demanding.

It is now 2 a.m. and Intern B is again called to see Mrs. A, who is becoming increasingly lethargic. It is obvious that she is in respiratory failure, and will probably die before morning if she is not given a respirator.

However, hospital policy requires that respirators be used only in the ICU, where the required supporting staff and facilities are available. There is only one bed open in the ICU. The residents like to save one bed for an emergency. As Intern B approaches, Mrs. A's sons are waiting. He knows their questions: What's wrong now? What will you do?

What should the intern do? And on what basis should he make his decision?

COMMENTARY

R. B. Schiffer

Mrs. A's sons, speaking for her, may ask for the respirator and ICU intervention. Should this request be granted?

There are a number of reasons why decisions concerning medical interventions for the seriously ill should be made by the patient, or by the patient's representative. But they do not apply in this case. Although Mrs. A's family has the right to refuse the ICU transfer and respirator, they do not have the right to demand it. Self-determination with regard to medical care is one thing, but a just allocation of scarce resources is another. The first right belongs to the patient, but the second is a claim which society makes upon the use of its health care resources.

Shall the physician decide? This would be an odd way to decide such questions (although in fact many are decided by physicians). Physicians, like families, have vested interests in some patients compared to others. And little in their educational background qualifies them as experts in the just allocation of scarce life-saving medical resources.

Still, I believe the physician has an important contribution to make. In this case, there is a single patient and an available, but costly, resource. We must first ask whether the scarce resource at issue *can* justifiably be used by the patient. We can separate this question from that of whether the resource *should* be so used. The physician might be in the best position to answer this first question.

Logically, there are two steps in deciding the allocation of a scarce medical resource for a seriously ill patient. The first is medical or clinical in nature; the second moral. The principle which guides the first step is usefulness; where there is no benefit, there is no obligation to intervene. Indeed, in a setting of scarcity, there may be a moral obligation not to expend resources from which a particular patient has no reasonable expectation of benefiting. The principle which guides the second step is that of justice; the fair allocation of scarce resources when not all who might benefit can be treated.

Suppose the family in the case had heard of the wonders of coronary artery bypass surgery, and demanded it for Mrs. A. This request would be denied for medical, and not moral, reasons. Such a procedure would be irrelevant for her, and would not improve her pulmonary dysfunction.

If it is the physician's responsibility to distinguish a useful from an irrelevant intervention, how should this be done? The case illustrates how difficult this problem can be. Is this woman medically eligible for the respirator/ICU intervention? Can we say that she has a reasonable expectation of clinically benefiting from this intervention? This I find a real dilemma.

Although medical eligibility is usually explained in terms of "usefulness" or "fruitfulness," it is difficult to find a clear statement of what this means clinically. An intuitive view of this concept might include the notion of an increased span of survival, that is, improved mortality. This view, however, raises the quality-of-life issue. The patient group for which these decisions are made is usually very ill. If the ICU machinery should prolong Mrs. A's existence, without clinical improvement, would we really describe her as having benefited?

Is clinical morbidity, then, the yardstick by which we should measure usefulness? If the contemplated intervention in this case held reasonable promise of improving level of consciousness, or of restoring respiratory function, should we say that the patient is medically eligible without regard to questions of mortality? This seems odd as well. What if she also had a metastatic malignancy, which augured death in days to weeks? Under these conditions it would not seem that she was clinically eligible for the expenditure of a scarce medical resource.

If there are problems with either significantly improved mortality or morbidity taken separately, perhaps their *conjunction* should guide physicians in determining medical eligibility. That is, for a mortally afflicted patient to be medically eligible for a specific scarce life-saving medical resource, there should be in the responsible physician's judgment some reasonable expectation of significant clinical improvement in both mortality and morbidity. From the few details we know in Mrs. A's case, she does not seem medically eligible for the ICU transfer, and it should not be offered to the family. Although her life span might be prolonged, there is no ground for expecting any significant improvement in her condition.

COMMENTARY

Benjamin Freedman

It is often said that questions of medical ethics fall into two categories: some concern procedures for decision, others the substance of decisions. The distinction, while intuitive, is not easy to sustain. How can we determine which procedures ought to be followed unless we know what values out to be sought? On the other hand, what means are permissible in seeking to implement values?

The issue of procedure pervades the case of Mrs. A with five decision-making agents entering the stage, each with a special claim:

1. *The hospital* has arrived at a policy judgment that respirators may be used only in the ICU. The reason for arriving at this policy—that the necessary superstructure for effective use of the respirator is available only in the ICU—seems to be an instrumentally rational policy. For such a policy to be followed, what requirements ought to be satisfied? Clearly, the empirical judgment which dictated the policy should be supported by the best data and technical judgment available. We cannot be certain that this is the case here; "hospital policy" can be made by physicians, health-care personnel, hospital administrators, or other groups.

Even assuming that the best available empirical investigation has been heeded, two further questions for instrumentally rational policy arise. Are the means morally acceptable? Is the end desirable? Both questions are ethical in nature. If the end sought in the ICU regulation is the efficient use of respirators, we quickly smoke out value judgments lurking in factual language. What do we mean by "efficient"? Is efficiency to be sought at all costs? If there are no more respirators available than ICU beds, then it may make sense to limit their use to the ICU, but if additional respirators are available and a patient will die if one is not used, then the refusal to use one under less than ideal conditions seems morally questionable.

2. *The residents* "like" to leave one bed in the ICU open for emergencies. This preference has the flavor of something approaching a gentleman's agreement; for reasons which may be too obvious to require examination, a practice has developed. We often speak of some practice as our "policy." Yet this kind of policy differs crucially from more formal policies in that it need not have been, prior to establishment, publicly debated and announced. The unfortunate result is that what seemed not to require examination often turns out not to stand up under examination. In any event, "practice as policy" does not *bind* those adopting it. In contrast to other kinds of policies, informal agreements may be informally broken. The intern need not feel bound by it. He is an independent moral agent, and should evaluate both the general worth of this policy and the appropriateness of applying it here.

3. *The intern* takes policies of the hospital and the residents and finds himself bound to interpret them. As courts have occasionally acknowledged, interpretation of a policy is an act of policy making in itself. If, for example, the intern decides against admitting Mrs. A to the ICU, giving as his reasons the policies of the hospital and the residents, he must himself have decided that Mrs. A's condition is not an emergency. In spite of the fact that without the respirator she will die, this decision could be acceptable—in the case when, for example, she would die despite its use. But without such a circumstance, the rights and wrongs of the matter should not be decided upon in the heat of action by the intern alone.

Some elements of the decision must be decided by the intern and/or his supervisors: Mrs. A's prognosis at the moment, for instance. But other questions would profit by more public examination in which invidious presuppositions, biases, and idiosyncratic views would, it is hoped, disappear. In this case the medical facts alone cannot tell us what is morally required. Even if the respirator will only prolong the patient's uncomfortable life, it is still a moral question whether that prolongation is of sufficient value that the treatment is morally required or permissible.

4. *The relatives* may wish to be involved in, and not merely informed of, the decisions being made in this case. Certainly the relatives' wishes should not necessarily be definitive in deciding what should be done in this case. If the agents responsible for hospital policy (rather than just the intern) decide that treatment that will only prolong life in a diseased state does not qualify one for a respirator (either in or outside the ICU), and if the patient and family are made aware of this before entering the hospital, their views about treatment should not override that policy. Furthermore, the script, curiously, has left out the main protagonist. What are Mrs. A's views? If she is totally unable to

communicate, the relatives may have a more significant place in the decisions, but if she is able to communicate and there has been no formally announced hospital policy against treatment in her case, then surely she should have some say in the matter.

5. *The patient* has been in this situation before. Has any effort been made to uncover what she feels about the aggressive efforts made in the past to maintain her in her morbid state?

Assuming that we may find out—possibly from the relatives—Mrs. A's wishes, I believe those ought to be respected. At worst, this would put her in conflict with the intern's individual judgment that her case does not constitute an emergency. A person's right to treatment should not be invariably subject to a physician's opinions, even when those opinions are based upon a mixture of medical and value judgments. It may be true that only a physician can assess the weight of the medical factors; it does not follow that the physician will do so correctly. If we must err, let us err on the side of individual dignity and autonomy.

The larger moral is that no quick delineation of policy in the heat of a medical crisis is likely to prove adequate for solving moral problems.

49

Refusing an Amputation: Who Should Pay for the Extra Care?

Otis Simmons, a fifty-eight-year-old derelict, walked barefoot in bitter cold through the streets of Manhattan shortly before Christmas, in order to reach Roosevelt Hospital. "I froze," he said later. "I sat in one place fifteen hours." After he was hospitalized, he developed gangrene in his badly frostbitten feet. The doctors wanted to amputate the infected portions, noting that otherwise the condition could become "life-threatening." Simmons refused the treatment: "My two legs got to stay on. I won't have the operation. I got to cure my own self."

Soon after, despite objections from hospital physicians, a State Supreme Court justice ruled that Simmons was legally competent and had the right to refuse the amputation.

Antibiotic treatment helped to stall the infection. However, Simmons finally lost two toes on his left foot and part of his right foot. The bill for his three-month hospitalization amounted to $29,000 and has been submitted to Medicaid. A hospital spokesman has said, "We don't know how much they will pay or when they will pay it."

Assuming a competent patient has the right to refuse medical treatment, does he have the right to have Medicaid funds pay for additional care required by the refusal?

COMMENTARY

Willard Gaylin

We have been dealt a bad hand. Anyone who would stand against Otis Simmons puts himself immediately into opposition to that grand tradition of rugged individualism so highly respected by modern American culture. One might just as well take on John Wayne, Billy Martin, and Kojak (three symbols, come to think of it, I wouldn't mind tackling).

Mr. Simmons, a derelict with dignity, demands the right to take his own risks and suffer his own consequences. The result—in the limited amount of data presented to us—seemed to place him not in the category of a crank, but of a medical conservative. He postpones surgery, preferring antibiotic treatment, until such time as partial amputation is ultimately necessary. It is true that this cost the taxpayers $29,000. On the other hand, it seems like a bargain when compared with the $16,000 bill (exclusive of special nursing and physicians' fees) presented to a friend of mine for a seven-day hospitalization. Hospital bills these days seem to bear no logical relationship to services rendered. Mr. Simmons acted within his rights.

Having said all this, a problem remains. Sooner or later, we are going to have to confront the relationship between autonomy and responsibility in health care. "Responsibility" is not a fashionable word these days; "rights" is the preferred language of current moral discourse. I have never viewed "rights" and "responsibilities" as essentially contradictory or mutually exclusive concepts; others do.

"Rights," of course, refers to two distinctly separate concepts: being left alone, and a claim against the government. It is specifically that latter interpretation of rights that is going to demand a reevaluation of responsibility. Claims against the government inevitably demand limits; limits demand comparisons; and forcing consideration of a just distribution of resources—I suspect—will lead us once again to the concept of personal responsibility.

The current popular concept of autonomy—autonomy without responsibility—is at best a peculiar one. I think specifically of a colleague of mine who is evangelical in the defense of adult autonomy. An adult ought to have the right to ride without seat belts, if he so prefers; to purchase any dangerous drugs at his own risk; and, it goes without saying, to commit suicide; in effect, to be the total executor—even a bad one—of all of his interests, provided he causes no harm to others. At the same time, this same colleague is outraged at the idea of penalizing in any way a person whose reckless irresponsibility leads to his own illness. This champion of autonomy argues that it is absurd, for example, to penalize the cigarette smoker, since that is to assume that he has some voluntary control over his smoking. This strict autonomist, it seems, is at the same time a psychic determinist in the manner of the early Freudians.

This peculiar concept of autonomy without responsibility strikes me as identical to the early adolescent's view of independence: "When it comes to decision making, I am my own master; the consequences of my behavior had best be handled by my parents." This view ignores, among other things, the fact that the knowledge that one must pay the piper becomes a significant factor in determining our behavior—unconsciously motivated as well as volitional behavior.

There are also those of us who believe that the concept of an "individual" is meaningless independent of the community that supports his very being as a human. To elevate autonomy to a point where the state legitimates self-destructive and dehumanizing behavior also defines the quality of the state. While the paternalistic state can be a tyrant worthy of dread, the "indifferent" state, by ignoring the biological and sociological concept of "community," can be equally destructive. Beyond that, in a time of limited resources, where spending a dollar in one area inevitably will mean *not* spending it in another, we have transcended the bounds where autonomous behavior ceases to impinge on the rights of others.

By considering the subject of personal responsibility, we immediately enter that dreaded bioethical locale, the "slippery slope." If the cigarette smoker is responsible for his cancer, is not the obese, the obsessive worker, or the physically inactive responsible for his heart attack? There is, I submit, a distinction between ordinary and extraordinary risk, direct responsibility and indirect responsibility. In questions of voluntariness the law has a long-standing, respectable expertise in drawing those distinctions. So have we all. If one believes in the moral right to abortion—and I am not here arguing that point—one can still see the distinction between abortion for a diabetic tendency and abortion for Tay-Sachs. In the latter, there is a greater urgency, a greater predictability, and a greater responsibility. Similarly, we ought to be able to begin to draw distinctions along lines of responsibility for our own health—not to the point of excluding forgiveness and decency, care and kindness; not to establish a pariah stature for the "offender," but at least to begin to introduce penalties and prices that encourage responsibility to oneself, to others, to the community. At a time of scarcities, when one person's irresponsibility may deprive someone else of health care, the question of autonomy takes on new meaning.

COMMENTARY

Charles Fried

Medicaid must pay. This conclusion bothers me, but I do not see how it can be avoided. The best way to understand it is to see it as an example of a general point: indigency does bestow certain immunities that people with resources do not enjoy.

It is quite clear on the facts as given that it would have been improper for the medical authorities to perform the amputation against the wishes of the patient; and I also have no quarrel with the court's conclusion that the refusal of the amputation was not in and of itself a proof of incompetency. To deny Medicaid reimbursement could only be justified on one of two grounds: (a) that Roosevelt Hospital should itself bear the cost of Simmons's hospitalization, or (b) that once Simmons refused the amputation he should have been discharged and denied further care. If Roosevelt Hospital acted properly in this case, there is no more reason it should end up without reimbursement than in the case of any other indigent with an expensive ailment. So there is no reason to expect the hospital to absorb the cost.

Did the hospital act properly in incurring these expenses? Since I assume that it could not have performed the amputation against Simmons's will, to say that it acted improperly must mean that Simmons should have been discharged when he refused the recommended course of care. Moreover, to say this commits one to the conclusion that no other hospital should have admitted him after such a discharge, since a successor hospital would just be in the same position as Roosevelt Hospital was in initially. And that would mean that having refused the care, the only proper course for a hospital (*any hospital*), the only course that would not result in a charge against its own resources, would have been to allow Simmons to die without further care. This is absurd. Therefore, I conclude that what Roosevelt Hospital did was proper, and that it should be reimbursed.

This conclusion becomes more acceptable when we realize that it is forced upon us principally because of Simmons's status as an indigent. If Simmons had been a person with resources, then a private insurer (or for that matter a government insurer) would quite properly have treated Simmons's choices as inappropriately increasing the cost of his care, an increase for which no coverage was provided. This would be viewed as a kind of uninsured option that Simmons could make, but at his own expense. If Simmons had been a wealthy bachelor with no dependents or relatives, nothing would be more reasonable than to charge him for the additional cost of his care. If he had had dependents, presumably they could put pressure on him not to deplete resources to which they might have some claim; but if they did not succeed, then he would still be required to pay the excess out of his own pocket.

The problem, therefore, is only difficult because he has no resources. It seems unfortunate that he should be able to cast such burdens on the public treasury, but the same situation would obtain had he attempted suicide, or become ill because of alcoholism or excessive cigarette smoking. And I do think it would be appropriate to charge higher health insurance premiums or to demand larger contributions from persons with selected, bad health habits—smokers, for example.

50

Two Cardiac Arrests, One Medical Team

George Burnham and Donald Mattison were patients in adjoining rooms in the rehabilitation division of a state medical center. George was a thirty-three-year-old, severely retarded man who had lived in state institutions since the age of three. His family had had no contact with him for over twenty years. George had been trained to feed himself and to keep himself reasonably clean, but at the age of twenty-five he had suffered a cardiac arrest that left him with some paralysis. After rehabilitation he only occasionally lacked bowel control. A second recent cardiac arrest left him semi-paralyzed and totally incontinent. The chances of his regaining even his former level of continence, the staff felt, were hopeless.

Donald Mattison, a forty-eight-year-old businessman, active in community and church affairs, married, and the father of four, had suffered a minor stroke, which left him slightly paralyzed. In his six weeks on the rehabilitation ward he had regained almost total use of his arm and leg. His prognosis for full recovery seemed excellent.

The hospital has at least one cardiac arrest team on duty twenty-four hours a day, and one crash cart in every patient area at all times. The possibility of simultaneous cardiac arrests seemed remote. If it were to happen, there would not be time to transfer an additional crash cart from another patient area, since the rehabilitation ward is served by an extremely slow elevator.

But in this case the improbable happened. George had a cardiac arrest at 3:00 one morning. Within four minutes the cardiac team had arrived in his room and was ready to begin work. At that very moment Donald also had a cardiac arrest. Knowing of the simultaneous cardiac arrests, every team member hesitated. Two also knew both patients' histories; the others, including the team leader, did not. After a moment, the team leader said, "First come, first served. Let's go to work." With no further hesitation, the team began to resuscitate George.

Without the emergency aid, Donald died. George was resuscitated, but suffered yet another cardiac arrest at 8:20 the next morning. This time another team was unable to revive him, and he too died. Did the team leader make the right decision in resuscitating George instead of Donald? Is "first come, first served" the proper principle to apply in such cases?

COMMENTARY

Kevin M. McIntyre and Robert C. Benfari

The most painful of all medical care decisions concerns life-preserving measures which, because of limited resources, require certain individuals to be excluded in favor of others. How does one weigh the relative rights of individuals to such care? Whenever possible, decisions to withhold lifesaving therapy should be made in advance. But in the absence of a clear expression that lifesaving care should be withheld, the person in charge must assume that care was intended. Should incompetency, the patient's family status, capacity to contribute to society, and related considerations be woven into the decision-making process? Let us consider each case on its own merits, then look at the priorities so as to answer the troubling question: "Who shall we permit to die?"

George has just suffered his third cardiac arrest. Since there was sufficient clinical information from two prior arrests to anticipate that cardiac arrest might occur again, in the absence of directions not to resuscitate we must assume that care should be initiated, as it was. George's severe retardation does not per se justify withholding resuscitative efforts, nor does his additional brain damage and total incontinence. The courts have indicated (in the *Dinnerstein* and *Spring* cases) that cardiopulmonary resuscitation (CPR) as well as other forms of lifesaving and life-prolonging therapy can be withheld in appropriate circumstances. But an appraisal by either care-provider or family of the "quality of life" of the life-long incompetent as a basis for withholding such therapy has been specifically rejected (in the *Saikewicz* and the *Storar* and *Eichner* cases).

Recently, the highest court in the State of New York ruled without equivocation that there exists in some circumstances a positive obligation to provide lifesaving treatment to the terminally ill life-long incompetent based on the common law requirement that a guardian act only in the best interest of the ward. While some may disagree, that decision supports the conclusion that there existed an obligation to treat George unless a court had already determined that withholding CPR was in George's best interests.

As for Donald, there are no indications that he had refused or would refuse resuscitation. He had a good prognosis for full recovery. He was young, married with four children, and employed.

Assuming that George would have received the full attention of the CPR team had Donald not arrested, how is one to proceed fairly? With a single crash cart and one cardiac arrest team, if we attempt to initiate CPR for both men, it is likely both will die. Donald's prognosis is better than George's. In addition, Donald's wife and children are emotionally and economically dependent on him so that there are broader societal costs were he to die. On balance, the choice clearly favors full commitment of CPR to Donald. Should we then abandon poor George? Or is it possible to allocate care in such a way that he may survive without seriously compromising Donald's chances?

One approach would be to initiate basic life support (artificial ventilation and external chest compression) immediately for Donald, using a single member of the team, and, as quickly as possible, attempt to defibrillate George. If initial attempts at defibrillation were unsuccessful, or if the attempt took more than thirty to sixty seconds, we would abandon efforts with George and concentrate totally on Donald. If George were in asystolic cardiac arrest (no electrical activity, as opposed to chaotic electrical activity in ventricular fibrillation) we would terminate efforts on his behalf because the likelihood of successful resuscitation would be very small and the time required would very likely preclude Donald's resuscitation.

This approach is based on the following considerations: (1) both George and Donald have a right to lifesaving treatment; (2) George's immediate prognosis is poorer than Donald's; (3) the societal costs of Donald's death would be substantially greater than those of George's; (4) George's best chance of returning to his previous state is immediate defibrillation.

Even the brief delay to defibrillate George may decrease the likelihood of successfully resuscitating Donald. But if Donald could be effectively ventilated (providing adequate air exchange in and out of the lungs of a patient whose breathing has ceased) and receive effective external chest compression (for the purpose of circulating blood in a patient whose heart has stopped beating) for a period not to exceed thirty to sixty seconds before all energies were directed toward him, the delay should not entail great additional risk. The small increase in risk to Donald must be balanced against the alternative, which would be to withhold all chances of survival from George. Would that conscientious decision making were as simple as ". . . first-come, first-served!"

COMMENTARY

Margaret Battin

To consider what would have been the right course of action for the crash cart team leader, let us look at two aspects of the case: first, the distributive principles to which one might appeal in order to honor fundamental moral commitments, and second, the procedural strategies one might use to put them into practice.

Of the many possible principles, at least three are plausible in this case:

Better prognosis. "When both cannot live, treat the one with the better prognosis." This principle, similar to that used in military triage, would clearly have preferred Donald. It reflects a moral commitment to maximizing the preservation of life. It should be applied only where the disparity between prognoses of competitors for treatment is relatively great: it will decide between two individuals when only one is likely to survive if treated, but it will not decide cases where the disparity is uncertain or small (for instance, which patient will receive a kidney, if one's recovery would probably take five weeks and the other's six). This principle can be applied without reference to George's retardation: if the medical history of arrests had been reversed, he would have been preferred.

Social worth. "When both cannot live, prefer the one who has greater value for other persons." This principle, although often attacked as inviting racism, sexism, and bias against the elderly, retarded, and mentally ill, may also be understood without bias: it prefers the person whose continuing life is of greater importance to others. This need not automatically mean Donald. Though George was seriously retarded, he might have contributed significantly to the life of the patients and staff of the ward; conversely, though Donald had prominent public status, he might have been a vicious abuser of relationships with his wife, children, and associates. However, we have no evidence for any such claims, and it is highly likely that Donald had greater value for other persons. Like "better prognosis," this principle is also to be applied only where the disparity between competitors is great; it will not decide, for instance, between saving the parent of two children and the parent of three. Correctly applied, it reflects a fundamental moral commitment to protecting important human relationships.

First come, first served. "When both cannot live, treat the one who is presented for treatment first." This principle, which the leader of the team chose to follow, is blind to the particular characteristics of competing individuals; since George's arrest occurred first he is to be saved, but it could have happened the other way around. Insofar as the principle is neutral to persons, it is similar to random selection, and seems to reflect a moral commitment to the equality of all.

We might praise the team leader's choice as reflecting a primary commitment to the equality of persons. But is this what the team leader's choice really shows? Note that both the other principles—"better prognosis" and "social worth"—would have required the team leader to make a comparative judgment about the conditions and circumstances of Donald and George. But the person-neutral "first come, first served" principle requires no background information about the competitors, presupposes no disparity except time of presentation for treatment, and will decide every hard-choice case except genuinely simultaneous ones. Did the team leader's choice (and do "first come" institutional policies) actually reflect a commitment to human equality, or the fact that this distributive principle is easier to apply? The fact that every member of the team "hesitated" before treating George suggests that other bases for decision were evident to all; is it sheer convenience that gives priority to this one?

Because non-neutral principles require judgments about conditions and circumstances, they are subject to bias when the disparities between competitors are small. Between Donald and George, however, the disparities in prognosis and social worth were very great; hence, bias would have been much less likely to arise.

To say that medicine might well pay greater attention to non-neutral distributive principles is not to deny that there will be disagreements over these principles, or occasions when relevant information is not available, or cases in which there are multiple disparities, some of which favor one competitor and some the other. But these are the hard cases. The case of Donald and George is *not* a hard case: both non-neutral principles could have been applied and would have favored Donald over George. Only a two-minute disparity in time of presentation favored George; a genuinely neutral principle would have permitted treatment of either one. In hard cases, retreat to neutral distributive principles cannot be avoided, but in this case the team retreated too soon. The society that resorts to easy strategies even before the choices become hard may fail to honor the fundamental moral commitments it makes.

51

The Doctor, the Patient, and the DRG

Jeffrey Wasserman

Lakeview Hospital has been reimbursed on the basis of "diagnosis related groups," or DRGs, since May 1980. The hospital's medical director, Jared Lapin, M.D., acts as a liaison between the hospital's managers and the medical staff. In addition, Dr. Lapin and Ellen O'Connor, director of finance, periodically review the performance of individual physicians from a financial viewpoint.

At a recent meeting, Dr. Lapin and Ms. O'Connor analyzed a lengthy computer report that matched, for each physician, the revenue the hospital received with the costs incurred for treating patients in each of the DRGs in one month. While studying the fifteen DRGs under Major Diagnostic Category number 14 (Pregnancy, Childbirth, and the Puerperium), they noticed that Dr. Daniel Weiner admitted seventeen patients who were later determined to be in DRG 373 (vaginal delivery without complicating diagnosis) but only two in DRG 371 (cesarian section, without complication and/or comorbidity). Yet for the other three obstetricians on staff, fifty-eight came under DRG 373 and nineteen under 371. Across all deliveries, the costs of treating Dr. Weiner's patients exceeded the revenue received from the DRG rates. But the total cost incurred in providing care to the other obstetricians' patients was considerably below revenue and hence the hospital was able to earn a "profit."

The computer report also revealed that the reimbursement rate the hospital received for routine deliveries fell just short of covering all the incurred expenses, whereas the rate paid for cesarian sections was substantially greater than the actual cost to the hospital. The reason for Dr. Weiner's comparatively poor overall "financial performance," Dr. Lapin and Ms. O'Connor concluded, was that he performed many fewer cesarians than did his colleagues.

Dr. Weiner explained that he did not agree with his colleagues that once a woman had a cesarian delivery, all subsequent deliveries must be cesarian; he felt that most of these women could have normal deliveries. He cited a number of recent studies that found no differences in outcomes (in terms of health risks to both mother and child) associated with the different delivery modes. Dr. Lapin countered that the tradition of performing repeat cesarians was strong and that more time and research were needed before large numbers of physicians changed their practices. He noted too that, if a complication were to arise, the attending physician would likely be faced with a malpractice suit.

Finally, he pointed out to Dr. Weiner that the hospital was losing money on almost every patient he treated. "Dan," he said, "it's in all our interests to look out for the financial health of the hospital. And since it is unclear which of the two approaches benefits the patient more, I urge you to reconsider the way you handle these cases."

Was it ethical for Dr. Lapin to approach Dr. Weiner if there was no indication he was delivering poor quality care? How should financial considerations, both those related to the hospital and society at large, be weighed against physician judgment? What if Dr. Weiner could convincingly demonstrate that his patients were actually at less risk than those of his colleagues?

COMMENTARY

J. Joel May

The ethical question raised in this case is: what considerations are appropriate in making medical decisions? Certainly the question of what is good for the patient in the opinion of a competent physician is, and will continue to be, an important ingredient in making such decisions. Thus, Dr. Weiner's belief that, given no difference in outcomes, it is desirable not to expose obstetric patients to the trauma of surgery is a justifiable part of the calculus. Also, when outcomes are similar, patient preferences with respect to alternative forms of treatment should be considered. Finally, what the regimen of care will cost the patient (but not what it will cost the insurance carrier) is frequently a part of such a decision.

But, this case asks, is the financial impact of the chosen mode of care on the *hospital* an admissible ingredient? Hospitals, by virtue of their social purpose and their tax status, are expected to provide "charitable care" (that is, care that is not financially profitable to the institution) to those in need. But if a hospital were to provide "too much" such care, it would fail financially. Potential future patients would suffer reduced access to care. The hospital's obligation to all present and potential patients must be weighed against its obligation to provide "charitable care" in a particular instance. In this case, the hospital is faced with either losing a little money on each patient delivered normally or making "substantial" money on each patient delivered by cesarian. The hospital does have an obligation to point out that fact to its physicians and to urge them to consider including it as a relevant dimension of their decision-making process. Thus, it was not only ethical but appropriate for Dr. Lapin to call Dr. Weiner's "poor financial performance" to his attention.

The ultimate decision of how to treat patients, on the other hand, should remain with the physician. Were Lakeview Hospital to order Dr. Weiner to deliver such patients by cesarian section in order to improve its profitability and thereby reduce the options available to him, it would be acting unethically. The question raised in the case (of how financial considerations should be weighed against the physician's judgment) is therefore moot.

Financial considerations should be a part of a physician's judgment. Financial issues important to the individual patient (such as out-of-pocket expenditures for the procedure) have always been a part of such judgments. Because new financial dimensions of the question are related to institutional, community, or societal concerns, rather than individual patient concerns, does not preclude them from consideration. Nor should they be treated as if they were juxtaposed to medical judgment. Instead they should be incorporated into the decision-making process.

The final question concerns a hypothetical situation in which Dr. Weiner was able to demonstrate that his patients, delivered normally, were actually at less risk than those delivered by cesarian section. Herein lies a real ethical dilemma. The amount of reduction in risk to the patients is associated with a cost to the hospital. But if the patients (or the physicians on their behalf) are willing to incur additional risk, the hospital makes a profit. From the hospital's perspective, the decision must revolve around the cost it is willing to bear in order to reduce the risk. Since outcomes of medical treatment are never certain, and since risk can never be totally eliminated, a common denominator must be chosen to measure the extent of risk that is "appropriate" given the cost, and that, in turn, must be weighed against the relationship between the financial impact on the hospital and its ability to serve future patients.

Probably in the situation presented in this case, the fact that only a small financial loss is associated with the reduced risk would (and should) lead the hospital to encourage the least risky approach, even in the face of a loss of income.

In the past, financial considerations have played a small part in shaping or constraining physicians' judgments, and this has contributed to the inflation in hospital costs. Absence of cost constraints has also led to the provision of unnecessary (too much) care for some, perhaps at the expense of limiting or denying care to others.

Factoring cost implications into the calculus of medical decision making is not only desirable but essential in deciding fairly and equitably who shall get how much of what kind of care. Dr. Lapin should continue to identify such circumstances and bring them to the attention of the physicians. Dr. Weiner and his colleagues have an obligation to include such considerations when making medical judgments.

COMMENTARY

Daniel H. Schwartz

Some fifty years ago my professor of ethics drew two circles on the blackboard—a large one representing the common good, and a smaller one the individual good. Arrows pointed from each circle to the other, indicating conflict. The problem in ethics, he said, was to put the small circle inside the large one, so that the individual and common good could both be achieved.

The hospital administrator has the responsibility of putting a number of smaller circles—patients and physicians, students and researchers in a tertiary hospital, the hospital and its community—inside the larger one of societal good.

Case studies like this are designed to present hard choices for the hospital administrator in fulfilling that responsibility. But perhaps the choice in this case is not so hard after all. There is no reason why a hospital cannot provide quality care to patients and survive under a well-constructed DRG or other prospective payment system. Assuming that the hospital is doing a good job, it should both survive financially and permit Dr. Weiner to continue his practice of preferring normal deliveries over repeat cesarians. Physicians should be aware of the fiscal impact of their activities. They should also, in my opinion, practice the best medicine as determined by the leaders of their profession.

Changes in practice are familiar problems in the evolution of medical care and the DRG system is set up to adjust to medical advances. It is my understanding that the old view on repeat cesarians has changed and in most leading institutions it is no longer the rule. An NIH Task Force reached this conclusion a couple of years ago. In our own hospital about 70 percent of previous cesarians are handled by normal vaginal delivery. The original DRG is based on historical data but will change.

On the other hand, changes in cases designed to produce a "profit" under the DRG system would result in identifying the change in the particular hospital and physician's case mix. The hospital would get into more trouble by insisting that Dr. Weiner alter his approach than it would by permitting him to continue to avoid repeat cesarians. The State Health Commissioner, during the DRG demonstration, tells me that if Dr. Weiner changed his practice, it could result in a penalty to the hospital.

All of us in hospital administration (and many other fields) know that you win some and you lose some. A creative administrator will find an ethical way to compensate for the financial loss in Dr. Weiner's case by a variety of actions that will help, not harm, patients: more precise coding of complications and comorbidities; getting doctors to do better documentation in medical charts (which will improve patient care); reducing unnecessary laboratory tests; and other measures that will be stimulated by the DRG system. One of the ways we expect to deal with this problem is discharging patients earlier to our Home Health Agency, providing appropriate therapy in the home at less than a tenth of the cost of hospital care.

Finally, speaking of ethics, it should be noted that Dr. Weiner would receive a bigger fee from Blue Shield for a cesarian yet he prefers to do normal deliveries in these situations. Furthermore, Dr. Lapin is right that Dr. Weiner exposes himself to a greater possibility of a malpractice suit, since our legal system lags behind medical advances. The plaintiff's attorney is certainly going to say: "Why didn't you do a cesarian?" Dr. Weiner's ethical courage should be commended.

COMMENTARY

Joy Hinson Penticuff

Dr. Lapin asserts that "it's in all our interests to look out for the financial health of the hospital." Yet in this case he put one interest, the financial health of the hospital, ahead of other, more important interests, the physical and psychological health of women. The DRGs will produce bad medical care—that is, some mothers will be subjected to needless cesarian sections—if "traditional" medical practice is maintained despite scientific evidence that innovations produce improved patient outcomes. Dr. Weiner can convincingly demonstrate that vaginal delivery is just as safe for selected mothers and infants as repeat cesarian section. In spring 1982, the American College of Obstetrics and Gynecology published guidelines that described medical indications for trial of labor and vaginal delivery after previous cesarian section. The ACOG studies concluded: "As many as 50 to 75% of a carefully selected group of patients may achieve vaginal delivery after previous cesarian section."

Furthermore, a cesarian section is not just a surgical procedure. It is a birth experience, and as such, carries much symbolic meaning. There may well be a psychological trauma associated with cesarian section because the mother may consider it as a failure. Most mothers feel a sense of disappointment when they are unable to deliver their infant normally, and they frequently feel that what should have been a natural process has taken on a sterile, technical quality. Indeed, many mothers seek out cesarian support groups to cope with their feelings of inadequacy and frustration.

Cesarian sections are painful and interfere with the mother's initial interactions with her newborn infant. Breastfeeding techniques must be modified, since the usual positioning of the infant against the mother's abdomen causes discomfort. To subject the mother to this needless stress for the purpose of preserving the "financial health" of the hospital is outrageous.

In attempting to persuade Dr. Weiner to perform more cesarian sections Dr. Lapin was clearly in the wrong. The real problem here is that the reimbursement for vaginal deliveries in this hospital is too low, and the inducement to perform cesarian sections is too great. It is Dr. Lapin's duty in his role as liaison between the hospital's managers and the medical staff, to correct the faulty calculation of the DRG reimbursement schedule. He is incorrect in taking coercive action toward Dr. Weiner, which would increase the already alarming intrusion of medical intervention into what is a highly significant family process: the birth of a new baby.

Ironically, DRGs are being forced on consumers just when consumers are demanding that health care professionals consider the whole person, not just an affected body part. DRGs do exactly what consumers fear most—they categorize patients according to diagnosis. A patient does not want to be viewed as "the gallbladder in room 312," but as a unique individual with a particular medical condition.

And individuals do respond to illness in distinctive ways. While two mothers may stay in the hospital for the same number of days following cesarian sections, one mother's psychological experience and her need for support following that cesarian birth may be vastly different from that of the mother in the next bed. She may need assistance from her physician and nurses which cannot be calcuted by a DRG.

DRGs were designed to decrease the cost of medical care. In this case, the faulty DRG reimbursement (giving incentive for performance of cesarian section over vaginal delivery) will drive up the cost of medical care because third-party payers will be paying for surgical deliveries rather than the less expensive vaginal deliveries. If one carries this logic to its natural conclusion, hospital administrators will coerce physicians into encouraging their patients to enter the hospital for a variety of unnecessary procedures just to ensure its own "financial health."

This case also shows the pressing need for consumers to be involved in the formulation of DRG reimbursement schedules. The best interests of individuals seeking health care *must* be the priority. Health care professionals who put the institution's financial interest above the best interests of the patient have sold their ethics to the highest DRG.

52

The HMO Physician's Duty to Cut Costs

William Edwards was thirty-nine when a serious, potentially life-threatening ventricular heart arrhythmia (irregular contractions) was diagnosed during a routine physical examination. The cardiologist first prescribed quinidine, but it failed to control the arrhythmia.

Diisopyramide was successful, but Mr. Edwards complained of severe blurred vision and dry mouth. When the medication was reduced, the side effects disappeared but the arrhythmia returned. At this point the cardiologist decided to combine the diisopyramide with propranolol, a common beta-blocker known to be effective in certain arrhythmias. This controlled the problem, without side effects.

Mr. Edwards continued with this medication regimen for five years until moving to a new town, where he joined a Health Maintenance Organization (HMO). He immediately consulted Dr. Sam Forester, a cardiologist.

Dr. Forester agreed that medication was needed, but he was concerned about diisopyramide, since severe problems had been reported in some patients. Moreover, Mr. Edwards and his original physician had never tried the obvious approach of using propranolol alone.

Both Dr. Forester and Mr. Edwards concluded that there were also risks in shifting to the single drug. Although it was generally safer than diisopyramide and probably should have been tried originally, there was a small chance of a fatal heart attack. On balance both agreed that the status quo was slightly better for the patient.

Dr. Forester then noticed the financial ledger for Mr. Edwards's care, which included the cost of the medication paid for in full by the HMO. The yearly cost of the diisopyramide was $430; the propranolol cost $26. He realized that even a significant increase in propranolol dosage, something that would involve little risk, would still reduce the HMO's medication bill by about $400.

Should Dr. Forester consider a change in medication, taking into account cost-saving for the HMO, or should he work solely on the basis of the welfare of the patient? If he should take into account the costs to the HMO, should he try to persuade the patient to agree to the change or should he simply refuse to authorize any further prescriptions for the diisopyramide? Does Mr. Edwards have any moral obligation to take costs to the HMO into account in choosing a medication regimen?

COMMENTARY

Robert M. Veatch

The traditional professional ethics of physicians—reflected in the Hippocratic Oath, the Declaration of Geneva, and elsewhere—is that the physician should always strive to do what he or she thinks will benefit the patient.

In this case that traditional ethical commitment is challenged. In effect, the question is: Should the physician divert his attention from the single-minded pursuit of the patient's welfare where the institution's or other subscribers' interests would be served by slightly compromising the patient? Specifically, a very small, but real increment of benefit is purchased for a very substantial cost. Does the patient-benefit principle apply in such cases?

Two ethical options are available, neither of which is very attractive. First, we could amend the Hippocratic commitment so that physicians should, at least in certain circumstances, take into account the welfare of others. We might give the physician the mandate to try to maximize total benefits instead of simply benefit to the patient.

That strategy produces at least two serious problems, however. First, physicians (like any other special social group) have unique notions about the comparative value of resource expenditures. In deciding whether to use Medicaid funds to pay for drugs, for example, a physician should have to compare the value of providing the drugs with the value of some remote nonmedical uses of the money. Asking health professionals to take these social trade-offs into account could introduce serious biases.

Second, if physicians include benefits to others in their calculations, patients have to be told that their physicians have conflicting agendas. The Hippocratic Oath would have to be removed from the waiting room wall and replaced with a sign that says, "Warning all ye who enter here. The physician will at times abandon your interests in order to benefit others and save them money." It is not clear that rational patients or physicians in an HMO would prefer this new mandate.

The other alternative is to give the HMO physician—in fact all clinicians—a special role-related ethic that exempts them from the general ethical duty to promote fair and reasonable distribution of resources. They would then be free to single-mindedly pursue the welfare along with the rights of the patient.

Then, however, someone else must decide to eliminate marginally beneficial care. Surely, in planning the HMO or insurance coverage, no rational persons would want all such care included. Assuming marginal care was eliminated for others as well as themselves, they would opt for a lower premium so they could spend the money on something they valued more. Mr. Edwards would reasonably prefer not to have the diisopyramide and other marginal treatments covered, if he could spend the savings somewhere else.

The most acceptable arrangement, therefore, would actively involve members of the HMO plan in decisions about whether certain marginal medical services are covered. Members might, for example, exclude heart transplant coverage, as Medicare does. They might decide to cover routine physical exams only every five years for people between twenty and forty even though they might reasonably benefit marginally from more frequent exams. They might cover only ten days of hospitalization for myocardial infarction even though a few more days would be marginally beneficial. These decisions should be made by the patients (the subscribers), however. Clinicians should not be put in the position of ruling on how much to compromise their patients.

The drug case poses an interesting problem. To the extent that the decision can be handled as a policy matter, it should be—like the physical exam frequency. Judgments like the one in the diisopyramide case, however, do not lend themselves to policy. No obvious solution is apparent. Administrators, especially in profit-making HMOs, are not in any better position to make such decisions than clinicians.

An ethics committee comprising a representative sample of patients might be given the authority to rule based on the facts presented by the HMO professionals. In doing so the group would be acting as agents for their fellow subscribers with a mandate to eliminate marginally beneficial care. Theoretically, they might be asked to eliminate all care where the cost exceeded the benefit. That, however, would create serious tensions among members and would be unfair to the sickest members, exactly the group that has the greatest claim of justice for care, even inefficient care. If this ethics committee of HMO members cannot make these judgments, we may be forced to the bizarre conclusion that no one is in an ethical position to decide to eliminate such care.

That brings us to the role of Mr. Edwards. Does he have any moral responsibility to consider that the best drug regimen for him is one that offers only marginally more benefit for a much greater cost? Surely, it is both moral and prudent for Mr. Edwards to take all of this into consideration in endorsing, promoting, or participating in collective arrangements by which members establish policies that eliminate marginally beneficial, expensive care.

Does he have any obligation, however, to suggest eliminating his diisopyramide—in order that others may benefit from the savings? I am not convinced he has a strict moral obligation to do so. Such a contribution to his fellow subscribers seems supererogatory.

I am thus forced to conclude that, although the expensive drug should be eliminated, neither Mr. Edwards nor Dr. Forester is the proper person to make that decision. Surely the administrators of the HMO are in no better position to do so. If that decision can be made ethically at all, it should be made by the HMO members as a whole—at the policy level if possible, and by a committee of the members if not.

COMMENTARY

Morris F. Collen

In almost every patient encounter, a health care practitioner must consider first the quality of care he or she is prescribing—that is, whether a particular clinical decision will achieve an accurate diagnosis and/or bring about the desired benefit; and second, the costs resulting from this decision to the patient and/or to the organization financing the care. Thus, a very common problem in the practice of medicine is balancing the quality with the costs of medical care.

The physician often provides professional services on a fee-for-service basis to a patient with a disease for which there are alternative acceptable methods of treatment. The physician always considers the relative effectiveness of each treatment mode and should also consider the comparative total costs associated with each treatment. The physician should attempt to assess whether the patient can afford the most expensive treatments, and should discuss with the patient the comparative costs and effectiveness of the alternative treatments available, ideally to arrive at a mutually agreeable decision. As the fee-for-service practitioner knows, if the costs for the prescribed treatment exceed the immediate financial resources of the patient, then payment of the physician's fee may be delayed. Thus the financial success of fee-for-service practitioners is intimately linked to the financial solvency of their private patients.

Similarly, if the patient has prepaid for medical care services in a Health Maintenance Organization, the HMO physician knows that the immediate cost consequences of his or her clinical decision will have a direct impact on the HMO's finances. Furthermore, if the overall HMO costs exceed those that had been budgeted by the HMO for the year, then in the following year the prepayment dues (premiums) as direct costs to the patient and to all other subscriber-members of the HMO, will proportionately need to increase to restore the HMO's positive economic balance. If the HMO excessively increases its annual premiums, it will no longer be competitive with other health insurance programs in the community, its membership will likely decrease, and it will need to compensate by reducing personnel or decreasing the comprehensiveness of its prepaid services. Thus the financial success of the HMO physician is intimately linked to the financial solvency of his or her HMO.

Only under arrangements where the patient has no obligation to pay for any medical treatment (as in the Veterans' Administration hospitals or a charity clinic) and where the physician's salary is independent of revenues generated from professional services can individual physicians consider the effectiveness of care without taking into account the treatment costs. However, increasing budgetary restraints and public support for cost containment are introducing economic questions even into these medical practice arrangements.

Thus, in any doctor-patient encounter, under any financing arrangement, the doctor has some financial incentive—in addition to a moral obligation—to consider both the quality and the costs of the care being prescribed and to attempt to arrive at a good balance that can be justified and defended to other physicians and the doctor should try to persuade the patient to agree to that treatment which is acceptably effective at the lowest cost. Rarely, in a case such as this one, is any treatment 100 percent effective in curing the disease, so rarely is the choice clear-cut or simple. The physician should not refuse to authorize a treatment that the physician and the patient agree is best. Finally, physicians should be prepared to defend their judgment before their peers in the community within which they practice; and before a jury in court if their decision varies from the comunity's standard of practice.

ORGAN PROCUREMENT AND TRANSPLANTATION

53

In Organ Transplants, Americans First?

Luiza Magardician, a twenty-year-old Rumanian citizen, arrived in New York in June 1985 in the hope of obtaining a kidney transplant. According to Reverend Dumitru Viorel Sasu of the Rumanian Orthodox Church of St. Dumitru in Manhattan, before her arrival here "all available methods of treatment were tried unsuccessfully in her country." The director of the National Kidney Foundation of New York-New Jersey says Ms. Magardician's chance of finding a kidney donor are bleak since "there is a bad shortage of donors in the United States, and U.S. citizens would usually come first." In addition, Ms. Magardician has reportedly exhausted her funds and could not afford hospital costs even if a donor were found.

In 1984, more than 8,500 Americans were waiting for kidney transplants; only half were expected to receive one that year. Should the decision to offer Ms. Magardician a transplant be made strictly on the grounds of her medical needs or should her country of origin or financial situation influence the decision? Should such decisions be made by individual hospitals or at the state or national level? Given the shortage of usable kidneys, what place should compassion, medical need, and justice play in allocating organs?

COMMENTARY

Jeffrey M. Prottas

Despite substantial improvements in the effectiveness of organ procurement efforts, the waiting lists for all transplants grow continually. More people wait longer for a transplant; some of them die waiting. All must accept medical treatments that are inferior in their own view and that of their physicians. Because organs are both valuable and in short supply their allocation among patients is a matter of important public concern. But only when two identifiable patients are candidates for the same organ does the issue of the treatment of nonimmigrant aliens arise.

When only one suitable recipient exists for a given organ there is no allocation problem; if Ms. Magardician is that recipient, no one denies that she should receive it. Her right of access to an organ is called into question only when a U.S. resident is also a medically suitable candidate. The issue is not one of citizenship, but of residence—membership in the community of potential organ donors. Unfortunately, with over 8,500 U.S. residents on lists awaiting a kidney transplant and thousands more awaiting nonrenal transplants, direct competition for an organ is more the case than the exception. The harsh fact is that, often, someone must be denied. On what grounds should that decision be made? I believe that membership in the community that supplies the organs is a legitimate criterion.

Every cadaveric organ available for transplantation in the United States is obtained through the generosity of members of the American community. Only the death of a young healthy person can make a suitable organ available, and only the willingness of family members to put aside their own grief can result in the organ retrieval. Every organ transplant starts in tragedy and kindness.

Organ procurement also requires a large investment in organizational, human, and financial resources. Over 110 organizations are at work locating and obtaining transplantable solid organs. These organizations represent the efforts of perhaps 1,000 men and women and over $100 million of public money.

In short, the American community (all those who live here) has committed resources and, more important, has demonstrated the altruism necessary to make organ transplantation possible. Under these circumstances members of this national community have a right not to be denied an organ transplant because that organ is being sent overseas or offered to a person who has traveled here specifically to obtain it.

An alternative to this policy that can be defended on the highest ethical grounds is that every individual be treated the same and that all nonimmigrant aliens seeking a transplant be placed on the nation's waiting lists without discrimination. But no nation operating an organ procurement system has seen fit to institute this practice. There is a sense that humanitarianism does not extend so far as to require a nation to share, to its own detriment, a scarce and lifesaving resource.

But what of Ms. Magardician? Even if we admit that she must take that kidney from a resident, isn't her need greater? The resident can in all probability remain on dialysis. And, if dialysis is a second best treatment for him or her, it is preferable to dying. Can we not set aside a percentage of organs on compassionate grounds?

First, I am very suspicious of generosity at the expense of other people. I will not have to go to dialysis treatments three times a week as a result of a decision to set aside a percentage of organs for immigrant aliens. But other residents will, and I would not ask that kind of unselfishness from anyone. Second, Ms. Magardician's situation is the same as that of most nonresident aliens. Since only the very rich can afford to treat end-stage renal disease without government support, almost all foreigners who come here explicitly for a transplant have as much claim on our compassion as she does. We cannot transplant them all. If some are more deserving of life than others, the solution is not a quota system but a decision-making process. This process would have to operate in a public manner, with explicit criteria and on a national basis. It is inappropriate to set aside a number of organs and ask individual hospitals to use them as they see fit.

Sending organs overseas or transplanting them into nonimmigrants is not sharing America's bounty but diverting its scarcity. As long as a shortage of organs continues in the United States, some individuals in need must be denied a transplant. Members of the community that make transplantation possible have a right to expect that their medical needs will be addressed and that allocation decisions will not adversely affect them.

COMMENTARY

Olga Jonasson

In North America, Europe, Australia, South Africa, and Japan, well-established programs in organ transplantation provide state-of-the-art therapy for highly selected patients with end-stage kidney failure. Transplantation is, however, unavailable in developing countries and in most of the impoverished areas of the world.

American medicine has a strong tradition and long history of generously sharing its medical technology and therapies. Foreign patients come to our medical centers in large numbers to obtain complex surgical procedures or medical treatment. It seems inconsistent with all our previous practices to exclude access to cadaver organ transplantation for patients from foreign countries.

Yet the reasons for reserving cadaver organs for American residents are compelling. Grossly insufficient numbers of organs are available for Americans who need transplantation; maintaining a patient awaiting kidney transplantation on dialysis is expensive, and thousands of patients wait for months or years until a kidney becomes available. Patients awaiting heart or liver transplantation, where no maintenance therapy is available to keep them alive, frequently die before an organ can be found. It is also commonly assumed (though unproven) that the public expects that the organs donated upon the death of a family member will be transplanted into an American resident. Lastly, the costs of public education campaigns encouraging organ donation and much of the costs of acquiring the organ are supported by tax dollars.

It is also probably true that several countries could mount adequate organ transplantation programs if necessary; the outlet provided by the centers in America and Europe that accept their citizens for transplantation removes the local incentive to establish centers, change laws, and educate the public.

Luiza Magardician came here with the expectation that she would find help in this generous country. In my experience, most of the foreign nationals who have come here for transplantation are like Luiza; they are ordinary folk, with no particular wealth or status and certainly without political clout or influence. Others have come with wealth and influence, and considerable pressure has been applied by institutions in this country and by our government to see to it that they receive a transplant, and as promptly as possible. This, of course, is completely unacceptable. But even people who are rich or powerful can be very sick. Organs should be distributed to rich and poor alike, on the basis of medical need.

Dealing with these issues has not been easy for the transplantation community. To close the doors to all foreign patients seeking transplantation is uncompassionate; to have a completely open policy is unfair to American residents. The Transplantation Society, an international multidisciplinary society with a broad membership from medicine and science, and the American Society of Transplant Surgeons (ASTS) have recently adopted similar positions condemning the commercialization of transplantation, wherein organs could be bought and sold. The ASTS also adopted a position, supported by a large majority of the membership, that at most 5 percent of all kidney transplants done in any center be in foreign patients, and that those patients be selected on the basis of the same medical criteria as all others.

The National Task Force on Organ Transplantation also addressed this issue, and was divided in its recommendations; the majority recommended the establishment of a quota (10 percent rather than 5 percent), but several members of the Task Force as well as many others in the field feel strongly that no organ should be given to a foreign patient unless no American resident is available as a recipient. I cannot agree with this view. It is inhumane to treat nonresidents as second-class patients, even if they voluntarily accept that status in order to gain a slight chance for an organ. They remain in this country, away from home and family, and often spend every asset they possess in the vain hope of obtaining treatment. Moreover, I am convinced that the public wants organs to be fairly allocated to sick patients, whether the recipient is or is not an American.

These decisions rest squarely with the transplantation community. It is their responsibility, as trustees of these precious organs, to develop and implement policies to provide organs to patients with equity and fairness; these policies must be publicly stated and defended, and carefully monitored.

The fact that Ms. Magardician has exhausted her funds poses another problem. Kidney transplantation costs about $30,000, if all goes well. She has no right to expect free care from any transplant center. Her government should be asked to fund her care; failing this, she must appeal to the Rumanian community in New York or elsewhere for support. Again, in my experience Americans are generous when faced with real need.

Clearly, a major reason for the serious discrepancy between need and availability is the failure of hospital personnel to identify potential donors and to offer the family the opportunity to give the gift of the organs. Policies of routine inquiry, guaranteeing that the families will be given this chance, would be important steps in meeting the needs of all deserving recipients.

COMMENTARY

John I. Kleinig

Ms. Magardician's situation is complicated by two factors: (1) she does not appear to have been accepted for assessment or treatment prior to leaving for New York; (2) she did not make adequate financial preparations (might she not have organized community or church support?). We get a whiff of moral extortion—though perhaps she shouldn't be singled out unfairly: a "nag factor," advantaging the importunate, seems to influence even routine decisions.

More important is whether she should be eligible for any consideration, given the shortage of kidney donors and the understandable tendency to feel that "U.S. citizens [better:residents] would usually come first." Should Ms. Magardician's medical needs determine her eligibility, to the extent of putting her ahead of a U.S. resident who might also benefit from the same donor kidney? How might we decide?

At a general level we could, I guess, ask donors (or those who agree to donation for others) to specify whether—given the scarcity of the resource—they would be willing for the kidney to be made available to a nonresident. But without some principled reason for allowing this discretion, donors could claim a more extensive discretion about recipients (regarding color, sex, and the like).

Should it then be left to individual hospitals or states to determine the scope of eligibility? The constraints on arbitrary and invidious discrimination might be stronger, but if nonresidents as such are to be excluded from access to scarce resources, some argument will be needed to deflect the charge of medical jingoism.

What reasons might we have for exclusivism? We might answer differently for private and public transplant units: allowing the former to take whomever they wish, perhaps influenced by ability to pay. This *could* result in a large foreign clientele. Publicly funded units, being taxpayer supported, could argue the reasonableness of a "citizens first" policy.

A problematic assumption underlies both approaches, insofar as they disqualify nonresidents on the basis of their lack of residency. The assumption is that medical facilities and technology are "owned" in some morally strong sense by those who operate or finance them, justifying them in an exclusivist policy.

But like many sophisticated human products, transplant technology is the child not of local or even national effort, but of internationally shared endeavor. That U.S. residents are now able to receive relatively successful treatment for kidney failure owes a good deal to the work, among others, of French and Dutch researchers. A "this is for us alone" policy in scientific research would (and, where it occurs, does) greatly inhibit human progress; there is no overriding reason for its introduction at the point of application.

Of course, there are some reasons for favoring one's own, even as one might agree to donate only because the recipient is a close relative. National bonds, cultural and economic, count for something. Residents have a reasonable expectation that their contributions to their social environment will be reflected in services—particularly of a lifesaving kind. An open-door policy (whether in immigration, education, or medicine) would be destructive to much that has been labored for and is counted dear.

But the alternative to an open door need not be a closed one. In a world of scarce resources, a quota system, safeguarding for resident use perhaps 90 percent of donated organs, would be consistent with the conservation of national resources and values. At the same time, providing some foreign access to transplant units would acknowledge the transnational character of beneficent technology.

As a consequence some U.S. residents will miss out on lifesaving treatment because nonresidents have been given the use of scarce organs. Thus, there is surely some argument for viewing the quota system as only an interim solution, and for developing less problematic alternatives: International kidney donations? The export of successful transplant technology?

Where does this leave Ms. Magardician? If fairness in allocation is the issue, her way of pressing her case does not create a helpful precedent. If a quota system were already in place, we could determine whether, under its terms, she would have qualified for admission. In the absence of a quota system, any decision would probably be clouded by political factors. Whatever is decided, her case will constitute a strong argument for developing general criteria for nonresident eligibility.

54

The Anencephalic Newborn as Organ Donor

Mrs. Z, a young, pregnant woman with no children underwent an ultrasound examination. Her baby girl was overdue and the ultrasound revealed that she was anencephalic. There appeared to be no brain tissue present except for portions of the brain stem. The parents were told of this tragic diagnosis and immediately decided to volunteer the baby as an organ donor. The obstetrician in charge of Mrs. Z's care decided to contact a large, tertiary care facility nearby in order to ascertain their interest in utilizing the child as a donor.

Two-thirds of children who suffer from anencephaly are stillborn. Many of the organ systems in such children are underdeveloped, but it is possible to utilize both the heart and kidneys for transplantation to other children. The obstetrician and the pediatrician agreed that it would soon be necessary to induce labor. However, if organ procurement was to be undertaken, it seemed reasonable to transfer her to the large tertiary care hospital and to induce labor there.

The rest of the medical staff was uncertain whether to proceed. If they accepted the mother's wish to have the baby be an organ donor, were they under an obligation to try to resuscitate the infant if it was stillborn? What steps should they take to try and support the child considering that babies born with this condition normally receive no aggressive treatment in the neonatal nursery? Perhaps most confusing was the question of when death should and could be pronounced.

Should Mrs. Z be transferred to the large medical center? Should the physicians accept the wishes of Mr. and Mrs. Z to have their child serve as an organ donor? If they do, what steps would be morally permissible to help increase the chances of allowing the child to serve as an organ donor?

COMMENTARY

Michael R. Harrison

Mrs. Z's case is problematic because there are ethical and legal obstacles to taking organs from a prenatally diagnosed anencephalic newborn. Her case is also promising because the use of fetal organs may be a biologically sound and cost-effective treatment for otherwise hopeless childhood diseases, and because use of organs from this category of newborns could alleviate or solve the growing shortage of vital organs appropriate for children.

Under present definitions and laws, organs cannot be taken from a person who does not meet the currently accepted "whole brain" definition of death, which requires "irreversible cessation of all functions of the entire brain, including the brain stem." The liveborn anencephalic does not meet this definition; it is not "brain-dead" even though the cranial vault is incomplete and most of the cerebral cortex is absent. Even with this devastating and completely hopeless anomaly, the residual lower brain stem can maintain vital functions, although precariously, for hours or days. However, if vital functions are allowed to deteriorate until cardiorespiratory arrest, vital organs are irreversibly damaged, making them useless for transplantation.

The "whole brain" definition of death was adopted to protect the comatose patient whose injured brain might conceivably recover function. Obviously, this precaution need not and should not apply to an anencephalic who never had and can never have the physical structure necessary for higher brain activity or cognitive function. Failure of the brain to develop is clearly different from injury to a functioning brain, and was not considered when the brain-death definition was formulated.

One possible approach is to consider the anencephalic "brain-absent." By creating a new category, which is limited exclusively to anencephalics, we may be able to avoid revising presently accepted "brain-death" criteria to include anencephalics. I believe "brain-absent" will come to have the same medical-legal implications as "brain-dead." That is, life support can be withdrawn and organs can be retrieved. Of course, this will have to be recognized by society and confirmed by the courts.

There are advantages to treating the anencephalic fetus and newborn as a person who by virtue of biologic deficiencies (the absence of a brain) is analogous to brain-dead. First, this category can be narrowly defined, and cannot be expanded to include individuals with less severe anomalies or injuries. Any attempt to make it possible to use organs from anencephalics should not relax or compromise the protection of fetuses and newborns with other, less devastating anomalies.

Another advantage is that an anencephalic fetus is considered a person, albeit one who is dying, a process that will be completed at or shortly after birth. Like the comatose patient on artificial life support, the anencephalic fetus requires maternal life support for maintenance of vital functions; but birth is inevitable, and birth will be death. If we accept the anencephalic as a person who is "brain-absent," we can recognize his devastating anatomic and functional deficiency without demeaning his very existence. Then it is easy to stipulate that organs can be taken only if this can be accomplished in a way that would not conceivably cause suffering, and would not detract from the dignity of dying or abridge the right to die.

Prolonging gestation to get more mature organs or prolonging extrauterine survival to maintain organ perfusion would be inappropriate. In this setting removal of organs must be carried out with compassion, sensitivity, and respect for the anencephalic donor and the family; this is best accomplished in the operating room as is presently done for the brain-dead heart-beating cadaver. Finally, this approach makes sense of the presently accepted practice of allowing termination of anencephalic pregnancy at any gestational age.

Another approach to organ procurement from anencephalics might be to consider the anencephalic a product of human conception incapable of achieving personhood. Although it might be argued that the anencephalic lacks the biologic structure (forebrain) giving the potential for characteristic human activity, there are several reasons to avoid this approach. First, it is difficult to reach a consensus about personhood and what constitutes humanness, especially when the issue of gestational age is involved. Second, denying personhood denigrates the pregnancy itself and may lead to a less respectful approach to the grieving family and to medical care of the fetus and newborn. Finally, this approach raises a specter of abuse in which other fetuses or newborns, possibly with less severe handicaps, might be denied personhood. This frightening potential would require the most stringent safeguards, and is probably best avoided altogether.

If the anencephalic fetus were to be considered "brain-absent" and thus equivalent to "brain-dead" for legal purposes, Mrs. Z would be ethically justified in allowing organ procurement after delivery. She and her physician should be able to arrange the timing and place of delivery to facilitate transplantation. After all, Mrs. Z's pregnancy provides fetal organ preservation and transport that is far better biologically and far cheaper than anything yet devised by the most accomplished organ harvest team.

Of course, the decision to end the pregnancy must be independent of and prior to any decision about using the organs for transplantation. The aim of perinatal management in this case is to evacuate the uterus as safely as possible for the mother and to allow fetal demise without discomfort. The newborn should be cared for by physicians independent of the transplant team and the condition of anencephaly (and therefore brain absence) confirmed by an independent team including a neurologist, bioethicist, and neonatologist. Prenatal diagnosis allows the family to choose beforehand whether they wish to see and hold the newborn as part of their grieving, and if and how organs can be procured.

If organ procurement from prenatally diagnosed anencephalics can be accomplished with safety for mother and respect for the fetal donor, Mrs. Z should be able to salvage from the inestimable tragedy of fetal anencephaly the consolation of offering the gift of life to a dying child.

COMMENTARY

Gilbert Meilaender

There is in principle no reason why parents should not—after the death of a child—donate the child's heart and kidneys to suitable recipients. But how much we would like to know that this case does not tell us—in particular, what the parents were told, and what they think they are doing.

Having heard the diagnosis, they "immediately" decided to donate the baby's organs. What does this mean? Do they perhaps imagine that they are simply aborting a fetus—even though the child is already overdue? Do they feel guilt that, however irrational, causes them to want to *use* the baby to wrest some good from terrible circumstances? Have they thought about whether they will want to hold their child at least briefly and say goodbye to the infant who occupied their thoughts (and, who knows, perhaps their prayers) for nine months?

Questions . . . none answerable at the moment. We can only reflect on the case and the questions. I presume that Mrs. and Mr. Z and the health care professionals involved all wish to respect the life of Baby Z. This baby cannot live for long even if born alive. She will never have the "higher" human capacities of consciousness and self-awareness. But if born with brain stem activity she will be a living human being, though one born dying.

We can know human beings, whatever their cognitive capacities, only in their bodies, and that is the way we will know this baby—one of the weakest members of our species. She rightfully claims our care. But, of course, potential organ recipients also need care. Can we meet their needs while also caring for this child and respecting her humanity? If we can, we will surely want to do so, but from the outset we should be aware that this may not be possible. Our obligation is not to achieve all the good we can, as if our responsibility were godlike. It is, rather, to effect what good we can within the limits morality places upon us. Not only what we can *accomplish* but what we *do* counts.

One question the case raises admits, I think, of a fairly straight-forward answer. Is there any reason why Mrs. Z. should not be transferred to the larger medical center nearby? *If* there is no other ground for objecting to the proposed organ donation, this need not be an obstacle. Transfer is primarily a matter of logistics. Were it feasible, it would be equally permissible to move potential recipients to the hospital where the donor is located. In this case the other direction of movement is called for, and that in itself does not seem objectionable.

As a guide to the more troubling issues raised by the case, we may take our cue from the first report published (in 1975) by the National Commission for the Protection of Human Subjects of Biomedical and Behavioral Research. That report dealt with the subject that had led to the formation of the Commission:

research on the fetus. A different topic from the one in our case, to be sure, but related in certain ways.

Among the issues discussed and reported on by the Commission, one of the thorniest concerned research on the aborted, nonviable fetus *ex utero*. On the one hand, the Commission held that such dying subjects could not be harmed in the sense of "injured for life." Since this altered the meaning of "harm" in subtle but very significant ways, the report suggested that the class of experiments carrying only "minimal risk of harm" might be larger for these nonviable fetuses than for other experimental subjects. On the other hand, the Commission held that the integrity of the dying subject was not to be violated. It concluded that "out of respect for the dying subjects, no nontherapeutic interventions are permissible which would alter the duration of life of the nonviable fetus *ex utero*."

That particular recommendation did not receive the support of the Secretary of HEW [Health, Education and Welfare, the former title of the Department of Health and Human Services], but it was a sound moral instinct. A similar principle can guide us through the case at hand. We should care for Baby Z as we would normally care for an anencephalic child who is born dying. The anticipated organ donation should not lead us to prolong her life or subject her to medical interventions—unless we would do so in any case, apart from the desire to transplant her organs. That is what it would mean to respect her as a dying subject and not just to use her life as a means to someone else's good. But—subject to the instruction of those with more medical knowledge—I suspect that acceptance of this principle will create difficulties for the planned organ donation.

How would we ordinarily care for this baby at her birth? The case suggests a standard, and it seems to me the right one: she would receive "no aggressive treatment in the neonatal nursery." She is born dying, and proper care for her does not entail useless attempts to sustain her life. Ordinarily, then, we would not and should not provide respiratory assistance to her, assistance that could only prolong her dying. Ordinarily we would not and should not resuscitate such an infant if she were stillborn. And ordinarily, I suspect, we would rely on the normal clinical signs to determine death.

But if the heart and kidneys of this child are to be available for transplantation, we might want to resuscitate her even if she were stillborn. If her organs are to be suitable for donation, we might want to provide (while she still lives) exactly the sort of assistance we normally eschew—respiratory assistance, with death determined not by ordinary clinical signs but by absence of brain activity. In other words, the anticipated organ donation tempts us to treat in ways we otherwise would not—which is, I fear, a temptation to use this child simply as a means to another (admittedly desirable) end.

If the transplantation can be carried out without significantly altering the way we would otherwise treat this baby, I see no reason to disapprove and much reason to approve it. But if transplantation requires significant change in the normal care of Baby Z, we ought to have serious moral reservations. To intervene in this baby's living and dying in ways we normally reject (because we think it an indignity to a dying subject) would be to do here what we normally think it wrong to do—and to do so for reasons entirely unrelated to the care of Baby Z. What we *accomplish* thereby would be good; what we *do* would not.

55

Can the Fetus Be an Organ Farm?

Mr. R, a twenty-eight-year-old engineer, has been on dialysis for three years, and is growing desperate because of the restrictions it places on his life. He can not work regularly because of the amount of time he has to spend in a dialysis center, and he feels weak and is suffering from many of the debilitating side effects of the treatment.

Mr. R has already investigated the possibility of obtaining a transplant. However, he had been adopted as an infant and does not know his natural family. In addition, tests show that he has a rare tissue type that makes it highly unlikely that a suitable cadaver kidney can be found.

Mr. R's physical and mental state continue to deteriorate and his wife suggests a solution to the transplant surgeon. She will, she says, become pregnant, and after five or six months, have an abortion. The kidneys from the fetus could then be transplanted in her husband.

The surgeon knows that technically such a transplant could be performed, and that the graft would probably not be rejected. He also knows that Mr. R has threatened to commit suicide if he has to remain on dialysis for an indefinite period.

Should he agree to transplant the kidneys of a deliberately conceived and aborted fetus?

COMMENTARY

Mary Anne Warren

I would argue that if the relevant factors were only those described, then the surgeon ought to agree to the woman's plan to provide her husband with the kidneys of a fetus conceived for that purpose, and aborted at five or six months. I say "if" because I want to consider the morality of the action apart from any of the legal, professional, or personal complications that might arise if such a plan were actually carried out in today's world.

Even more than the typical abortion case, this case forces us to focus on the moral status of the (five- or six-month-old) fetus, that is, on whether or not it should be considered a human being with a full-fledged right to life. For none of the more plausible arguments intended to show that abortion is morally permissible even if the fetus has the same right to life as an adult human being apply in this case; it is not a matter of self-defense on the woman's part, nor an exercise of her right to retain control of her body by refusing to submit to an unwanted pregnancy. Unless, therefore, one supposes that mere biological parenthood confers the right to kill one's offspring, at any age, one must conclude that if a fetus of this age is a human being with full moral rights, then the woman's proposal is tantamount to murder. On the other hand, if a fetus does not have a significant right to life, then the plan raises no serious moral problem, and provided that the operation has a good chance of saving her husband's life without seriously endangering hers, it should certainly be performed.

It is clear that if we are to make a reasoned judgment about the moral status of fetuses, and of nonhuman animals, alien life forms, intelligent machines, and other problematic entities, we must develop a criterion for the possession of moral rights that is species-neutral. That is, it will not do to make "genetic humanity" (mere genetic affiliation to the human species) either a necessary or a sufficient condition for the possession of full moral rights. To make it necessary is to beg the question against all nonhuman entities, even those which may prove to have intellects and sensibilities comparable or superior to our own; while to make it sufficient is to beg the question against abortion, particularly in a case like this one.

My candidate for a species-neutral criterion for the possession of full moral rights is what I call *personhood*. A person, to speak very roughly, is an entity that has the (actual, not merely potential) capacity for consciousness, complex and sophisticated perception, rationality, self-awareness, and self-motivated behavior. Such entities have rights by virtue of the fact that they have definite, preconceptualized preferences with respect to their own present and future states; they have desires, hopes, plans, and fears. Above all, they normally desire to go on living, or at least not to be killed in a way not of their own choosing. This is why killing people against their will is intrinsically bad, and in most cases morally wrong.

But fetuses, one might say, as yet have no will; they do not desire life, or anything else, any more than trees or amoebas do. Neither the mere *potential* to become a person, nor preconscious organic existence, not even a degree of sentience unaccompanied by the other aspects of personhood, can generate a right to life comparable to that of a person. Hence I think that there can be no serious moral objection to killing a fetus, an entity far below the threshold of personhood, in order to save the life of an adult human being.

I realize, of course, that most people will resist such a conclusion. Fetuses, especially those as old as five or six months, elicit our sympathy, and tempt us to endow them with moral rights, not only because they are potential people, but because they look disconcertingly like people; their physical features are recognizably human. But this sympathy is misplaced, unless there is a good deal more conscious activity in the fetal "mind" than we have any reason to suspect. While a fetus of five or six months may, perhaps, possess some flickering of sensation, or some capacity to feel pain, this is equally true and probably even more true of creatures like fish or insects, which few would doubt the propriety of killing in order to save human lives. In such cases, a proper respect for the right to life requires that it not be respected where it does not exist.

COMMENTARY

Daniel C. Maguire

One of the most neglected ways to resolve an apparently irresolvable ethical dilemma is to ask: are there viable alternatives to that which is proposed? In this case, there is one alternative that seems to transform the dilemma of Mr. and Mrs. R, making the intentional abortion for a transplantable kidney morally out of order. The alternative is: allow the baby to be born, and then see whether its tissue type is a suitable match. Since the mother's genes enter into the baby's genetic endowment, it is possible that the kidney will be incompatible with the father's rare type.

If the match is good and if the baby has two kidneys, one could be removed and given to the father. The greater maturity of the organ would likely enhance the prospects for successful transplant. Allowing the baby to be born changes the *what* of the case significantly, making the transplant proposal medically and morally more promising. The mother's plan to conceive a baby who might or might not have the right tissue type and to terminate the life of the fetus in any event is not the same case as bearing a baby who might, among other things, be a suitable donor for its father.

There are many reasons for having a baby, and, of course, the baby makes its own sweet case for living when it arrives. But, having a baby as a potential donor does not appear either evil or frivolous. And, medically, a born baby seems to have more realistic credentials as a donor. Even if the baby were not the right tissue type, its birth might possibly give Mr. R more zest for life helping him to bear his terrible affliction.

But suppose Mr. and Mrs. R insist that they do not want to have a baby, they only want to have a kidney. In reply I would point out the difficulty of having one without the other. More technically, I would say that they do indeed want a baby, but as a means not as an end. This is not self-evidently immoral.

In addition to these points against the abortion, I confess an extreme uneasiness in contemplating the very idea of the uterus as an organ farm or the fetus as an organ bank. Maybe my uneasiness is simply a shrinking before the unaccustomed, a horror of the new, or weakness of the masculine mind in the face of a tragic but moral option. Maybe the death of the fetus makes sense in a world where laying down one's life for a friend is the supreme moral achievement. The death of the fetus might be more easily entertained since it is preconscious, and not in the same human situation as a fully personalized adult.

On the other hand, my uneasiness may be the yield of moral intelligence. Ethics begins in awe and moves on to articulation, argument, and debate. Even in the midst of debate, the mind of the moralist should be attentive to the awe that is its foundation. In this case, my uneasiness, plus the facts and alternatives, conspire to make me very certain in offering a negative moral judgment on the proposed abortion.

One question remains: what right have we to presume the permission of the baby in donating its kidney to its father? Shouldn't the autonomy and privacy of the baby be protected until it grows to adulthood and can consent to such a dramatic donation?

A baby is not born outside the pale of human solidarity. It is a horrid individualism that sees the baby born into a "state of nature" with no debts or beneficent relationships to the social body until it "consents" to participate in the social contract. A baby is not an alien untouchable or a mere candidate for human communal existence. "Person" is a relative term and even baby-persons are intrinsically related to other persons.

Relationship to the other and the capacity for sharing are present before we are aware of them, since they relate to our elementary humanity and not just to our subsequent maturity and volition. Part of the awesome grandeur of parental care is the right and duty to interpret sensitively what a baby's humanity entails. And it may entail the surrender of a paired organ when that surrender is "a gift of life." The inability to permit this has its roots in an isolationist-individualist anthropology that ostracizes the baby from genuine humanness under guise of protecting its nonadult status.

Notice that the issue here cannot be discussed merely at the level of consent—whether personal or proxy. It involves the foundation upon which one's entire ethics is based.

COMMENTARY

Carol Levine

The conception and birth of a wanted child have always been among humanity's most powerful affirmations of life and its intrinsic value. When a pregnancy is unwanted, and abortion is contemplated, it is usually because of some serious reason—contraceptive failure, rape or incest, severe medical problems in the mother, probable genetic defects in the offspring, or economic deprivation. In these cases the rights and interests of the already existing person must be weighed against those of the fetus. Abortion in such cases need not be condemned; neither, of course, should it be celebrated.

The scheme proposed in this case study, however—planned conception followed by planned abortion for the sole purpose of producing a body organ—is a perversion of both acts. Creating life in order to destroy it mocks both religious and humanistic concepts of the value of an individual. Manipulating the procreative process in this way transforms it from a natural and positive act to a callous and calculating one that transcends the permissible limits of human interference.

And one need not be opposed to abortion in all cases to be opposed to it in this one. The fetus is not an adult or even an infant; neither is it a chicken or a carrot. As what I would consider a potential person, it has at the very least the right to be treated with respect and dignity, and not as a source of spare parts for another's body. In carrying out this scheme, Mrs. R would not only be using her unborn child solely as a means and not as an end, but she would also be permitting herself to be used in the same unethical way.

But would this violation of the moral imperatives of valuing life and treating persons as ends and not means be acceptable because of another, more compelling principle—saving the life of another human being? There may be situations in which it is the highest form of altruism to sacrifice one's life to save another's, but that is not at issue here. It is harder to imagine situations in which one person may be allowed to sacrifice the life of another, even potential, person, to save a third, but even that is not at issue.

Consider the facts. Mr. R is not dying—he is only threatening to kill himself. Two medically accepted therapies are available for his kidney disease. He has tried dialysis, and finds it too restricting. Now he wants a transplant, and no near relatives or suitable cadaver organs are available. But even if the aborted fetus's kidney were available, success is by no means guaranteed. With present medical knowledge, such a transplantation is technically feasible, but it is not certain that the kidney tissue will match or that if it does, the graft will take over his failed kidney function. Rejection rates for kidneys from related donors are much lower than for cadaver organs; even so, a third fail within five years.

Transplantation itself involves a not inconsiderable risk of death. Even the successfully transplanted patient faces the frequently serious medical and psychological effects of continuous immunosuppressive drug therapy. It is quite likely that the best Mr. R could hope for is a few years' respite from dialysis, and then what? Another conception? Another abortion? Another transplant?

Mr. R finds dialysis intolerable, but thousands of other patients like him have learned to accept it. For some it is even the treatment of choice: it is more predictable, safer, and less damaging to the body over the long run than repeated transplants.

But Mr. R does not feel his life on dialysis is worth living, even though he has a supportive wife to share his difficulties. In a desperate attempt to give her husband the reason to live that she alone apparently cannot provide, Mrs. R is willing to use her body to produce the kidney he wants. Can her offer be considered entirely voluntary, or must it inevitably be suffused with the guilt and bitterness she must feel knowing that her husband values her not as a marriage partner, or as the mother of his child, but as an organ incubator? Threats of suicide can be very persuasive, but they are at the same time coercive.

I believe that the transplant surgeon should refuse to participate in the abortion scheme. Instead, he should try to help Mr. R to understand and adjust to the practical alternatives. Some psychiatric counseling seems in order for Mr. R as well as marriage counseling for the couple. Adding the burden of a morally unacceptable act to a serious medical problem and a troubled marital relationship would only deepen their despair.

56

A Prisoner in Need of a Bone Marrow Transplant

JB, who is serving a prison term for third-degree murder, is being considered for an early pardon and release so that he can undergo a bone marrow transplant. He is suffering from chronic myelogenous leukemia (CML). Without the transplant, doctors say he will probably die within five years. With a transplant, JB has a 50 to 60 percent chance of long-term remission.

Ordinarily, inmates who need medical care are hospitalized and then returned to prison. But officials would prefer to release JB before his transplant, because they say they cannot afford the $100,000 to $200,000 estimated costs of surgery. If JB is released, he will probably qualify for public aid, since bone marrow transplants for CML are no longer considered experimental in his state.

Should JB be granted an early release on the grounds of his medical condition? If an early release is not feasible, does the prison system have an obligation to pay for his care? In or out of prison, is it fair for him to receive a publicly funded transplant when others who need a transplant might have to pay for it out of their own pockets?

COMMENTARY

Robert L. Cohen

Does the fact that a prisoner has chronic myelogenous leukemia disease (CML) meet the criteria for medical parole? Assuming that JB was incarcerated for a crime that he actually committed, that he received due process in his trial and sentencing, and that he has more than five years left to serve, the decision to grant medical parole should be based on prognosis and current degree of debilitation.

Prognosis is a relative issue because a very long anticipated survival would moot the question of medical parole. The five years survival prognosticated in this case seems to me long rather than short in the context of medical parole, and would argue against early release. If JB's physical condition were marked by a severe degree of debilitation, and it seemed to the relevant officials that he was physically unable to pose any threat to the community, this would argue for medical parole. Continued incarceration would no longer serve the "correctional goals" of deterrence and punishment effectively (a severely debilitating terminal illness being punishment enough). However, from the record we are given, JB does not appear to be in a state of terminal debilitation. An early release therefore would not be appropriate.

Indeed, the chance of prisoners to receive medical parole is determined by other factors as well. Prisoners' social status, their access to influential legal and political supporters, and the perceived "seriousness" of the crime for which they have been incarcerated are the most critical issues. It may be that the aging of the prison population, as well as an increase in the number of terminally ill prisoners secondary to cancer and AIDS will result in expanded availability of medical parole. If such were to occur, driven by the economic pressures upon State Departments of Correction caring for terminally ill people, it would be a good thing.

Based on the principle that all individuals deserve equal access to medical care, which prison officials in this case seem to support, the question of who should pay for JB's transplant is a real one. In practical terms, the state is obligated for the cost of care, since an incarcerated individual has no effective way of paying for his or her own medical services. The fact that JB would be eligible for Medicaid as a medically disabled person if released from prison, whereas he is not as a State prisoner, is a cost sharing problem, not an ethical one. These questions could be raised only in a system in which medical services are not universally available and where payment precedes the provision of necessary care. It is to our country's dishonor that universal access to care that is free at the point of delivery has not been codified as law.

The final question raised is the fairness of JB's receiving a bone marrow transplant while incarcerated. Such a transplant would be publicly funded, and might place him at an advantage to others equally in need of a bone marrow transplant but who might have to pay for it "out of their own pockets." The normal course of events is in the opposite direction: availability of scarce and expensive medical technologies is often determined by market forces. Those with the greatest economic resources have the greatest access to these expensive and scarce procedures. In any case, the availability of bone marrow transplantation as a treatment for CML represents the fruit of publicly funded research and should be available to all, regardless of their ability to pay. I do not think it will be unfair for JB to receive a bone marrow transplant if that were clinically indicated.

COMMENTARY

Jeffrey Paul

Presuming punishment for a crime necessarily involves forfeiture, temporarily or permanently, of some of the criminal's rights (personal liberty, for example), which rights ought to be circumscribed by the state and to what extent? To determine what degree of circumscription is appropriate for a certain category of criminal, we must first assess the moral seriousness of the crime and analyze the social purposes that are to be served by assigning punishment. Such purposes have traditionally included retribution, incapacitation, reform, and deterrence.

Given the deliberate character of third-degree murder, a suitably severe punishment may deter some prospective criminals from committing it. Any punishment that deters others from unjustifiably taking an innocent life and does not *inappropriately* transgress the rights of the criminal should be incorporated into his sentence.

What counts as an appropriate transgression of those rights? Where deterrence, reform, incapacitation, and retribution are collectively employed to determine the requisite punishment, the retributive component must set the morally appropriate boundaries for such transgressions.

Thus, to ask what rights the perpetrator of third-degree murder surrenders is to ask what retribution is morally appropriate for a certain type of criminal. Because the crime involves violation of the victim's right to life, it can be argued that the criminal surrenders the right to life, or at least the right to life at liberty, by committing it. But because the crime here is murder in the *third degree*, the moral culpability of JB is less than that of someone who commits murder in the first or second degree. JB thus has surrendered neither his right to life nor the whole of his right to liberty. The punishment assigned to him therefore should not involve taking his life or permanently abrogating his liberty (in the form of life imprisonment, for example). However, given that his crime involved violation of another's right to life, neither is the state obligated to do everything in its power to sustain his life while he is incarcerated.

Against this it might be claimed that JB has only been denied a life at liberty temporarily, that his punishment assumes his eventual release, and, thus, that provisions must be made to maintain his existence until that time. Yet this does not address the goals of retribution, deterrence, and reform. Arguably, imprisonment for third degree murder requires the state to take only technologically and economically *ordinary* measures to assure the criminal a life at liberty after he serves his term. One of the rights the third degree murderer surrenders by his crime is that of access to extraordinary care for disease that, untreated, would be fatal.

This argument for retribution is further supported by one that appeals to the deterrence value of denying such criminals access to extraordinary lifesaving treatment. If prospective murderers know that, should they contract a potentially fatal disease during their prison terms, they may die because they may be denied extraordinary treatment, some murders may be prevented. Moreover, those who contract such illnesses during their terms but survive their sentences to seek treatment when released may learn something from such a harrowing experience. Denying extraordinary care might, that is, also reform such criminals.

Clearly a punishment that includes both a temporary denial of liberty and access to technologically or economically extraordinary lifesaving measures precludes a criminal's entitlement to a publicly funded transplant of the kind contemplated in this case. Having partially surrendered his rights, the criminal may justifiably be denied access to public funds for treatment. If the goals of deterrence and reform are also served, this increases the moral desirability of denying access.

Thus JB should not be granted an early release on the grounds of his medical condition, nor should the prison system pay for his care. The severity of his crime militates against either, and should preclude his eligibility for any publicly funded treatment.

HEALTH CARE POLICY

57

Regulating an Anti-Aging Drug

Thomas Lockhart is the president and chief executive officer of Lockhart Pharmaceuticals. His company has been doing basic pharmacological testing on a series of compounds attempting to identify an agent that will affect the basic processes of aging.

In its early work the company tested procaine analogues, vitamin E, BHT, and a series of other compounds reported to have life-span-extending properties. They found, however, that the most promising was a compound that would be marketed under the trade name of Sinemort. The drug would be very inexpensive to produce, and promises to be a money-maker for the company as well as, in Lockhart's view, a great help to mankind.

The compound has proven promising in animal testing, and Lockhart is now considering human trials. In fact, he himself has been taking the drug on an experimental basis and is enthusiastic about its promise. The drug being tested is already marketed for use in humans as an antidepressant. Although it has not been widely used for this purpose because there are other, more effective drugs available, the compound has been demonstrated to be safe in humans at dosage levels above those contemplated in the clinical trial. In fact, it has been found safe for use in children.

Lockhart is working with Wilson Jeffers, his medical director, to prepare the IND (investigation of new drug) application for the Food and Drug Administration. They have reached the point where they have to list the possible harmful effects of the drug. According to Jeffers, the side effects are mild, rare, and immediately reversed upon discontinuing the drug. Dr. Jeffers remarks jokingly, "We could say that the drug will also change the life style of the population, increase the size of the labor force, bankrupt the Social Security Administration, create new and unknown family relationships, possibly make the country more conservative politically, and make drug taking routine from puberty on."

The FDA is charged with evaluating potential risks and benefits before approving an IND and eventually establishing that the drug is safe and effective before approving it for general use. It is staffed with pharmacologists and lawyers to review applications.

Should Lockhart Pharmaceuticals be obliged to include the social, political, and life-style risks of their drug in the IND application? If not, who should take on that task?

COMMENTARY

Sidney Callahan

As usual, in debates over bioethical questions one issue concerns *who* should decide possible risks and benefits; in this case, who should control the anti-aging pill? There is also the substantive problem of *what* ought to be decided: should we legitimate anti-aging medication?

In answer to the first question, I can see no justification for leaving the decision solely in the hands of Mr. Lockhart, Dr. Jeffers, or the FDA's pharmacologists and lawyers. Ethical and social decisions that will affect the general public for better or worse should not be decided by a few persons whose training and interests may be very narrow.

Nor would the problem be solved by hiring an in-house ethicist who could give a Good Housekeeping seal of ethical approval, in case the consumers complain. One ethicist does not guarantee wisdom. It is equally hopeless, of course, to look for guidance from "the people" or the mythical man in the street.

In such a dilemma, I think, important bioethical decisions should be put before an appointed interdisciplinary group of persons specifically charged with considering the ethical and social ramifications of medical technology. (The National Commission for the Protection of Human Subjects is a prototype.) This group should include many who have had extended ethical training in different traditions.

But once the group is created, the problem remains: what should they decide about anti-aging research? If called to testify, I would say, "Let's go ahead with this work for the following reasons based on the following affirmations."

My first affirmation is that it is good to live and bad to die. Life, like pleasure, health, and plenty, is a good thing; and death, like pain, disease, and poverty, is an evil to be avoided. My second affirmation is that technology, rationality, and science are both liberating and essential. The fact that technology has been misused does nothing to deny the great benefits that it has brought to human life, from irrigation to vaccines.

The objections offered against the anti-aging pill in this case do not seem convincing. Changing American lifestyles and reorganizing the labor force and the Social Security Administration are long overdue items on the nation's social agenda. I also doubt that increasing the age of the population will automatically make the country more conservative; instead it will create a force to struggle with discrimination against the aged, one of the last unacknowledged prejudices.

As for the problem of making drug-taking routine from puberty on, surely that tendency already exists. Who among us doesn't already depend to some degree upon caffeine, alcohol, soft drinks, tobacco, marijuana, vitamins, and aspirin? Mild antidepressants, from wine to a spot of tea, have relieved human anxieties for a long time.

A more serious question and difficulty would concern the way in which the drug worked. If it simply prolonged life after deterioration was extensive and succeeded only in producing chronic debilitation, there would be little progress. To be a real anti-aging agent it would have to produce a higher level of vigor for a longer time. This version of the drug would be better named Convital rather than Sinemort. Another important factor would be whether its action was continuous or discontinuous. Would one age suddenly, as did the natives of Shangri-la when they left the valley? Some might still choose a sudden decline, but others would not.

The availability and distribution of such a drug would raise other ethical problems. Surely it would be unfair for only the rich to have access, since they already live longer and look younger. The question of how family patterns would be changed is also a serious ethical concern. While it would be wonderful to live longer and know one's forebears and descendants, it would be disastrous to have one's children take the pill first, especially if it slowed down the whole maturation process. The prospect of living out a present life span while still supporting one's slowly aging dependent children would produce a new kind of oppression.

The overall trend in evolution has been to delay human maturation, but at the same time the life expectancy of the parenting generation has also been extended. The empty-nest period could be seen as the reward of the increased social and economic investment in rearing children.

It is well to remember that the objections to anti-aging research have been raised about every technological change in history. After all, the neolithic revolution in agriculture also increased the life span, changed lifestyle, changed the family, and created a lifelong dependence upon the daily intake of an artificially created substance, that is, food from agriculture. Surely there are problems in managing progress, but we can be hopeful about the abilities of humans to cope. For one thing, with the successful introduction of anti-aging measures, we will all have a lot more time in which to think.

COMMENTARY

James F. Childress

The question "who should control the anti-aging pill?" is subordinate to the question "what ought we to do about this possible technology?" The answer to this second question depends on "technology assessment," which, as William James said of pragmatism, is only a new name for an old way of thinking. Technology assessment, as Joseph Coates has argued, is an "art form," not a science.

Any technology assessment may have different implications at different stages of decision making. Consider three questions that might be asked. First, should we give research on aging or on some specific anti-aging technology high or low priority in the allocation of public resources? Second, should we conduct or permit research on human subjects in order to determine the safety and efficacy of a technology? Third, should we prohibit, allow, or control the implementation, distribution, and use of a technology? We could, for example, decide not to fund research on aging but to permit research, implementation, and use of any technologies that are developed. The ethical and public policy issues may vary at these different stages.

The third question, which is important in this case, cannot be answered without examining the probable positive and negative consequences of anti-aging technology. The consequences indicate why this technology is or should be a matter of public interest. While our society has not yet provided a high quality of life for the elderly, society's failures can be distinguished, in part, from such quality-of-life factors as power and vigor of body and mind. An anti-aging technology could increase the length of life (1) with an increase in the period of physical and mental vigor or (2) without an increase in the period of physical and mental vigor. While the Lockhart Company assumes that Sinemort will be "a great help to mankind," it does not mention the quality of life that individuals whose lives are expanded can expect. To retard the aging process without an increase in the period of vigor would hurt rather than help. All the problems of quality of life that the elderly now face would be extended, and the broader social problems of caring for health and welfare would be dramatically increased.

Let us take the category emphasized in the National Academy of Sciences report, *Assessing Biomedical Technologies:* "Longer life with parallel increase in vigor (i.e., an 'addition' of extra years of vigorous maturity without any increase in the period of adolescence or decline)." Suppose that these extra years could be provided easily (for example, by drug rather than by diet or discipline) and inexpensively. While such a prospect is no doubt very attractive for most of us, its overall social consequences may not be so attractive.

What about the positive consequences? For the most part, they are very speculative. Albert Rosenfeld argues that if we extend the life span, people will then have the motivation to care about what happens to posterity; it will be in their self-interest to do so since they will be around long enough to experience the consequences. And Zhores Medvedev suggests that if the life span were longer, "People might savor it in less haste, and perhaps with more altruism." Such speculations feature the language of possibility—what might happen—but it is very difficult to base public policies on such flimsy possibilities.

What about the negative consequences? Some commentators fear that people would be less willing or able to carry out projects with "alacrity and promptitude" since they would not feel the pressure of time and impending death. Others fear that people would be less willing to take risks—survival would be more important since people would not want to risk so many years of life. The result could be stagnation, or a society of control.

In the light of these speculative consequences, what should we do? We do not yet know enough in this area to override the presumption in favor of inquiry, research, and commercial implementation. Yet public controls and regulations are in order. Lockhart should be permitted to proceed with carefully controlled research on human subjects and controlled implementation that would be monitored so that the society could make necessary adjustments as it learns more about the aging process and the effects of anti-aging technology on the quality of life and society. Regarding social impact, the possibility of negative effects on social security, and so on, raises important caution flags, but societies and conditions do change, for better or worse. Hence, we should develop policies that keep options open. In this scenario we are not yet at the point where prohibition is justified.

Lockhart should include social risks in its application and FDA should consider these broad effects. But the public's participation in the assessment of anti-aging technology is indispensable and should be maximized through public hearings, publicly funded workshops, and congressional hearings.

58

Drinking on the Job

Boyd Anderson was a company man. He started working at Tone Master Radio in 1945, just as it was beginning to expand. Over the next twenty-five years the company became a huge conglomerate. Anderson worked his way to the top, becoming vice-president of the western division in 1970.

Shortly thereafter the company brought in an aggressive young president to revive lagging sales. He lasted only a year, but in that time he replaced Anderson and transferred him back to the company's main office, where he was given only limited responsibilities, a small office, and a part-time secretary.

Anderson had become accustomed to meeting clients at lunch and having a few drinks. When he had to face the humiliation of being useless to the company, he began to drink more heavily. He lobbied for new positions within the company but failed. Month after month the mail brought only rejection letters from other firms. His drinking became more and more uncontrollable.

Offered a minor overseas post with the firm, he refused it, in part because his family was not able to go with him, but largely because he was afraid his drinking would become known. By this time his self-confidence was gone. The company had been his life, and it was clear that his career was over.

In 1973 at the age of fifty-eight he was told to accept special early retirement. Within a month he was found in an alcoholic convulsive coma. He went through several episodes of drying out and drinking again. Nothing worked.

At this point he sued the company for $1.1 million for retroactive medical disability, claiming his job had made him an alcoholic. He claimed not only the disability pay, but payment of his medical and psychiatric expenses and back pay. He argued during a hearing, "My God, you give your life to the company, then you discover that they think you're washed up. The mental strain is just too much. Drinking was part of my business life. The company should bear the responsibility."

What kind of responsibility, if any, should the company bear for Anderson's drinking problem? If it is not found legally liable for his expense, does it still bear a moral responsibility?

COMMENTARY

Herbert Fingarette

Insofar as Anderson's problems were caused by his excessive drinking, he is morally responsible for them. He should also be legally liable for their costs unless he is specifically insured.

Until he was demoted, Anderson voluntarily accepted his company position, including (presumably without protest) the custom of luncheon drinks. Over a period of many years he drank at lunch without drinking to excess.

What changed things? The company president reassigned him to a less important position. Understandably, he was unhappy. He then began drinking excessively. Plainly, it was the demotion and resulting unhappiness that were decisive in triggering his excessive drinking, not the long-established custom of drinking at lunch.

Can Anderson reasonably justify his claims against the company? He can claim that his alcohol abuse was job-related. But the risks and damages at issue here are not specific to a particular job. They are risks associated with working for hire generally—one risks being demoted or fired, either of which is likely to make one unhappy. So Anderson's drinking is not "job-related" in any specific way that would entail company responsibility or financial liability. After all, an employer cannot be held responsible for keeping an employee happy or for the untoward consequences of the imprudent actions of an unhappy employee.

Anderson could try to base his claim on the fact that he is an "alcoholic," that "alcoholism" is a "disease" that he acquired while on the job, that his self-damaging behavior is a "symptom," and that therefore he is not responsible for his behavior or its consequences.

But even if Anderson has a "disease" and so is not responsible, meaning in this context "at fault," this does not imply that the *company* should be held responsible or liable. Anderson's vulnerability to disappointment and the resulting "disease" are his bad luck, if they are not his fault. Why should the company automatically have to pay?

Moreover, the assumption that Anderson is not responsible, because diseased, is unsound. We often hold a person responsible for imprudent conduct that brings about a disease; additionally, we may hold a person responsible for failing to take steps to prevent the disease from doing damage to oneself or others, or for taking steps to limit or cure the disease. The word "disease" is not an incantation that gives blanket relief from all responsibility for the damages it does.

However, one might assume that "alcoholism" is a very special disease in that it destroys one's "will power" and renders one incapable of acting responsibly. But this is contrary to the assumption shared by medically oriented treatment programs, as well as by such major alcohol-abuse programs as AA. Such programs rely on the alcoholic's initiative in seeking and entering treatment, or they use inducements to elicit voluntary entrance and then rely on the alcoholic's self-discipline which requires a large amount of "will power."

Finally, is it true that "alcoholism" is a "disease"? Consider the following facts: there is no scientifically accepted basic understanding of the origins, causes, or nature of "alcoholism"; nor is there a scientifically demonstrated method of "cure"; nor is there even any generally satisfactory analysis of what is meant by "alcoholism." The slogan "alcoholism is a disease" represents not a scientific discovery or a generally accepted scientific hypothesis; it represents the *faith* of many health professionals that a "solution" to the problems of alcohol abuse will someday be found by medical science.

But not every social problem is rooted in physical disease. At present, the evidence to be found in the enormous literature on alcohol and drug abuse reasonably allows one to suppose that there is not a single causal process, but a complex set of problems having biological, psychological, social, and cultural dimensions.

More to the present point, no one can satisfactorily explain in specific and scientific terms why Anderson started to drink excessively, why he kept it up, or what would get him to stop. He is to be pitied. It is a misguided pity, however, that assures him that he is a helpless victim, with no responsibility for his drinking problems. It is morally corrupting, and legally unsound, to assure him that it is the company's fault. It is simple deception to give him to understand that these assurances are grounded in a modern scientific understanding of alcohol abuse.

COMMENTARY

Luther A. Cloud

Alcoholism is a disease, and has been accepted as such by the American Medical Association and by virtually every major medical and scientific body in the world. Criteria for the diagnosis of the disease of alcoholism were published in 1972 by the National Council on Alcoholism, and are in use by the medical profession.

Boyd Anderson's claim, however, is being made on a faulty premise. Since alcoholism is a physiological disease entity, it would be manifestly impossible for the company to have "given" Anderson that disease, just as it would have been impossible for them to have given him a cancer or have caused him to have a weak heart.

Anderson's job *did not require* him to drink. He was required to take out clients and entertain them. His drinking was a matter of his own choice. About one out of ten individuals who drink appears to have a biochemical or physiological "predisposition" to alcoholism. Obviously, Anderson was one of these individuals.

He contracted alcoholism, not as a result of his drinking per se, but because of a physiological difference which, coupled with his drinking, gave him the disease of alcoholism. The company can hardly be blamed for this situation.

Anderson might have had a valid claim if he had based it on the manner in which the company handled the situation that resulted from his alcoholism. Instead of telling him "to accept early retirement," the company would have been better advised to offer him a firm but fair choice between accepting treatment for his disease (alcoholism *is* treatable), or accepting the alternative early retirement.

Treatment for the disease of alcoholism should have been covered by the group health insurance policy just as it would cover treatment for any other disease.

Many firms have programs which offer alcoholic employees a choice of accepting the disciplinary consequences of the poor job performance caused by their alcoholism. These companies consistently report long-term, stable recovery rates from 70 percent to 85 percent and occasionally even higher. Any company that does not have such a program leaves itself open to suits like Anderson's, which can be extremely costly to the company, even if it wins in the end.

COMMENTARY

Sally Guttmacher

The issue of legal liabilities is the least interesting raised by this case. It seems unlikely that many courts would recognize Anderson's claim. Anderson, it can be argued, accepted the rules, and willingly took risks for the possibility of substantial rewards. Yet he claims that in the course of his work he became damaged by as well as dependent on the company. In effect, Anderson declares illegitimate the rules he had previously accepted and seeks compensation through the only means possible—the legal system.

His case is weak. Unlike occupational disease such as black lung where the line of causality is clear, self-destructive behavior (suicide, drug addiction, chronic excessive eating, drinking, or smoking) is generated by a combination of factors—some work-related and some not. In addition, most would argue that chronic excessive drinking is to some extent voluntary. Perceiving the alcoholic simply as a victim of his "disease" denies the notion of his autonomy, an approach that may actually impede rehabilitation.

The more subtle and engaging questions emerge from viewing self-destructive behavior as a response to, or even sometimes a rebellion against, the inhumane and pathological conditions of our lives. How does self-destructive behavior become a commonly selected option for dealing with stress or failure? And who bears the moral responsibility for this situation? How are such disorders related to work in our society, and how might work be restructured to decrease the risk of such outcomes? Finally, why are there so few real options outside the work situation through which an individual can develop self-esteem and taste success?

Even though it may be difficult to argue that an individual corporation should be held *legally* responsible for a pattern of behavioral response that is clearly a product of broadly based social habits, these habits are not mere accidents. They are covertly encouraged, for example, by being presented as a legitimate way for adults to deal with stress. (One needs merely to note in one evening of commercial television viewing the proportion of scenes involving social interaction in which alcohol and cigarettes are common props.) Through a myriad of such linkages—each perhaps weak in itself, but powerful in the aggregate—the corporation acquires responsibility in its broader role as part of the ruling segment of the society that establishes "the rules of the game" and even creates and encourages life styles for its own benefit.

Therefore, a given corporation cannot be permitted to retreat conveniently behind the claim that it, too, is the victim of the iron laws of the market. This may be a legal defense, since laws are codifications of the rules of the game, but it fails as a moral defense given the rudimentary facts that modern corporations exist chiefly to make profits. To the extent that these profits are at the expense of the well-being of workers or of consumers, corporations can be charged with behaving immorally.

Certainly, within the current rules many will argue that the corporation acted fairly, even humanely, in its dealings with Anderson. While there is some merit in this view, the motivation behind the corporation's action is another question. With relatively high levels of unemployment many workers carry the status of expendable, easily replaceable commodities. That Anderson was offered other options by the company is not simply testament to corporate compassion, but rather an indication that he belongs to a special class of workers who, because a substantial investment goes into their training, are perceived as (human) capital. Thus, as with fine-tooled machinery, some trouble is taken to see that they continue to function in some productive capacity. At the very least, the company will make an effort to see that those with problems, such as Anderson, are handled in ways that do not demoralize the others.

Because Anderson must bring the case to court and bear the burden of proof, the issue becomes depoliticized. Accepting this way of proceeding, moreover, ratifies the view that problems such as alcoholism simply represent the unintended, unforeseen, and unwanted consequences of an essentially well-functioning system. This is a curious response to a problem that now affects 10 percent of our work force, a statistic that may be interpreted as an indicator of a serious malfunction in our way of life.

With these rates in mind, we must ask who bears the risks in our society, and, if these risks are too great, who has the power to restructure the system and decrease the risk? By presenting the problem as a question of individual corporate responsibility, we lose sight of its broader implications. And by permitting corporations in general to shift the price and responsibility for the human wastage that is a by-product of our whole economic system onto public institutions, we ignore the need for a basic reorganization in the structure of work.

59

Mentally Retarded Hepatitis B Carriers in Public Schools

In compliance with a court order that requires placement of mentally retarded residents of a state institution into less restrictive community settings, New York State officials have begun to place a number of school-aged children in family and foster homes and other community residences in New York City. They have also arranged for these children to attend special education classes in public schools.

In 1977 a teacher of several of these children became infected with type A hepatitis. An investigation by the New York City Department of Health concluded that the teacher's type A hepatitis did not appear to present a serious health problem. However, a hepatitis B problem might exist because of the infectious nature of this disease, which almost all the children in the institution had contracted.

Hepatitis B is a virus which may have a debilitating effect upon the liver and has been linked to cancer. After a several-month period of incubation the virus, in a susceptible person, may reach the acute state. In some of these cases, involving jaundice and inflammation of the liver, the disease is very serious and can even lead to death. In other cases, especially among children, the acute phase may be very mild, and is often mistaken for flu and a fever. There is no known cure for hepatitis B, although a vaccine is being tested and may be available within four years.

After the acute phase has passed, there may be one of two outcomes. If the patient has built up sufficient antibodies, the virus will be eliminated; and the individual will be immune from the disease indefinitely. If, however, the patient does not create sufficient antibodies, he or she may appear clinically healthy but, upon careful examination, will be found to be "carrying" the virus (antigen) in his blood. This carrier can transmit the virus to another, who may also become a carrier, without either of them showing clinical signs of illness. For example, approximately 30 percent of the residents of the state institution are now immune, and about 60 percent are carriers.

As a result of the Health Department's report, a task force was formed to conduct a study to determine the extent of the hepatitis B problem. All children in special education programs where known hepatitis B carriers were present were included in the study—a sample of about 450 students. Of that number, forty-four were already known carriers, because they had come from the institution, where they had already been tested. The tests on the remaining children identified five additional carriers. There was no way of determining how they contracted the virus, but suspicion immediately focused upon contact with the already known carriers.

This explanation seemed likely because of the unhygienic behavior displayed by many of the identified carriers. The virus is transmitted through body fluids—saliva, blood, etc. Among the students there was hand-to-mouth contact, drooling, bleeding gums, biting, and scratching.

As a result of this study the Department of Health recommended that the Board of Education test students at regular intervals, and classify them as "carriers," "immunes," or "susceptibles." Susceptible children were to be grouped separately from carriers, in classrooms and lunchrooms, and were to receive special supervision to avoid contact with carriers. (Some of these children are particularly susceptible because of poorly developed immune systems.)

Some parents, as well as representatives of the teachers' and the staff's unions, opposed these guidelines. They claimed that it was unfair to subject the "susceptible" group to restrictions. They also argued that the plan could never be implemented because there was insufficient personnel to provide the required close supervision. They believed that the "carriers," not the "susceptibles," should be segregated. They proposed removing the forty-four identified carriers from the public school and sending them to education programs at the state institution. Because children in special education classes have so little contact with normal school children, this group urged, the complete absence of such contact would have a minimal effect, if any, upon them.

The staff at the state institution opposed this idea. They argued that contact with society, even in a limited way, is essential to the development of a mentally retarded child. Moreover, they were not convinced, given the uncertainty of the data about the susceptibility to infection of persons with hepatitis B antigens, that restrictions upon either the susceptibles or the carriers were justified. They maintained that control measures should focus upon good hygiene practices, prohibitions against sharing toilet articles, and special handling of blood-contaminated items.

Should the Board of Education segregate the carriers from other students? Or should they maintain them in the classrooms? On what grounds can either decision be justified?

COMMENTARY

Robert Plotkin

This case presents a classic problem in contemporary terms. Forty-four former residents of a mental retardation institution who now live and attend school in the community have been identified as hepatitis B carriers. Should the Board of Education segregate them from the rest of the special education students in the public schools by returning them to the institution for their education? The forty-four assert their right to live and be educated in the most normal environment appropriate to their individual needs. Their claims are in apparent conflict with the Board's public duty to protect the health and welfare of other students, the teachers and staff who have a right to avoid exposure to a communicable and possibly fatal disease. Which of these competing interests should be accorded the higher priority, and for what reasons?

Where there are competing liberty claims, the task is to determine the relative worth of the interests. One must choose which interest represents the greater good by comparing the degree of risk to the public health with the extent of the proposed restrictions upon individual liberty. Where known risks to the majority present an imminent and substantial threat to the public, it is more likely that restrictions upon individual autonomy will promote the greater good. But where the potential risks are unclear and the threat to the public is speculative, interference with individual liberty becomes the lesser good. A comparative analysis of the risks and rights at stake in this problem leads to the conclusion that the forty-four identified carriers should *not* be segregated from their fellow students.

The public health risk is not sufficiently clear to justify exclusion. Although hepatitis B can be fatal, death is statistically rare. It is not a readily communicable disease; it is transmitted primarily by blood contact. While other modes of transmission may exist, the evidence for the probability of contagion remains ambiguous. Whatever the dangers, the degree of risk appears to be related inversely to the cleanliness of the affected environment and the participant's personal hygiene—factors that in this case are controllable through the provision of proper educational programming, staffing, and classrooms.

The degree of risk that is actually involved in contacts with hepatitis B carriers is also uncertain, because it is not now possible to separate carriers who will transmit from those who will not. Interestingly, the incidence of hepatitis B—either active cases or carrier cases—among the institutional staff where these students resided is not unusual or significant. This demonstrates that even prolonged exposure in an area highly concentrated with carriers does not necessarily result in infection. The forty-four identified carriers could easily go through their entire lives without infecting a single person.

Moreover, even if the formerly institutionalized students are returned to the facility, the risk of infection, whatever it may be, is not significantly lessened because carriers also appear in the students who were never institutionalized. In other words, identification as a hepatitis B carrier is not synonymous with one's status as a former resident. It is just as likely that, if the larger group of students were subjected to the same intensive screening devices, it too would include a number of carriers. While one might speculate that in the larger group carriers resulted only from contact with one or more of the forty-four former residents, there is simply no way to be sure that they were not undetected carriers prior to that exposure. Removal of the forty-four may alleviate somewhat the already minimal risks of continuing exposure, but it is surely impossible to quantify the level of that reduction.

Thus, the public health rationale advanced to justify the segregation of the formerly institutionalized carriers is at best tenuous, and in any event the solution proposed for protecting the public's health is inadequate because some carriers will still remain in the public schools. Arguments favoring the segregation of the minority group are more likely based improperly upon real-world economic and administrative concerns: it is cheaper and easier to isolate than to accommodate.

Balanced against these public welfare concerns are the principles of autonomy and respect for persons. The rights infringed by a decision to again segregate the formerly institutionalized persons—rights of liberty, association, and free expression—are among the most fundamental components of individual autonomy, and the severe restrictions on their physical liberty are self-evident. In addition, these students will be deprived of positive emotional and environmental influences, their future intellectual and social growth will be stymied, and already developed life skills may atrophy. The speculative "risks" to the public health pale when balanced against this enormous loss of individual liberty and personal growth.

Significantly, numerous court decisions and federal and state laws mandate that handicapped children live and be educated in the environment that is most normal and appropriate to their individual needs. Placement in the public schools had previously been determined as legally proper for these forty-four students, and a subsequent decision to override those assignments must be based upon evidence more compelling than that presented here.

Finally, there is an additional, important argument against the segregation of these particular students. Principles of social justice demand that their right to live in the community be accorded special deference because the comparative value of their freedom is greater than that of the general student body. They were involuntarily placed in a state-operated facility, ostensibly "for their own good." While there, they were actually exposed to harms such as the hepatitis B virus, and their human and medical needs were neglected. They never agreed to these arrangements, and while some elements of society-at-large may have "benefited" from their confinement, they certainly did not. The public has unreasonably interfered with their pursuit of a normal life. It must now redress that injustice by demanding particularly convincing justification before they are again excluded and stigmatized anew as "carriers." Thus, not only must general principles of ethics and law forbid any segregation based upon so flimsy a public health rationale, but the renewed institutionalization of these children deserves special resistance.

The enormous discrepancy between the speculative "good" to the public that may be achieved by isolation, and the actual harm that will likely be experienced by the forty-four identified carriers, prohibits excluding the carriers from the public schools. The Board of Education must devise alternative preventive health methods that will better accommodate these competing interests.

COMMENTARY

H. Tristram Engelhardt, Jr.

If there could be a general moral maxim for attitudes towards the mentally retarded, it should be this: they should not on principle be treated differently from other humans. However, the term "mentally retarded" misleads as much as it informs, gathering together in one category individuals of diverse abilities, interests, and difficulties. Moreover, like the medical terms syphilitic and leper, it tends to alter radically social reality, casting its bearers in sick roles that often lead to unwarranted isolation. Of course, all disease language is evaluative and to some degree performative. That is, disease language places a value upon a particular human state and assigns individuals in that state a place in a social world of cure, care, prevention, and quarantine. Thus, being called mentally retarded is like being deputized by the sheriff: the people in the world around you at once are authorized to look at you in a different fashion. At times such evaluations are inappropriate in the sense that they lead to the loss of important human goods. Moreover, as one would expect in all complex human situations, it often occurs that human goods are put at jeopardy in a fashion that not all can be realized, even given the best choices. Such appears to be the case here.

The case of the deinstitutionalization of these mentally retarded individuals raises at least the following ethical concerns:

1. One wishes to treat the previously institutionalized mentally retarded individual as fairly as possible, giving him as normal a life context as feasible.

2. One wishes not to expose unconsenting teachers and children to the dangers of hepatitis B or perhaps, in addition, cancer (if such be a sequela).

3. One is concerned as well not to expose unconsenting foster parents to the risk of hepatitis B and the possibility of cancer.

4. Similarly, one has an interest in protecting the public against dangers of increased exposure to hepatitis B and cancer.

5. With reference to points 2–4, one should out of regard for concerns of fairness wish to determine what the implications of any policy choices with regard to the mentally retarded would be for relevantly similar populations (e.g., nurses working on hemodialysis units who may become active carriers of hepatitis B virus).

This constellation of issues is similar to the concerns with regard to maximizing value over disvalue, and of protecting the innocent against unconsented-to injury raised by the disputes concerning the safety of nuclear power plants, recombinant DNA research, and industrial pollution. There are disputes concerning the actual risks involved. There are arguments with regard to the rights to forebearance of individuals who might be subject to injury. One in short is confronted with a scientific issue with a heavy ethical and political overlay, so that the questions appear in part to turn upon empirical issues and in part on ethical questions. With respect to the latter the basic issue concerns determining the point at which the interests of one group to exercise their rights or to pursue their goods is defeated either (1) by the injuries caused to another group by the first group, or (2) by the rights of the second to the forebearance of the first. This determination, in turn, will at least in part be a function of the facts of the matter. What indeed are the possible injuries?

I believe that an answer can only be reached given a better appreciation of the empirical data involved, as well as of their softness. Such demurral is, I believe, appropriate in that there appear to be possibilities of two forms of technologically resolving at least some elements of the controversy. As a result I will for the most part simply attempt to clarify the geography of the problems.

The only major point I will forward is that whatever conclusions one reaches with regard to quarantining the mentally retarded should be explored with regard to their implications for our conduct with respect to other similar populations who are likely to be active carriers of serum hepatitis B virus (e.g., dentists, nurses working in renal dialysis units, etc.). In many such cases, it might, however, be properly rejoined that such individuals, given their general level of cleanliness, and so forth, do not represent a public health menace of the same proportion as the mentally retarded children in question.

To resolve this issue one would need to have made judgments on the following points:

1. How soon will a vaccine for hepatitis B virus be available and how safe and effective will this new vaccine be?

2. What are the actual benefits to the mentally retarded children of deinstitutionalization?

3. What would the consequences be of delaying deinstitutionalization until a vaccine is available?

4. Can antigen tests be used to identify the actual active carriers of hepatitis B virus and therefore decrease the number of individuals concerning whom one need have concern that they might transmit the disease to others? If this group is small enough, can they then be adequately "quarantined" in special classrooms in the regular school system without losing the benefits of deinstitutionalization? (See question 2 above.)

In short, one has a case of different groups each concerned that it not be forced to cede its rights, on the one hand to develop its potentials, on the other hand not to be exposed to the risk of serious disease or death. One has, in short, a head-on conflict between rights. However, here there is the possibility of a technological fix, a test for true, active carriers and the possibility in the relatively near future of a vaccine. In short, the problems focus upon the question of a delay or of a compromise through some halfway procedures in an interim period.

In any event, one will need to give to all foster parents full information about their potential exposure to risk. Moreover, one will need to be assured that high-risk school personnel are adequately protected before they are exposed to a substantial risk of morbidity and mortality. This would include, for example, teachers who are older, have diabetes, congestive heart failure, or are post-menopausal. For such individuals there are good grounds for believing that exposure to such a risk is an exposure to a substantial danger of serious illness and death. There are probably few who would contest their rights to be protected. It is in other populations, where the risks are more remote and less severe, that the answers are not as clear. In short, as in most complex bioethical quandaries, the problems are as much questions of fact as of principle.

60

Health Risks and Equal Opportunity

Robert E. Stevenson

Mark Dalton, a thirty-two-year-old technician, was hired six months ago by a large chemical company. He has proven to be highly skilled and works at a rate exceeding his co-workers. Recently, after he took a sick leave, the employee health department nurse was surprised to learn that he is suffering from chronic renal disease. His entrance medical questionnaire did not mention any problem.

Since his job requires exposure to chemical solvent vapors at levels permissible by OSHA regulations, the company physician counseled him that continuing exposure to the vapors could exacerbate the disease.

Company management found a job for which he would qualify at the same rate of pay; but two current employees, one of whom is female, who are eligible for promotion are interested in the job. Both have better training and longer service with the company than Dalton.

Management has grounds for dismissing Dalton on the basis of false representations about his health. If he is given the available job to protect his health, it is likely that the woman employee who is better qualified will file a complaint charging discrimination with the Equal Employment Opportunity Commission.

Should Dalton be fired? Given the safer job? When three workers have a valid claim to a job, one based on health, one on seniority, and the third on equal opportunity, which should prevail?

COMMENTARY

Deborah G. Johnson

This case raises a set of questions about the relationship between employers and employees. Just what rights and obligations each party has with respect to the other is a matter that is only vaguely understood and only partially defined by law. Nevertheless, assumptions proliferate on both sides. Employers assume, for example, that employees should have a certain amount of loyalty to their employers; and employees assume that they should have the right to an appeal if they are treated unfairly in evaluation and promotion.

In this case, if Dalton knew of his condition and failed to report it on his application form, then he falsely represented himself and the company's commitment to him is voided. In a sense, the application form becomes part of the tacit contract between employer and employee. The company agrees to employ the individual, to provide certain benefits in exchange for work of a certain type and quality, but the employer agrees to do this on the assumption that information given by the applicant is true. The company would not have hired Dalton if they had known of his condition; thus, it does not have a duty to continue to employ him. But, this does not mean that they must or should fire him. Since he misrepresented himself, it is morally permissible to fire him, but continuing to employ him does not violate a moral norm.

Companies that hire individuals to work in environments that are unsafe or pose a threat to health have a duty to inform those workers of the risks involved. Failure to inform workers whose health is at risk or will be at risk is a violation of employees' bodily integrity. Violating employees' rights to control what is done to their bodies is roughly the same as placing people at risk in an experiment without their consent. However, companies should not make decisions for their workers. To do this would be to deny the autonomy of individual workers and to disregard their ability to judge what is in their best interests. Each worker should decide for himself or herself whether or not to take the risks involved. Workers can do this only if they are given information about the risks, and therefore companies have an obligation to so inform workers.

In this case, since levels conform to OSHA standards, the company has fulfilled its obligation by counseling Dalton that continuous exposure to the vapors would be dangerous to his health. If Dalton is a mature, sane individual and wants to continue working, the company may continue to employ him. Of course, if Dalton chooses to take the risks and his condition worsens subsequently, the company should not be considered liable for compensation. Dalton would have accepted the responsibility for his condition by accepting the job knowing the risks.

If Dalton prefers another job in the organization, the company may provide such a job but, as already indicated, they are not obligated to do so. It might be good for Dalton and might be good for the company but morality does not demand that these goods be brought about. The company would have an obligation to find an alternative position for someone who developed a renal problem while working for the company, and this obligation would be even stronger if the condition was caused by the work environment, but this is not the case with Dalton. In this instance, if people already employed by the company are qualified for an available job, then the company has a stronger obligation to promote these employees according to rules that are operative in the company.

This analysis suggests that companies have obligations to their employees but that these obligations are voided if workers misrepresent themselves. It suggests that the company has no obligation to act paternalistically, that is, to protect employees from themselves (which is what the company would be doing if it refused to let Dalton work at a job of his choice, even when he knew the risks involved). Rather, the obligation is to provide information to employees so that they can make autonomous decisions. But circumstances might arise when the claims of individual employees would compete.

While Dalton's claim to the job does not compete with the claims of the other workers, the rights of a worker with seniority may well conflict with those of a woman. I do not think we can decide in advance how companies should resolve all such cases. The merits of each claim must be weighed in the light of given circumstances. Who has the stronger claim will depend on such matters as the type of job available, the merit of the employees, the company's past record on discrimination, and the firm's stated policy on seniority. This does not mean that companies should disregard a claim to equal opportunity. On the contrary, a commitment to equal opportunity means an obligation to consider the strength of an applicant's claim on the basis of relevant criteria.

COMMENTARY

Knut Ringen

English and American common law traditionally have held that the employer is responsible for the conduct of work, including the provision of a safe and healthy workplace. This common law principle underlies the Occupational Safety and Health Act of 1970.

However, absolutely safe and healthy workplaces do not exist today, and they will not exist in the future. Given the reality of residual risks, particularly associated with chronic diseases, safety and health in the workplace must be a responsibility shared by employer and worker.

How can this responsibility be shared fairly? Employers through their associations continue to insist that they should have absolute control of the workplace, including the right to restrict information about hazardous substances. For this reason, many workers, who are forced to be responsible to some extent for their own health, are not informed about the hazards that they are exposed to in the workplace.

However, we can assume that Dalton was knowledgeable about the risks. This case therefore raises the following issues of responsibility:

- Did the worker act irresponsibly in not revealing the chronic renal condition at the time of employment, and should he therefore be fired?
- Should the worker be moved to another job for health reasons?
- If moved, should he be given precedence over other candidates for the available alternative job?

Legally, a worker is required to give truthful answers to preemployment medical questions. In reality, however, the worker should be allowed some leeway, just as the employer is given leeway in providing a safe and healthy workplace. Most workers know that they will not be employed if they provide information about having a chronic disease, because the employer does not want to risk being held liable if the worker gets sick. Thus, even where there is no association between type of work and the worker's chronic disease, the mere presence of the disease (or even a personal disease risk factor) may preclude employment. We must expect that some workers who understand this situation will not be totally candid in answering their preemployment medical questionnaire. However, we would expect the technician to be more responsible for assessing the risk and potential hazard than a less informed worker.

Justification for firing the technician on these grounds thus may or may not exist. We cannot know for sure if the worker knew of his renal condition at the time of employment. We also cannot be sure that he knew the condition could be exacerbated because of his work. The company physician seems to acknowledge that the contribution of workplace exposure to the disease progression is potential, but not certain. Given this caveat, justification could exist for the worker not to admit his chronic disease. It would be unreasonable to expect him to jeopardize a specialized career by revealing medical conditions that he might judge unrelated to his work.

Medical removal protection is central to the current debate on occupational health regulations. This principle was legally promulgated for the first time in OSHA's initial occupational safety and health standard for asbestos exposure and it is an essential element of the recent standard to protect workers from exposure to lead (43 *Federal Register* 52952, 1978). Under the lead standard, a worker may be removed from his or her regular employment on the basis of an examining physician's medical opinion or when the measured level of lead in the worker's blood is high enough to indicate a "material impairment to health or functional capacity." When removed under this provision, the worker will receive compensation in the form of maintained earnings, seniority, and other benefits.

Although the lead standard requires only temporary removal of the workers and may not necessarily apply to permanent displacement, it clearly signals a new direction for the protection of worker rights. It represents a means of last resort to protect individual workers where the established permitted level of exposure to risks is inadequate. OSHA standards, including the lead standard, allow some exposure because it is not feasible to achieve a zero level and they may be fairly adequate for most workers. However, individuals who are especially susceptible to a given toxic effect will suffer disease even when exposure falls within accepted limits. It is these individuals that the medical removal provision will protect.

A few employers voluntarily offer job security and medical removal. In a few union contracts (notably the Steelworkers) medical removal is part of the benefit program. However, most workers know that they will lose their jobs and suffer other adverse employment effects because of an abnormal medical finding. The workers realize that once fired for medical reasons they will have a very hard time obtaining similar types of work and may even be investigated by companies that monitor workers' compensation claim files (see *Business Insurance*, June 9, 1980, p. 27). And workers have long known intuitively what was documented recently by the Department of Labor Interim Report to Congress on Occupational Diseases. According to that report, only 1 to 5 percent of job-related diseases are covered under current workers' compensation programs.

The ethical employer should also recognize the limitations of existing OSHA standards and the inequity of firing for medical reasons the worker who is denied general health protection under existing standards because of unique susceptibility. In other words, the same latitude that is allowed the firm in operating at levels of exposure that will fail to protect everyone should apply to the workers who cannot tolerate those exposures. In this case, the employer acted correctly in voluntarily providing medical removal protection.

Finally, the case raises the issue of preferential treatment. If the lead standard is cited as the precedent, preferential treatment would probably favor the worker with the medical condition. The worker is not at fault for the medical condition, and to deny alternative employment would be to place the burden on him. Also, various medical problems today qualify for affirmative action under federal law, and medical removal could fall into this category.

Selected Bibliography

Part VI: Allocation and Health-Care Policy

Aaron, Henry J., and Schwartz, William B. *The Painful Prescription: Rationing Hospital Care.* Washington, DC: Brookings Institution, 1984.

Bayer, Ronald, Caplan, Arthur L., and Daniels, Norman, eds. *In Search of Equity: Health Needs and the Health Care System*. New York: Plenum Press, 1983.

Callahan, Daniel. *Setting Limits: Medical Goals in an Aging Society*. New York: Simon and Schuster, 1987.

Childress, James F. "Who Shall Live When Not All Can Live." *Soundings* 53 (Winter 1970): 339–55.

Churchill, Larry R. *Rationing Health Care in America: Perceptions and Principles of Justice*. South Bend: University of Notre Dame Press, 1987.

Daniels, Norman. *Just Health Care*. New York: Cambridge University Press, 1985.

Evans, Roger W. "Health Care Technology and the Inevitability of Resource Allocation and Rationing Decisions." *Journal of the American Medical Association* Pt. I 249 (15) (April 15, 1983): 2047–53; Pt. II 249 (16) (April 22/29, 1983): 2208–19.

Fried, Charles. "Equality and Rights in Medical Care." *Hastings Center Report* 6 (February 1976): 29–34.

Fuchs, Victor R. *The Health Economy*. Cambridge: Harvard University Press, 1986.

Outka, Gene. "Social Justice and Equal Access to Health Care." *The Journal of Religious Ethics* (Spring 1974): 11–32.

President's Commission for the Study of Ethical Problems in Medicine and Biomedical and Behavioral Research. *Securing Access to Health Care*, Vols. I–III. Washington, DC: U.S. Government Printing Office, 1983.

Task Force on Organ Transplantation. *Organ Transplantation: Issues and Recommendations*. U. S. Department of Health and Human Services, Public Health Service, Health Resources and Services Administration, April, 1986.

Winslow, Gerald R. *Triage and Justice*. Berkeley: University of California Press, 1982.

Glossary

Advance Directive An advance directive is a declaration by a person that stipulates the forms of medical treatment to be provided by caregivers and/or designates someone to act as a proxy should the person at some future date lose decision-making capacity. In written form, an advance directive is often referred to as a "living will."

Autonomy Derived from Greek words meaning "self-rule." In bioethics, autonomy typically refers to the patient's right of self-determination concerning medical care. Autonomy may be used in various senses including freedom of action, effective deliberation, and authenticity. It supports such moral and legal principles as respect for persons and informed consent.

Beneficence The principle of beneficence involves duties to prevent harm, remove harm, and promote the good of another person. In bioethics, beneficence refers to the obligation of health care professionals to seek the well-being or benefit of the patient.

Best Interests A decision-making standard used in the absence of an advance directive or when a substituted judgement is not possible, best interests involves more objective, societally shared criteria about what reasonable persons would probably choose in a particular situation.

Competence Competence refers to a patient's capacity to make decisions about the provision of medical care for him or herself. It is an element of informed consent, and involves comprehending information, choosing in accordance with one's values, and communicating a decision. The decisions of competent patients are usually respected, while a determination of incompetence may warrant paternalistic and coercive measures, such as involuntary commitment.

Conscience Moral agents often appeal to conscience in making ethical judgements about particular cases. The content of conscience is informed by basic moral values. In medical ethics, health care professionals may refuse to perform certain procedures, for example, abortions, sterilizations, or withdrawal of life-sustaining treatment, based on fidelity to conscience, a phenomenon known as "conscientious objection."

Deontology Derived for the Greek *deon* or "duty," deontological moral theories (along with utilitarianism) form the philosophical basis for contemporary bioethics. A deontological position holds that the moral worth of acts is not limited to assessing the character of the agent of the consequences or the performance of the act, but that there are intrinsic features of acts that are at least as relevant and may even be decisive for moral deliberation. The principles of autonomy, respect for persons, and distributive justice are typically grounded in a deontological theory.

DNR Orders Do-Not-Resuscitate orders are directions not to initiate cardiopulmonary resuscitation (CPR) in the event of cardiac or respiratory arrest. DNR orders raise ethical questions about when life-sustaining treatment should be withheld and who should make that decision.

Ethics Ethics is systematic reflection on the norms, principles, or values that do or should guide human conduct or action, and as such can be distinguished from morality, which is the practice or conduct itself. Bioethics is a form of *applied normative* ethics that involves the application of general ethical principles and rules to specific moral problems that arise in medical practice, the provision of health care, and scientific research.

Euthanasia Eytmologically, euthanasia means easy or gentle death. Contemporary usage is often ambiguous, and modifiers are used to make the intended sense clearer. "Active" euthanasia refers to the direct killing of a patient, and is typically contrasted with "passive" euthanasia, which involves the withdrawal of medical technologies in order to allow the underlying disease process to take its natural course. "Voluntary" euthanasia (either active or passive) means that the action is undertaken at the behest of the patient, and should be distinguished from "nonvoluntary" euthanasia where the patient has not made or is not capable of making such a request, and "involuntary" euthanasia, where the action is performed against the patient's wishes.

Extraordinary/Ordinary Means of Treatment Historically, extraordinary and ordinary means of treatment have been distinguished according to whether (a) a proposed medical intervention has a reasonable chance of succeeding, and (b) the benefits of the intervention outweigh the burdens. The distinction is based on a moral or professional obligation to provide ordinary treatments, but no obligation to provide extraordinary treatment. The "extraordinary/ordinary" distinction has been criticized recently for focusing attention on treatments for diseases rather than patient interests, leading to decisions about the provision of treatment based on what is routine or customary in medical practice. The terminology of "optional/obligatory" has been proposed as a preferable, patient-centered, standard for such judgments.

Informed Consent Except in emergency situations, physicians are morally and legally required to obtain the patient's informed consent to invasive medical procedures. The elements of informed consent include professional disclosure and patient comprehension of information, and patient voluntariness and competence to consent.

Justice As a general moral concept, justice requires that persons be given what they are due. Theories of justice have specified different criteria upon which such a determination can be made, for example, societal benefits might be distributed to persons based on equality, need, effort, merit, or contribution to society. In bioethics, distributive justice is especially important in decisions about the fair allocation of health care resources.

Nonmaleficence The principle of nonmaleficence prohibits the infliction of harm, injury, or death upon others, and supports more specific moral rules such as the prohibition of killing. Nonmaleficence is related to the maxim *primum non nocere* ("above all, or first, do no harm"), which is widely used to describe the duties of health care professionals. The duty not to harm others is typically considered more stringent than the duty to benefit others and it also imposes moral limits on autonomy.

Paternalism Paternalism assumes a parent (father)-child relationship in which an authority figure acts to benefit the subordinate party even against his or her desires or choices. Medical paternalism normally involves the refusal of a health care professional to accept the wishes, judgments, or acts of a patient on the grounds that the health care professional knows best. Paternalism is widely viewed as morally suspect because of its assumptions of moral inequality in the professional-patient relationship and because it violates patient autonomy. However, paternalism is usually considered warranted if the patient's capacity for autonomous choice and competent decision making is restricted or impaired.

Personhood Philosophers and theologians frequently propose criteria—for example, sentience, consciousness, or purposive action—that specify when a living entity is or becomes a person. The concept of personhood is critical in many bioethical debates. Divergent views of personhood are assumed in arguments over the moral status of the human fetus and animals, and over the determination of death.

Professional Ethics Ethical standards are important in defining the boundaries of a profession such as medicine or nursing. Most professions have developed codes of ethics that identify the responsibilities of the professional in special relations with patients or clients. These standards are viewed as obligatory upon members of the profession, and may not be applicable to nonmembers or to relationships outside the professional setting.

Proxy Consent When a patient has been determined to be incompetent and incapable of giving informed consent to the provision of medical teatment, a proxy may be appointed to make decisions for the patient. The proxy, frequently a family member or relative, may be appointed by the court or designated by the patient through an advance directive.

Quality of Life Quality of life is often contrasted with quantity or sanctity of life and indicates that there are moral limits to the use of life–prolonging medical interventions. It is portrayed as a patient-centered moral criterion, emphasizing the worth of the patient's own life to him or herself.

Respect for persons The moral principle respect for persons is based on the maxim that a person should never be treated simply as a means, but always as an end. At a minimum, it requires providing reasons or moral justification for actions that infringe upon the liberty and life plans of others. Respect for persons supports moral rules, such as privacy, confidentiality, and truthtelling.

Rights Rights are justified claims upon others for action or forebearance. "Negative" rights are rights to noninterference by others, such as the "right to life," to undergo an abortion based on the right of privacy, or to refuse medical intervention. "Positive" rights are claims on others for assistance, such as federal or state funding for access to abortion, or the right to health care.

Risk-Benefit Analysis Risk-benefit analysis weighs the probability and magnitude of potential harm against the probability and amount of potential benefit. Various measures of harm and risk are used. This form of analysis is widely used to set standards of safety and health for the workplace and to assess medical technologies.

Sanctity of Life The principle of sanctity of life assumes that the moral and religious value of life transcends judgments about its quality. In bioethics, the sanctity of life principle is associated with conservative, life-prolonging positions in debates over such matters as abortion, infanticide, suicide, and euthanasia.

Slippery Slope Argument A "slippery slope" or "wedge" argument raises questions about the precedents that may be set and the consequences that may follow if a particular practice is accepted. In its *sociological* version, the slippery slope argument suggests that if X is accepted, then Y will follow as a matter of due course. The legal acceptance of active, voluntary euthanasia, for example, is often predicted to erode society's respect for the value of life so that moral barriers against nonvoluntary or involuntary euthanasia would be undermined. In its *logical* version, the slippery slope argument suggests that the acceptance of X already contains an implicit justification of Y, even if in practice Y never occurs. For example, arguments that support the use of infants with anencephaly as organ donors might seem also to validate harvesting organs from patients in a persistent vegetative state.

Substituted Judgment In a case of substituted judgment, a proxy decision maker makes a decision about medical treatment for an incompetent patient based upon his or her understanding of what the patient would have decided if competent. The "substituted judgment standard" has been important in influential legal decisions and is typically contrasted with the "best interests standard."

Supererogation Supererogatory acts are those considered "above and beyond the call of duty." Such acts, like a rescue that imposes substantial risk to the rescuer, are not considered morally obligatory and failure to perform them would not be regarded as morally wrong. The moral agents who do perform them are often praised for their heroism. Judgments about supererogatory action are often role dependent: because of commitments to standards of professional ethics, the ethical expectations of lifeguards or physicians to save life are often higher than those imposed upon normal citizens.

Triage Drawn from a French term for "sorting," triage is important in emergency medicine and in procedures for determining which patients should receive scarce medical resources. Patients may be classified according to whether they will probably (1) survive without immediate medical treatment, (2) die even with immediate treatment, or (3) survive only with immediate treatment.

Utilitarianism Utilitarianism is a philosophical theory that assesses the moral worth of acts according to their extrinsic features, particularly their outcomes and consequences. In a utilitarian position, the morally justifiable act is that which produces the greatest amount of value over disvalue. Utilitarianism supports a range of ethical principles, including nonmaleficence and beneficence, and methods of moral assessment, such as risk-benefit analysis.

Acknowledgments, continued

11. *Vol. 15, No. 3, June 1985, pp. 17–18*
12. *Vol. 15, No. 1, February 1985, pp. 17–19*
13. *Vol. 14, No. 4, August 1984, pp. 26–27*
14. *Vol. 15, No. 5, October 1985, pp. 29–31*
15. *Vol. 16, No. 1, February 1986, pp. 24–25*
16. *Vol. 13, No. 1, February 1983, pp. 22–23*
17. *Vol. 6, No. 5, October 1976, pp. 10–15*
18. *Vol. 15, No. 2, April 1985, pp. 22-23*
19. *Vol. 10, No. 2, April 1980, pp. 25–27*
20. *Vol. 18, No. 1, February/March 1988, pp. 21–22*
21. *Vol. 11, No. 2, April 1981, pp. 25–26*
22. *Vol. 16, No. 6, December 1986, pp. 15–17*
23. *Vol. 12, No. 5, October 1982, pp. 27–29*
24. *Vol. 17, No. 4, August 1987, pp. 18–19*
25. *Vol. 8, No. 1, February 1978, pp. 13-14*
26. *Vol. 9, No. 4, August 1979, pp. 12–13*
27. *Vol. 5, No. 3, June 1975, pp. 9–10, 47*
28. *Vol. 10, No. 5, October 1980, pp. 21–22*
29. *Vol. 14, No. 1, February 1984, pp. 24–26*
30. *Vol. 17, No. 3, International Supplement, June 1987, pp. 23–26*
31. *Vol. 9, No. 5, October 1979, pp. 19–21*
32. *Vol. 17, No. 6, December 1987, pp. 33-35*
33. *Vol. 8, No. 4, August 1978, pp. 21–22*
34. *Vol. 7, No. 3, June 1977, pp. 13–15*
35. *Vol. 12, No. 4, August 1982, pp. 26–28*
36. *Vol. 14, No. 3, June 1984, pp. 22–24*
37. *Vol. 18, No. 2, April/May 1988, pp. 24–26*
38. *Vol. 11, No. 6, December 1981, pp. 21–23*
39. *Vol. 13, No. 3, June 1983, pp. 17–19*
40. *Vol. 11, No. 4, August 1981, pp. 20–21*
41. *Vol. 16, No. 4, August 1986, pp. 31–33*
42. *future Report*
43. *Vol. 5, No. 1, February 1975, pp. 49–51*
44. *Vol. 12, No. 3, June 1982, pp 18–19*
45. *Vol. 6, No. 2, April 1976, pp. 13–15*
46. *Vol. 14, No. 5, October 1984, pp. 52–54*
47. *Vol. 9, No. 3, June 1979, pp. 19–20, 26*
48. *Vol. 7, No. 6, December 1977, pp. 21–22*
49. *Vol. 10, No. 1, February 1980, pp. 23–24*
50. *Vol. 12, No. 2, April 1982, pp. 24–25*
51. *Vol. 13, No. 5, October 1983, pp. 23–25*
52. *Vol. 15, No. 4, August 1985, pp. 13–15*
53. *Vol. 16, No. 5, October 1986, pp. 23–25*
54. *Vol. 16, No. 2, April 1986, pp. 21–23*
55. *Vol. 8, No. 5, October 1978, pp. 23–25*
56. *Vol. 17, No. 5, October/November 1987, pp. 26–27*
57. *Vol. 8, No. 3, June 1978, pp. 19–20, 46*
58. *Vol. 8, No. 6, December 1978, pp. 16–18*
59. *Vol. 9, No. 6, December 1979, pp. 15–17*
60. *Vol. 10, No. 6, December 1980, pp. 25–26*